ON CALL
NEUROLOGY
Second Edition

Be ON CALL with confidence!

Successfully managing on-call situations requires a masterful combination of speed, skills, and knowledge. Rise to the occasion **with W.B. SAUNDERS COMPANY's On Call Series!** These pocket-size resources provide you with immediate access to the vital, step-by-step information you need to succeed!

Other Titles in the On Call Series

Adams & Bresnick: *On Call Surgery,* 2nd Edition
Bernstein et al: *On Call Psychiatry,* 2nd Edition
Bresnick & Adams: *On Call Procedures*
Chin: *On Call Obstetrics and Gynecology,* 2nd Edition
Dirschl & LeCroy: *On Call Orthopedics*
Henry & Mathur: *On Call Laboratory Medicine and Pathology*
Khan: *On Call Cardiology,* 2nd Edition
Lewis & Nocton: *On Call Pediatrics,* 2nd Edition
Marshall & Ruedy: *On Call: Principles and Protocols,* 3rd Edition

ON CALL
NEUROLOGY
Second Edition

Randolph S. Marshall, MD
Associate Professor of Clinical Neurology
Columbia University College of Physicians and Surgeons
Co-Director, Cerebral Localization Laboratory
Associate Attending Neurologist
New York-Presbyterian Hospital

Stephan A. Mayer, MD
Associate Professor of Clinical Neurology (in Neurosurgery)
Columbia University College of Physicians and Surgeons
Director, Neurological Intensive Care Unit
Associate Attending Neurologist
New York-Presbyterian Hospital

W.B. SAUNDERS COMPANY
A Harcourt Health Sciences Company
Philadelphia   London   New York   St. Louis   Sydney   Toronto

W.B. SAUNDERS COMPANY
A Harcourt Health Sciences Company

The Curtis Center
Independence Square West
Philadelphia, Pennsylvania 19106

Library of Congress Cataloging-in-Publication Data

Marshall, Randolph S.

On call neurology / Randolph S. Marshall, Stephan A. Mayer.—2nd ed.

p.   ; cm.—(On call series)

Includes index.

ISBN 0-7216-9221-4

1. Neurology—Handbooks, manuals, etc. I. Title: Neurology. II. Mayer, Stephan A. III. Title. IV. Series.
[DNLM: 1. Emergencies—Handbooks. 2. Nervous System Diseases—therapy—Handbooks. 3. Nervous System Diseases—diagnosis—Handbooks. 4. Neurology—methods—Handbooks. WL 39 M369o 2001]

RC355.M37 2001   616.8—dc21

DNLM/DLC   2001020108

ON CALL NEUROLOGY   ISBN 0-7216-9221-4

Copyright © 2001, 1997 by W.B. Saunders Company.

All rights reserved. No part of this publication may be reproduced or transmitted in any form or by any means, electronic or mechanical, including photocopy, recording, or any information storage and retrieval system, without permission in writing from the publisher.

Printed in the United States of America.

Last digit is the print number: 9   8   7   6   5   4   3   2   1

To the New York-Presbyterian neurology residents, past and present, who have helped us teach and learn.

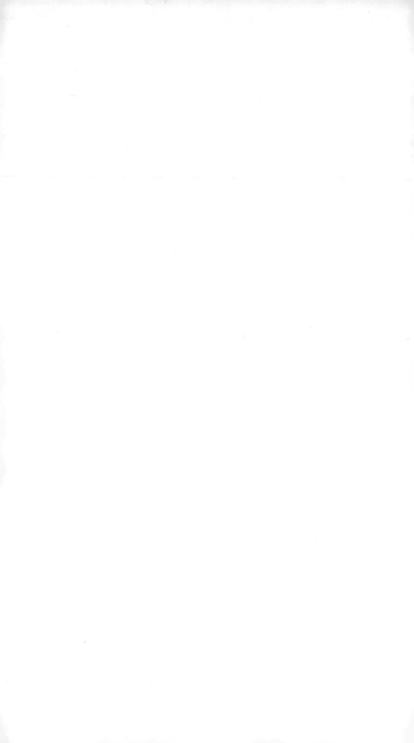

CONTRIBUTORS

Casilda Balmaceda, MD
Assistant Professor of Clinical
 Neurology and
 Neurosurgery
Columbia University College
 of Physicians and Surgeons
Assistant Attending
 Neurologist
New York-Presbyterian
 Hospital
New York, New York
Neuro-oncology

J. Torres-Gluck, MD
Attending Neurosurgeon
Our Lady of Mercy Medical
 Center
New York, New York
Neuro-oncology

Lawrence J. Hirsch, MD
Assistant Professor of
 Neurology
Columbia University College
 of Physicians and Surgeons
New York-Presbyterian
 Hospital
New York, New York
Epilepsy and Seizure Disorders

Elan D. Louis, MD
Assistant Professor of
 Neurology
Columbia University College
 of Physicians and Surgeons
Assistant Attending
 Neurologist
New York-Presbyterian
 Hospital
New York, New York
Movement Disorders

Juan M. Pascual, MD, PhD
Clinical Fellow in Pediatric
 Neurology
Columbia Presbyterian Center
New York-Presbyterian
 Hospital
New York, New York
Pediatric Neurologic Emergencies

Louis H. Weimer, MD
Assistant Professor of
 Neurology
Columbia University College
 of Physicians and Surgeons
Assistant Attending
 Neurologist
New York-Presbyterian
 Hospital
New York, New York
Nerve and Muscle Diseases

PREFACE

This book is meant to serve as a pocket reference for medical students, house officers, and nonneurologist physicians who care for patients in the hospital. Neurologic problems are common and, by their nature, complex. The goal of *On Call Neurology* is to provide the reader with accessible, highly structured protocols for the assessment and management of neurologic disorders in the emergency room, the intensive care unit, the hospital floor, or the clinic. We have tried to emphasize treatment and have attempted to simulate the focused and goal-directed thought processes of an experienced clinical neurologist.

On Call Neurology is designed to be comprehensive in scope but is admittedly limited in depth. We acknowledge that much of the content reflects "our way" of doing things. It is our hope that the protocols presented in this book will stimulate the student of neurology (whether a medical student or an attending neurologist) to research the literature, analyze the available data, and reach independent conclusions about optimal patient care. In short, we have intended this book to serve as a starting point for clinical problems in neurology rather than as a definitive reference.

We are grateful to our patients, colleagues, and teachers at The Neurological Institute of New York at New York-Presbyterian Hospital, who taught us most of what we know about neurology. In particular, we would like to thank J.P. Mohr, John Brust, Matthew Fink, and Lewis P. Rowland. Their voices can be heard in many of the pages of this text, and their dedication to teaching and education has served as an inspiration to generations of young physicians like us.

Stephan A. Mayer
Randolph S. Marshall

STRUCTURE OF THE BOOK

This book is divided into four main sections:

The first section, Introduction, provides an overview of the clinical approach to the neurologic patient, including the neurologic examination, neuroanatomic localization, and neurodiagnostic testing.

The second section, Patient-Related Problems: The Common Calls, is a symptom-oriented approach to chief complaints that frequently require neurologic consultation in the emergency room, clinic, or hospital floor. Each problem is approached from its inception, beginning with relevant questions that should be asked over the phone, temporary orders that should be given, and the major life-threatening disorders that should be considered as one approaches the bedside:

■ PHONE CALL

Questions

Pertinent questions to assess the urgency of the situation.

Orders

Urgent orders to stabilize the patient and gain additional information before you arrive at the bedside.

Inform RN

RN to be informed of the time the housestaff anticipates arrival at the bedside.

■ ELEVATOR THOUGHTS

The differential diagnoses to be considered while the housestaff is on the way to assess the patient (i.e., while in the elevator).

■ MAJOR THREAT TO LIFE

Neurologic emergencies that can lead to death or neurologic devastation unless immediate action is taken.

■ BEDSIDE

Quick Look Test

The quick look test is a rapid visual assessment to place the patient into one of three categories: well, sick, or critical. This helps determine the necessity of immediate intervention.

Vital Signs

Selective History and Chart Review

Including pertinent negatives and neurologic review of systems.

Selective Physical and Neurologic Examination

A rapid, focused neurologic examination designed to assess the extent and degree of neurologic dysfunction.

■ MANAGEMENT

Provides guidelines for neurodiagnostic testing and gives access to indicated medications and dosages. When applicable, checklists and specific management protocols are provided.

The third section, Selected Neurologic Disorders, provides an overview of important neurologic diseases and their management not covered comprehensively in the "common calls" section, such as CNS infections, multiple sclerosis, neuromuscular diseases, movement disorders, and brain tumors.

The fourth section, the Appendices, provides neuroanatomic references and other materials helpful for managing neurologic patients.

The On-Call Formulary is a compendium of medications commonly used to treat neurologic disorders. Drug indications, mechanisms of action, dosages, routes of administration, side effects, and comments for optimal use are provided.

COMMONLY USED ABBREVIATIONS

ABG	arterial blood gas
ACA	anterior cerebral artery
ACE	angiotensin-converting enzyme
ACTH	adrenocorticotropic hormone
AFB	acid-fast bacillus
AIDS	acquired immunodeficiency syndrome
AION	anterior ischemic optic neuropathy
ALS	amyotrophic lateral sclerosis
AMN	adrenomyeloneuropathy
ANA	antinuclear antibody
ANCA	antineutrophil cytoplasmic antibody
APD	afferent pupillary defect
aPTT	activated partial thromboplastin time
AV	arteriovenous
AVM	arteriovenous malformation
BAER	brain stem auditory evoked response
bid	two times a day
BP	blood pressure
BUN	blood urea nitrogen
CAA	cerebral amyloid angiopathy
CBC	complete blood cell count
CBF	cerebral blood flow
CHF	congestive heart failure
CIDP	chronic inflammatory demyelinating polyneuropathy
CK	creatine kinase
CMAP	compound muscle action potential
CMV	cytomegalovirus
CN	cranial nerve

CNS	central nervous system
CPAP	continuous positive airway pressure
CPK	creatine phosphokinase
CPP	cerebral perfusion pressure
CPR	cardiopulmonary resuscitation
CRAO	central retinal artery occlusion
CSF	cerebrospinal fluid
CT	computed tomography
DDAVP	desmopressin acetate
DIC	disseminated intravascular coagulation
D5W	5% dextrose in water
D5WNS	5% dextrose in normal saline
D50W	50% dextrose in water
DVT	deep vein thrombosis
DWI	diffusion-weighted imaging
EBV	Epstein-Barr virus
ECG	electrocardiogram
EEG	electroencephalogram
EMG	electromyography
EP	electrophysiologic
ER	emergency room
ESR	erythrocyte sedimentation rate
EtOH	ethanol
FDA	Food and Drug Administration
FFP	fresh frozen plasma
FNF	finger-nose-finger
GBM	glioblastoma multiforme
GBS	Guillain-Barré syndrome
GCS	Glasgow Coma scale
GI	gastrointestinal
GU	genitourinary
HCG	human chorionic gonadotropin
HEENT	head, eyes, ears, nose, throat

HIV	human immunodeficiency virus
HKS	heel-knee-shin
HR	heart rate
HSE	herpes simplex encephalitis
HSV-1	herpes simplex virus 1
HTLV-1	human T-cell lymphotropic virus type I
Hz	Hertz
ICA	internal carotid artery
ICH	intracerebral hemorrhage
ICP	intracranial pressure
ICU	intensive care unit
IgG	immunoglobulin G
IM	intramuscular
IMV	intermittent mandatory ventilation
INO	internuclear ophthalmoplegia
INR	international normalized ratio
ION	ischemic optic neuropathy
IV	intravenous
IVIG	intravenous immune globulin
IVP	intravenous push
KVO	keep the vein open
LFT	liver function test
LCM	lymphocytic choriomeningitis
LP	lumbar puncture
MABP	mean arterial blood pressure
MAO	monoamine oxidase
MCA	middle cerebral artery
MELAS	mitochondrial encephalomyopathy, lactic acidosis, and stroke
MI	myocardial infarction
MLD	metachromatic leukodystrophy
MLF	median longitudinal fasciculus
MMN	multifocal motor neuropathy

MMSE	Mini Mental State Examination
MRI	magnetic resonance imaging
MS	multiple sclerosis
MSA	multiple-system atrophy
NCS	nerve conduction study
NCV	nerve conduction velocity
NPO	nil per os (nothing by mouth)
NS	normal saline
NSAID	nonsteroidal anti-inflammatory drug
OCB	oligoclonal band
OKN	opticokinetic nystagmus
ON	optic neuritis
PCA	posterior cerebral artery
PCNSL	primary central nervous system lymphoma
Pco_2	partial pressure of carbon dioxide
PCR	polymerase chain reaction
PE	pulmonary embolism
PEEP	positive end-expiratory pressure
PET	positron emission tomography
PLED	periodic lateralizing epileptiform discharge
PML	progressive multifocal leukoencephalopathy
PNET	primitive neuroectodermal tumor
PO	per os (by mouth)
Po_2	partial pressure of oxygen
PPD	purified protein derivative
PPRF	paramedian pontine reticular formation
PRN	as needed
PT	prothrombin time
PTT	partial thromboplastin time
PVS	persistent vegetative state
qd	every day
qhs	every day at nighttime
qid	four times a day

RA	rheumatoid arthritis
RAM	rapid alternating movements
RBC	red blood cell
RF	rheumatoid factor
RPR	rapid plasmin reagin
SAH	subarachnoid hemorrhage
SBP	systolic blood pressure
SC	subcutaneous
SFEMG	single-fiber electromyogram
SIADH	syndrome of inappropriate antidiuretic hormone
SIMV	synchronized intermittent mandatory ventilation
SL	sublingual
SLE	systemic lupus erythematosus
SMA	spinal muscular atrophy
SMP	sympathetically maintained pain
SPECT	single photon emission computed tomography
SPEP	serum protein electrophoresis
SSEP	somatosensory evoked potential
SSPE	subacute sclerosing panencephalitis
t-PA	tissue plasminogen activator
TCA	tricyclic antidepressant
TCD	transcranial Doppler
TENS	transcutaneous electric nerve stimulation
TFTs	thyroid function tests
TGA	transient global amnesia
TIA	transient ischemic attack
tid	three times a day
TMB	transient monocular blindness
VDRL	Veneral Disease Research Laboratory
VEP	visual evoked potential
VER	visual evoked response
WBC	white blood cell

NOTICE

Neurology is an ever-changing field. Standard safety precautions must be followed, but as new research and clinical experience broaden our knowledge, changes in treatment and drug therapy may become necessary or appropriate. Readers are advised to check the most current product information provided by the manufacturer of each drug to be administered to verify the recommended dose, the method and duration of administration, and the contraindications. It is the responsibility of the treating physician, relying on experience and knowledge of the patient, to determine dosages and the best treatment for each individual patient. Neither the publisher nor the editor assumes any liability for any injury and/or damage to persons or property arising from this publication.

THE PUBLISHER

CONTENTS

INTRODUCTION

1. Approach to the Neurologic Patient On Call: History Taking, Differential Diagnosis, and Anatomic Localization   3
2. The Neurologic Examination   12
3. Diagnostic Studies   31

PATIENT-RELATED PROBLEMS: THE COMMON CALLS

4. Seizures and Status Epilepticus   47
5. Stupor and Coma   58
6. Acute Stroke   76
7. Spinal Cord Compression   92
8. Delirium   102
9. Head Injury   113
10. Ataxia and Gait Failure   126
11. Acute Visual Disturbances   137
12. Increased Intracranial Pressure   150
13. Dizziness and Vertigo   161
14. Headache   170
15. Neuromuscular Respiratory Failure   185
16. Syncope   201
17. Pain Syndromes   213
18. Amnesia and Dementia   228
19. Brain Death   240

SELECTED NEUROLOGIC DISORDERS

20. Nerve and Muscle Diseases 249
21. Demyelinating and Inflammatory Disorders of the Central Nervous System 270
22. Infections of the Central Nervous System 285
23. Neuro-oncology 302
24. Cerebrovascular Disease 325
25. Movement Disorders 340
26. Epilepsy and Seizure Disorders 351
27. Pediatric Neurologic Emergencies 369

APPENDICES

A-1 Muscles of the Neck and Brachial Plexus 381
A-2 Muscles of the Perineum and Lumbosacral Plexus 384
A-3 Brachial Plexus 386
A-4 Lumbar Plexus 388
A-5 Sensory Dermatome Map 389
A-6 Mini-Mental State Examination 390
A-7 Surface Map of the Brain 393
A-8 Nuclei of the Brainstem 394
A-9 Surface Anatomy of the Brainstem 395
B On-Call Formulary: Commonly Prescribed Medications in Neurology 397
INDEX 419

INTRODUCTION

chapter 1

Approach to the Neurologic Patient On Call: History Taking, Differential Diagnosis, and Anatomic Localization

It's in the early morning hours. You get a call from a resident in the emergency room (ER). A 48-year-old teacher has headache, neck pain, and urinary incontinence, and, as of this morning, is no longer able to hold a pen in his right hand. How do you proceed? What do you tell the ER resident? What tests should be ordered? How urgent is this situation?

Neurology, perhaps more than any other field in medicine, demands familiarity with a wide spectrum of anatomic details and diagnostic studies. Electrophysiologic, serologic, genetic, pathologic, and a host of imaging techniques have enabled diagnoses to be made with a higher degree of accuracy and certainty than ever before. Yet all diagnostic puzzles, simple or complex, begin with the presentation of a symptom by a patient to a doctor.

It is often said that 90% of the neurologic diagnosis comes from the patient's history. Indeed, it is the exception when a diagnosis is stumbled upon after a "shotgun" approach of ordering diagnostic studies unguided by the patient's initial complaints. In the type of encounter for which this book was written, namely, a rapid response to an acute complaint, the single most important factor in the encounter is the initial interview with the patient. This book aims to guide you through a logical, focused, and effective approach to diagnosis and management of your patient's acute problem. After a discussion of general principles of managing patients on call, some key points about neurologic history taking are covered in this chapter along with principles of differential diagnosis and anatomic localization. The neurologic physical examination is outlined in Chapter 2. The basics of the most important initial diagnostic studies are covered in Chapter 3.

■ PRINCIPLES OF MANAGING PATIENTS WHEN ON CALL

1. **Obtain adequate information from the initial phone contact.**

   Establish the nature of the complaint, understand its

acuteness and its severity, and learn what has been done so far (Have vital signs been checked? Has any labwork been sent?).
2. **Establish a working differential diagnosis before you see the patient.**
   Some preparatory thought will produce a more efficient and directed interview and examination of the patient. Prioritize your diagnoses by placing the most potentially dangerous diagnoses at the top of the list, followed by the most likely diagnoses.
3. **Be focused in your bedside assessment.**
   Unlike the comprehensive examination that you perform when admitting a patient to the hospital or when seeing a patient for the first time in the clinic, your history taking and examination of the patient when you are on call needs to be focused and efficient.
4. **Know when to call for additional consultation.**
   Examples would be an ophthalmologic consultation for branch retinal artery occlusion versus anterior ischemic optic neuropathy, or a neurosurgical consultation to place an intracranial pressure monitor.
5. **Be accurate and concise in your documentation of the encounter.**
   Although it will be your responsibility to solve the clinical problem as completely as possible, many times you will be unable to make a diagnosis or complete a treatment during the time you are involved with the patient. You must document the patient's history and physical examination as precisely as possible. Make sure you date and time your note. If there was a delay in arriving at the bedside because of another emergency, document this. Include relevant laboratory data in your note. Your evaluation and formulation of the problem should be well integrated and transparent. The recommendations for treatment should be stated clearly and should be concordant with what was written in the orders. If discussions with family members took place, the content and outcome of the discussions should be documented.

■ PRINCIPLES OF HISTORY TAKING IN NEUROLOGY

Key features of the neurologic history include the following:
1. **Patient's demographics: age, gender, and race-ethnicity, if relevant**
   Age is often crucial in the initial consideration of the differential diagnosis. Disorders causing ataxia, for instance, would include multiple sclerosis and viral cerebellitis in

patients under 45 years of age, whereas cerebral infarction and alcoholic cerebellar degeneration would be higher on the differential diagnosis list for the same syndrome in older patients. Gender-specific neurologic conditions include benign intracranial hypertension and multiple sclerosis, which are more common in women.

Race-ethnicity differences include the higher incidence of intracranial atherosclerosis in African-American and Hispanic patients, whereas in Caucasians, extracranial atherosclerosis tends to develop with higher frequency.

2. **Temporal course of the disease**

   The temporal pattern of your patient's symptoms is one of the most important pieces of history that you will obtain. Many neurologic disorders can be differentiated by their temporal course. Precipitous onset suggests a vascular or epileptic etiology across a wide spectrum of complaints. Onset over minutes to hours suggests a toxic or infectious cause. Subacute or chronic progression of symptoms prompts investigation of metabolic, neoplastic, or degenerative disorders.

   The subsequent pattern of symptoms is also important. Symptoms that follow a paroxysmal course lead to a limited differential diagnosis: transient ischemic attack, migraine, and seizure are often considered when paroxysmal episodes are relatively short lived. Myasthenia gravis, multiple sclerosis, and periodic paralysis have a fluctuating or recurrent course as well, but typically with less rapid cycles.

3. **Characterization of the symptoms**

   It may seem excessive or inefficient to obtain a detailed description of your patient's symptoms, yet the initial disqualification of untenable diagnoses can be accomplished with confidence only when you are sure of the symptoms being reported. The mode of onset, prior occurrences, surrounding events, and character of the complaint—including what makes it better or worse—are important in establishing an initial differential diagnosis. You may need to ask more than once or use alternative terminology to elicit the details of a particular symptom. Notoriously ambiguous symptom descriptions in neurology include "heavy," which may mean weak, numb, or clumsy; "numb," which may mean decreased sensation or paresthesias; "dizzy," which may mean vertiginous, lightheaded, or confused; and "confused," which may mean disoriented, agitated, aphasic, or even sleepy. Be wary also of actual diagnoses that are presented in lieu of symptoms. The patient who keeps getting "seizures" in the arm or the one who presents with "trauma" should be redirected to a vocabulary of symptoms alone.

4. **Medical history**

Although a detailed medical history is not necessary in every interview, you will need to obtain information about any disease that could contribute to the patient's present complaint. For example, it is crucial to be aware of cerebrovascular risk factors including cardiac disease, hypertension, diabetes mellitus, and smoking if stroke is in the differential diagnosis. A history of carcinoma would be important if metastasis or paraneoplastic disease is being considered. Some systemic illnesses, such as sarcoidosis, systemic lupus erythematosus, and diabetes mellitus, may be associated with a spectrum of neurologic complaints. Information regarding current medications should be elicited in every case. Travel and occupational history may be relevant, for example, when toxic and infectious etiologies are under consideration. If the patient cannot provide the necessary information, you may need to interview a family member or caretaker or review the patient's medical record.

■ ESTABLISHING THE INITIAL DIFFERENTIAL DIAGNOSIS

Neurologic complaints lend themselves to categorization of the differential diagnosis based on **anatomic localization**. Acute visual dysfunction, for example, may be divided into unilateral loss of vision (suggesting pathology in the retina or optic nerve), binocular visual field defects (implying disease in the optic tracts or radiations), or diplopia (suggesting either neuromuscular or brain stem dysfunction). Other neurologic complaints are best categorized initially by the **rate of onset**. The likely diagnoses related to acute ataxia, for instance, are different from those associated with chronic or subacute gait failure. The differential diagnosis for many neurologic complaints, however, contains a wide variety of disorders that are not easily sorted until more information is obtained from the history and physical examination. For these complaints, we suggest that you develop a standard method of considering the differential diagnosis. One mnemonic, which appears in many of our patient complaint chapters, may be useful: VITAMINS, representing vascular, infectious, traumatic, autoimmune, metabolic/toxic, iatrogenic/idiopathic or hereditary, neoplastic, and seizure/psychiatric/structural etiologies.

■ ANATOMIC LOCALIZATION

The neurologic examination is presented in Chapter 2. Certain principles of anatomic localization warrant emphasis here, because establishing the correct diagnosis in neurology is often dependent on localization of the lesion. Listed here in tabular form are general principles of localization of lesions from the brain to the periphery. Most of these localizations are discussed within the pertinent chapters on **patient-related problems**.

Localization in the Upper Motor Neuron (Pyramidal) System

Principle: Tone is increased, causing spasticity and hyperreflexia.

Site	Symptoms	Signs
Cortex	• Differential weakness of limbs and face • Sensory symptoms • Language, visual, or attentional alterations	• Fractionated weakness (e.g., arm greater than face and leg) • Aphasia, hemianopia, or hemineglect • Cortical and primary sensory loss • Cognitive dysfunction
Corona radiata	• Differential weakness of limbs and face	• Fractionated weakness • Primary sensory loss
Internal capsule	• Weakness only	• Face, arm, and leg affected equally and densely
Brain stem	• Unilateral or bilateral weakness • Diplopia, vertigo, dysarthria, or dysphagia	• Dense hemiparesis • Ocular or oropharyngeal weakness
Spinal cord	• Difficulty with gait • Difficulty walking • Urinary incontinence	• No face involvement • Spastic quadriparesis (cervical) or paraparesis (thoracic) • Sensory level

Localization in the Lower Motor Neuron System

Principle: Tone is decreased, causing flaccidity and hyporeflexia.

Site	Symptoms	Signs
Anterior horn	• Progressive flaccid weakness	• Wasting, weakness, fasciculations • No sensory loss

Site	Symptoms	Signs
Root/plexus	• Single limb weakness and sensory loss • Pain in the neck, back, or limb	• Weakness in radicular/plexus distribution • Electromyogram (EMG) shows denervation in affected muscles
Nerve	• Focal weakness (mononeuritis) • Distal weakness (polyneuropathy)	• Focal or distal weakness • Atrophy in affected distribution • Fasciculations • Hyporeflexia • Slowing or low amplitude on conduction studies; denervation on EMG
Neuromuscular junction	• Fluctuating weakness • Diplopia	• Positive edrophonium test • Decremental response with repetitive stimulation on EMG
Muscle	• Proximal weakness • Difficulty climbing stairs and brushing hair • Muscle aches	• Proximal weakness • Normal nerve conduction • Polyphasic, low-amplitude motor units on EMG

Localization Within the Brain Stem

Principle: Specific cranial nerve involvement guides localization (Fig. 1–1).

Site	Signs and Symptoms
Midbrain	• Impaired vertical gaze • **CN 3 palsy** (plus contralateral abduction nystagmus suggests ipsilateral internuclear ophthalmoplegia [INO]) • **CN 4 palsy** • Contralateral motor signs (hemiparesis suggests Weber's syndrome; ataxia suggests Claude's syndrome; tremor or chorea suggests Benedikt's syndrome) • Alterations in consciousness, perception, or behavior (peduncular hallucinosis)

Approach to the Neurologic Patient On Call 9

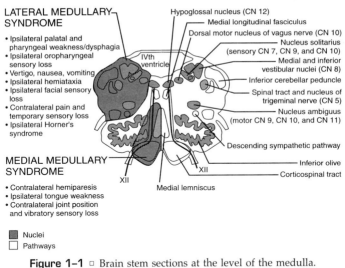

Figure 1-1 □ Brain stem sections at the level of the medulla.

Pons
- Dysarthria and dysphagia
- Contralateral hemiparesis or hemisensory loss
- Ipsilateral facial sensory loss **(CN 5)**
- Ipsilateral gaze palsy (paramedian pontine reticular formation [PPRF]) or one-and-a-half syndrome (PPRF and median longitudinal fasciculus [MLF])
- Locked-in syndrome (bilateral basis pontis; associated with ocular bobbing)
- Horizontal nystagmus (often brachium pontis)
- Ataxia

Pontomedullary junction
- Vertigo **(CN 8)**
- Dysarthria
- Horizontal or vertical nystagmus
- Contralateral hemisensory loss and hemiparesis

Lateral medulla (Wallenberg syndrome)
- Ipsilateral Horner's syndrome
- Ipsilateral limb ataxia
- Ipsilateral face and contralateral body numbness
- Gait ataxia
- Vertigo, dizziness, nausea **(CN 8)**

	• Dysphagia **(CN 9, CN 10, and CN 12 palsies)**	
Medial medulla (rare)	• Contralateral hemiplegia • Contralateral posterior column sensory loss • Ipsilateral tongue weakness **(CN 12 palsy)**	

Localization in the Spinal Cord

Principle: Localization is assisted by the combination of tracts involved.

Site	Signs and Symptoms	Common Causes
Hemicord (Brown-Séquard's syndrome)	• Ipsilateral hemiparesis • Contralateral spinothalamic sensory loss • Ipsilateral dorsal column sensory loss • Sphincter dysfunction	• Penetrating trauma • Extrinsic cord compression
Anterior cord	• Upper and lower motor paralysis • Spinothalamic sensory loss • Sphincter dysfunction • Sparing of posterior columns	• Anterior spinal artery infarction (often involves T4 to T8)
Central cord	• Paraparesis • Lower motor paralysis; wasting and fasciculations in arms • Sensory loss in "shawl" distribution (if in cervical region)	• Syringomyelia • Neck flexion-extension injury • Intrinsic tumor
Posterior cord	• Proprioceptive and vibratory sensory loss • Segmental tingling and numbness • Sensation of constricting "bands"	• Vitamin B_{12} deficiency • Demyelination (multiple sclerosis) • Extrinsic compression
Foramen magnum	• Spastic quadriparesis • Neck pain and stiffness • C2 to C4 and upper facial numbness • Ipsilateral Horner's syndrome	• Tumor (meningioma, chordoma) • Atlantoaxial subluxation

	• Ipsilateral tongue and trapezius muscle weakness	
Conus medullaris	• Lower sacral saddle sensory loss (S2 to S5) • Sphincter dysfunction; impotence • Aching back or rectal pain • L5 and S1 motor deficits (ankle and foot weakness)	• Intrinsic tumor • Extrinsic cord compression
Cauda equina	• Sphincter dysfunction • Paraparesis with weakness in the distribution of multiple roots • Sensory loss in multiple bilateral dermatomes	• Extrinsic tumor • Carcinomatous meningitis • Arachnoiditis • Spinal stenosis

chapter 2 | The Neurologic Examination

Clinical examination is of primary importance in the practice of neurology, even with the availability of advanced neuroimaging techniques. **This is because the neurologic examination provides critical information that no other test can provide: it tells you whether the patient's nervous system is working normally.** Unfortunately, many clinicians never master the neurologic examination because it is taught in a way that makes it seem time-consuming, excessively complicated, and of questionable relevance. In real on-call situations, however, expert neurologists almost never perform the type of comprehensive, top-to-bottom examination that is taught in medical school; rather, they focus on the problem at hand, eliminate those parts of the examination that are not relevant, and actively test hypotheses suggested by the history.

The intent of this chapter is to acquaint (or reacquaint) the physician with the basic components of the neurologic examination. Suggested problem-oriented examinations for specific clinical presentations (e.g., coma, back pain, or acute weakness) are provided in later chapters.

■ THE NEUROLOGIC EXAMINATION

The components of the neurologic examination are shown in Box 2–1.

Mental Status

The importance of the mental status examination cannot be overemphasized. In patients with suspected intracranial pathology (e.g., in those experiencing sudden severe headache), a change in mental status signals that the problem is more than just one of pain: it indicates that the brain is not working correctly. The implications for further workup and management are significant.

Human mentation is extraordinarily complex, and students of neurology frequently have difficulty with the mental status examination because they are taught to evaluate a "laundry-list" of mental functions (Table 2–1) without emphasis on how to integrate the findings. To simplify the mental status examination, we advocate a five-step approach that emphasizes five basic ele-

> **Box 2–1. COMPONENTS OF THE NEUROLOGIC EXAMINATION**
>
> For the beginner, even remembering all of the components of the neurologic exam can be difficult. Memorizing the first letter of the seven main sections of the exam (M C M C R S G) may be helpful for avoiding omissions when first learning the examination:
> Mental status
> Cranial nerves
> Motor
> Coordination
> Reflexes
> Sensory
> Gait and station

ments: (1) alertness and attention, (2) confusion, disorientation, or abnormal behavior, (3) language, (4) memory, and (5) other higher cortical functions.

- **Step One: Examination of level of consciousness, attention, and concentration**

  As illustrated schematically in Figure 2–1, the brain's arousal and attention mechanism (mediated by the diffuse cortical projections of the reticular activating system of the brain stem) serves as the foundation of all higher cognitive function. Level of consciousness, attention, and mental concentration can be conceptualized as three levels of a pyramid, because dysfunction at a more basic level (depressed level of consciousness) almost guarantees that functions at the top of the pyramid (attention and concentration) will be abnormal. Similarly, if a patient cannot remain alert or attend or concentrate, normal functioning of memory, language, or other higher functions cannot be expected. *Delirium* is characterized by severe attentional deficits in a patient with relatively preserved alertness (mildly lethargic to hyperalert).

  1. **Level of consciousness.** *Is the patient alert, lethargic, stuporous, or comatose? Lethargy* resembles sleepiness but with one important difference: the patient cannot be fully and permanently awakened. *Stupor* can be operationally defined by the requirement for painful stimuli to obtain the patient's best verbal or motor response. *Coma* indicates lack of responsiveness even to painful stimuli.
  2. **Attention.** *Is the patient attentive to you?* Global attention is impaired in patients who are lethargic or encephalo-

Table 2-1 □ MENTAL STATUS: EMOTIONAL AND HIGHER COGNITIVE FUNCTIONS

Behavior	Is the patient's behavior appropriate, hostile, or bizarre?
Abstract reasoning	Can the patient judge similarities and interpret proverbs? Poor abstract reasoning results in "concrete thinking."
Insight	Does the patient have an appropriate understanding of the current medical problem?
Judgment	Is the patient's judgment impaired? Ask what the patient would do if he or she found a wallet or smelled smoke in a theater.
Calculations	Can the patient add, subtract, and multiply?
Visuospatial ability	Can the patient copy figures, draw a clock face, or bisect a line?
Praxis	Does the patient have *apraxia*—the inability to execute motor tasks (whistle or blow out a match) in response to a verbal command or imitation (ideomotor apraxia) in the absence of a comprehension, sensory, or motor deficit?
Affect	Is the patient's affect (an immediately expressed and observed emotion) depressed, euphoric, restricted, flat, or inappropriate?
Mood	What is the patient's long-term emotional disposition?
Thought form	Does the patient display loosening of associations, flight of ideas, tangentiality, circumstantiality, or incoherence? When seen in the absence of impaired level of consciousness, attention, memory, or language, thought disorders are characteristic of psychiatric illness.
Thought content	Is the patient's thought content characterized by paranoia, delusions, compulsions, obsessions, phobias, or derealization?
Perceptions	Does the patient have hallucinations or illusions?

pathic. A normally attentive patient looks at you and responds to questions and commands immediately. Inattention is characterized by impaired visual fixation and pursuit, delayed verbal responses requiring multiple prompts, and motor impersistence. *Spatial hemineglect* results from large hemispheric lesions and is almost

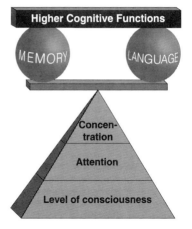

Figure 2–1 ◻ Schematic representation of the basic elements of human cognition. Arousal mechanisms (level of consciousness, attention, and concentration) serve as the foundation of all mental activity. Language and memory are anatomically localized, highly developed basic cognitive modalities. All other higher cognitive functions depend on normal function of these three basic elements.

always associated with impaired global attention as well.
3. **Concentration.** *Can the patient count from 20 to 1 and recite the months in reverse?* These are relatively overlearned tasks and are less susceptible to the effects of prior education than are serial sevens. Abnormal responses include long pauses, omissions, and reversals.
- **Step Two: Assessment for disorientation, confusion, or a behavioral abnormality**
  This step is initially based on observation during history taking. *Behavior* should be assessed in terms of psychomotor activity (agitation versus abulia) and emotional responses (elation, sadness, anger, or flattening).
  1. **Formally test orientation to name, place, time (date, day of week, month, and year), and situation.** Disorientation reflects abnormal *integrative functioning* of the brain. Unlike abnormalities of arousal, memory, or language, disorientation has no implications with regard to anatomic localization—there is no "orientation center" in the brain. *Remember that disorientation typically follows a sequential pattern, first involving situation, then time, place, and name.* Hence, a patient who is oriented to time and place but who does not know his or her own name probably has a psychiatric problem.
- **Step Three: Language testing**
  Focal lesions of the dominant hemisphere may lead to *aphasia,* defined as abnormal language production or comprehension. Four essential components of language should always be tested:

1. **Fluency.** *Is the rate and flow of the patient's speech production normal?* Dysfluency is defined by reduction in the rate of speech production. Speaking with effort, finding words with difficulty, losing normal grammar and syntax, giving perseverative responses, and making spontaneous paraphasic errors are characteristic.
2. **Comprehension.** *Can the patient perform one- and two-step commands?* If the patient is attentive, inability to follow commands implies impaired auditory comprehension.
3. **Naming.** *Can the patient name a watch, a pen, and glasses?* Check for *anomia* and *paraphasic errors.* Listen for *phonemic paraphasias* (substitution of one phoneme for another, e.g., "tadle" for "table") and *semantic paraphasias* (substitution of one semantically related word for another, e.g., "door" for "window").
4. **Repetition.** *Can the patient repeat "The train was an hour late" and "Today is a sunny day"?* Intact repetition in the presence of serious deficits in fluency or comprehension is diagnostic of *transcortical aphasia,* which implies a good prognosis for recovery.

With the preceding information—fluency, comprehension, naming, and repetition—you can diagnose and classify any aphasia (Table 2–2). Asking the patient to read aloud is also a sensitive screening test for aphasia and alexia. *Broca's aphasia* (localized to the dorsolateral dominant frontal lobe) results in nonfluent, effortful speech and is usually associated with hemiparesis. *Wernicke's aphasia* (localized to the posterior superior temporal lobe) leads to fluent, nonsensical speech with impaired comprehension, and in most cases, the patient is unaware of the problem (anosognosia). If an aphasia is present and more precise characterization of the deficit is desired, check reading and writing in detail. Don't confuse aphasia with *dysarthria,* which is a motor disorder.

- **Step Four: Memory testing**

  Memory is classified as **immediate, short term,** and **long term.** In neurologic patients, impaired immediate recall is usually due to attentional deficits rather than to pure amnesia. Short-term memory can be tested by asking the patient to recall three words (e.g., "Jane, red, elephant") in 3 to 5 minutes. Long-term (remote) memory is best tested by asking about famous politicians (e.g., Richard M. Nixon or John F. Kennedy), twentieth-century historical events (the Watergate crisis or World War II), or sports figures. *Confabulatory (incorrect)* responses occur with severe amnestic disorders.

- **Step Five: Testing for emotional and higher cognitive functions**

  These components of the mental status exam are listed in Table 2–1 and are usually not anatomically localizable and

Table 2-2 □ CLASSIFICATION OF APHASIAS

	Fluency	Comprehension	Naming	Repetition
Broca's aphasia (motor)	O	+	O	O
Wernicke's aphasia (sensory)	+	O	O	O
Transcortical motor aphasia	O	+	O	+
Transcortical sensory aphasia	+	O	O	+
Global aphasia	O	O	O	O
Conduction aphasia	+	+	O	O
Anomic aphasia	+	+	O	+

O, abnormal; +, normal.

not essential to test in all cases. They are primarily of value for identifying complex cognitive and neuropsychiatric disorders.

Cranial Nerves

CN 1 **Olfactory nerve**
Testing for olfactory nerve function is rarely needed and is usually omitted.

CN 2 **Optic nerve**
1. **Fundus**
    Check for papilledema, optic disk pallor or atrophy, retinal hemorrhages or exudates, spontaneous venous pulsations, and hypertensive microvascular changes (arteriovenous [AV] nicking and copper wiring) (Fig. 2–2).
2. **Visual fields**
    Stand facing the patient, instruct him or her to look at your nose, and have the patient count fingers in all four quadrants (Fig. 2–3). Test each eye separately. Check lateralized blink to threat if the patient is inattentive.
3. **Visual acuity**
    Test acuity with eyeglasses, one eye at a time, using a "near card."
4. **Color vision**
    This is usually tested only by an ophthalmolo-

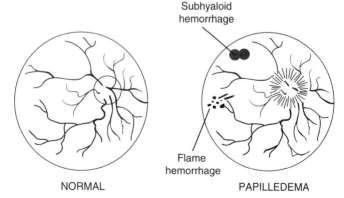

Figure 2–2 □ Common abnormalities found on examination of the optic fundus. Papilledema is characterized by optic disk congestion and the loss of distinct vessels crossing the blurred disk margin.

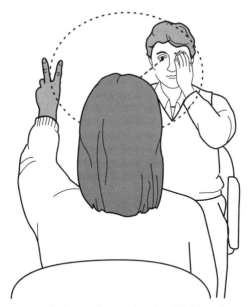

Figure 2-3 □ Technique for visual field testing.

gist. Color desaturation occurs with optic nerve disorders.

CN 3, **Oculomotor, trochlear, and abducens nerves**
CN 4, **1. Eyelids**
CN 6   Check for *ptosis,* defined as a drooping eyelid that does not clear the upper margin of the pupil. Ptosis occurs with oculomotor nerve (CN 3) injury or with *Horner's syndrome* (ptosis, miosis, facial anhidrosis), which results from injury to central or peripheral sympathetic nerve pathways.

2. Pupils

Check for shape, symmetry, reactivity to light, and accommodation. *Anisocoria* (pupillary asymmetry) can result from *miosis* (an abnormally small pupil) or *mydriasis* (an abnormally large pupil), and in some cases, examination in both light and dark conditions is necessary to determine which pupil is abnormal.

An *afferent pupillary defect* (APD, or Marcus Gunn pupil) results from a lesion of the optic nerve (e.g., optic neuritis in multiple sclerosis). It is elicited using the swinging flashlight test: as the light

swings from one eye to the other at 3-second intervals, the abnormal pupil will *dilate* rather than constrict when the light shines on it.
3. **Extraocular movements**

Ask the patient to fixate on and follow your finger in all directions of gaze. Unilateral impairment of ocular motility usually results from an isolated cranial nerve deficit. Besides checking for limitations of eye movement, look for abnormalities of *fixation* (square wave jerks, nystagmus, opsoclonus), *smooth pursuit* (saccadic pursuit), and *saccadic eye movements* (hypometric saccades, ocular dysmetria). Test saccades by asking the patient to rapidly switch fixation from one hand to the other.

Opticokinetic nystagmus (OKN) is a normal physiologic nystagmus that occurs when the patient is asked to fixate on a series of moving visual stimuli (e.g., striped OKN tape). Asymmetric loss of OKN results from frontal or parietal lobe lesions on the side to which the tape is moving.

CN 5 **Trigeminal nerve**

Sensory function of V1, V2, and V3 is evaluated by testing for deficits to light touch, pinprick, and temperature on the forehead, cheek, and chin, respectively (Fig. 2–4). Motor function can be tested by checking for asymmetry of lateral jaw movements. Lateral pterygoid muscle weakness results in ipsilat-

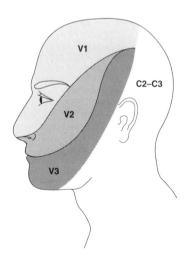

Figure 2–4 □ Sensory distribution of the trigeminal nerve.

eral deviation on jaw opening and weakness of lateral movement to the opposite side.

The *corneal reflex* (mediated by V1) is elicited by lightly touching the cornea with a cotton wisp, which results in contraction of the orbicularis oculi (CN 7). It usually needs to be tested only in comatose patients, or if focal brain stem or cranial nerve pathology (e.g., an acoustic neuroma) is suspected.

CN 7 **Facial nerve**

A *widened palpebral fissure* and *flattened nasolabial fold* are indicative of facial weakness. Ask the patient to grin and raise the eyebrows, and check the strength of eye and lip closure against active resistance. Upper motor neuron facial weakness tends to spare the contralateral forehead because it has bilateral upper motor neuron innervation, whereas the lower portion of the face does not.

Taste usually requires testing only when there is evidence of facial weakness. Dip a wet cotton swab in sugar or salt and apply it to the tip and side of the tongue with the tongue kept protruded. Absence of taste confirms a peripheral CN 7 lesion proximal to the junction of the chorda tympani.

CN 8 **Vestibulocochlear nerve**

Auditory deficits can be screened for by testing appreciation of *finger rub* in each ear. If unilateral hearing loss is present, sensorineural and conduction deafness can be differentiated using a 512-Hz tuning fork:

- *Weber's test* is performed by striking the tuning fork and placing it against the middle of the forehead. Ask the patient if the tone is equal in both ears. Diminution in the affected ear indicates sensorineural hearing loss. A louder tone in the affected ear results from *conduction deafness* (disease of the ossicles in the middle ear). In conduction deafness, a pure tone transmitted through the skull is appreciated in the affected ear, whereas the tone sounds softer in the normal ear because of competing ambient noise transmitted via the tympanic membrane and ossicles.
- *The Rinne test* is performed to confirm the presence of conduction deafness in the affected ear. Strike the tuning fork, place it on the mastoid process, and ask the patient when the tone can no longer be heard. Then place it over the external auditory

meatus—normally, the patient will hear the tone again; if not, conduction deafness is present.

CN 9, CN 10 **Glossopharyngeal and vagus nerves**

Ask the patient to say "ah," check for symmetry and adequacy of soft palate elevation, and listen for hoarseness or nasal speech (all motor functions of CN 10). The gag reflex, tested by lightly touching the posterior oropharynx with a cotton swab (CN 9 sensory, CN 10 motor), is often absent or depressed in older patients. *Dysphagia* and risk for aspiration are best screened for by asking the patient to swallow a small quantity of water (3 oz); coughing indicates aspiration and inability to protect the airway.

CN 11 **Spinal accessory nerve**

Have the patient flex and turn the head to each side against resistance (tests the sternocleidomastoid muscle). Contraction of the left sternocleidomastoid muscle turns the head to the right and vice versa. Have the patient shrug the shoulders against resistance to test the trapezius muscle.

CN 12 **Hypoglossal nerve**

Have the patient stick out the tongue and push it into each cheek. Unilateral CN 12 dysfunction results in deviation of the tongue to the weak side upon protrusion and in inability to push the tongue into the opposite cheek.

Motor

1. **Inspection**

   Look for *muscle wasting* (atrophy), *fasciculations,* and *adventitious movements.* Preferential spontaneous movement of the limbs on one side suggests paresis of the unused limbs. If the patient is comatose, check for a preferential localizing response to sternal rub.

   Tremor should be evaluated at rest (rest tremor), with sustained posture (postural tremor), and with active movement (action or intention tremor).

2. **Tone**

   Have the patient relax; check muscle tone by passively moving the elbows, wrists, and knees.

   a. **Hypotonia** occurs with acute paralysis, lower motor neuron disease, ipsilateral cerebellar lesions, and chorea.
   b. **Hypertonia** comes in three varieties:
      (1) **Spasticity** develops as a consequence of upper motor neuron lesions. It is generally characterized by a sudden

increase in tone (a "catch") as the limb is passively flexed or extended. The clasp-knife phenomenon is a particular form of spasticity sometimes encountered in the legs; muscle tone is greatest at the beginning of movement and slowly decreases until there is a sudden loss of resistance.

(2) **Rigidity** occurs with disease of the basal ganglia. Increased resistance is present throughout the full range of motion. *Cogwheel rigidity*, characterized by a regular ratchet-like loss of resistance, is especially characteristic of parkinsonism. Cogwheel rigidity at the wrist can often be accentuated if the patient is asked to repeatedly open and close the opposite hand.

(3) **Gegenhalten** (holding against), or paratonia, occurs with dementia and frontal lobe syndromes. It is characterized by a variably and inconsistently increased tone that alternates with relaxation.

3. **Screening tests for hemiparesis**

In many instances, cerebral lesions lead to subtle hemiparesis with normal strength against resistance. Check the following to screen for subtle indications of hemiparesis (Fig. 2–5):

a. **Pronator drift**

Have the patient hold both arms forward, palms up, with eyes closed. Check for pronation and downward drift.

b. **Rapid finger taps**

Check thumb and forefinger taps in each hand separately. Although often considered a sign of cerebellar dysfunction, slowing of fine rapid finger movements also occurs with corticospinal tract lesions.

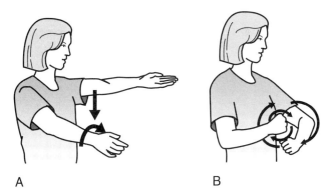

Figure 2–5 □ Screening procedures for mild hemiparesis. *A*, Pronator drift: the weaker right arm drifts downward and pronates. *B*, Arm-rolling test: the stronger left arm tends to "orbit" the weaker right arm.

c. **Arm-rolling test**
  Have the patient make fists and rotate the forearms around each other. With hemiparesis, the normal arm will tend to orbit the weaker arm.
4. **Power**
  Detailed testing of strength against active resistance in multiple individual muscle groups is usually unnecessary unless a peripheral cause of weakness is suspected. *For screening purposes, testing of strength at the shoulders, wrists, hips, and ankles will often suffice.* Be aware that estimates of lower extremity strength in bedridden patients are often unreliable and that walking is the best way to screen for leg weakness.
  By convention, muscle strength is graded as shown in Box 2–2.

Coordination

Disease of the cerebellar hemispheres leads to limb ataxia, whereas midline cerebellar lesions lead to gait ataxia. The following tests can be used to detect incoordination and ataxia.
1. **Finger-to-nose test**
  Have the patient alternately touch a fingertip to his or her nose and your finger. Check for intention tremor (irregular chaotic movements as the target is approached) and past pointing (often easier to elicit when the eyes are closed). Subtle dysmetria can be detected by holding the cap of a pen and having the patient slowly place the pen into the cap (Fig. 2–6).
2. **Rapid rhythmic alternating movements**
  Have the patient touch each of the fingers to the thumb in rapid succession, turn the hand over and back (pronation-supination) as fast as possible, and touch the toe and the heel to the floor in rapid succession. With cerebellar disease, these movements are slow and awkward (*dysdiadochokinesis*).

Box 2–2. MUSCLE STRENGTH GRADING SCALE

0 No muscle contraction detected
1 A barely detectable flicker or trace of contraction
2 Movement occurs only in the plane of gravity
3 Active movement against gravity but not against resistance
4 Active movement against resistance but less than normal strength (may be graded as 4+, 4, or 4−)
5 Normal strength

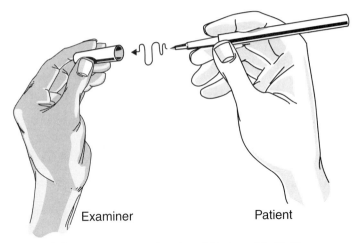

Figure 2–6 □ Screening procedure for subtle dysmetria. Hold a pen cap, and look for an intention tremor as the patient tries to guide the pen into the cap.

3. **Heel-to-shin test**
   Have the patient slide the heel up and down the front of the shin. Limb ataxia results in a side-to-side "tremor" as the test is performed.

Reflexes

1. **Deep tendon reflexes**
   Striking the muscle tendon with a reflex hammer normally leads to a reflex muscle contraction mediated by the lower motor neuron reflex arc. *Hyperreflexia* results from upper motor neuron lesions as a result of release from normal descending inhibition, whereas *hyporeflexia* results from lesions of the lower motor neuron. The principal deep tendon reflexes and their corresponding spinal roots are listed in Table 2–3. Severe hyperreflexia results in *clonus*—repeated rhythmic contraction elicited by striking a tendon or dorsiflexing the ankle.

   By convention, deep tendon reflexes are graded on a scale of 0 to 5 (Box 2–3).

2. **Plantar reflex**
   Firmly stroke the sole of the patient's foot with the handle end of your reflex hammer, beginning at the heel and following up the lateral margin and across the ball of the foot to the base of the big toe. Flexion of the big toe at the metatarsophalangeal joint is the normal response; extension

Table 2-3 □ DEEP TENDON REFLEXES

Reflex	Segments
Jaw jerk	Trigeminal nerve (CN 5)
Biceps reflex	C5 and C6
Brachioradialis reflex	C5 and C6
Triceps reflex	C7 and C8
Finger flexion reflex (Hoffman's reflex)	C8 and T1
Knee reflex	L2, L3, and L4
Ankle reflex	S1

(*Babinski's sign*) occurs with upper motor neuron lesions. If the patient is sensitive, lightly stroking the lateral heel alone is often enough to elicit a normal response.

3. **Cutaneous reflexes**

   These reflexes do not require routine testing, but their testing is useful when a spinal cord or a cauda equina lesion is suspected. They are frequently absent in otherwise normal elderly or obese individuals. The presence of these reflexes implies normal function of the spinal cord and corresponding sensory and motor nerves at the level tested.

   a. **Abdominal reflexes**

      Use a key, wooden stick, or reflex hammer handle to lightly stroke from the lateral to the medial section of the abdomen above (T8–T9) and below (T11–T12) the umbilicus. The normal response is local contraction of the ipsilateral rectus abdominis muscle.

   b. **Cremasteric reflex**

      Striking the medial thigh (L1–L2) results in ipsilateral retraction of the scrotum (S1).

   c. **Bulbocavernosus reflex and anal wink**

      Squeezing the head of the penis (S2–S3) or stroking the perianal skin (S3–S4) results in reflex contraction of the external anal sphincter (S3–S4).

Box 2–3. TENDON REFLEX GRADING SCALE

   0 Absent
   1 Diminished
   2 Normal
   3 Increased (may spread to adjacent muscles)
   4 Unsustained clonus (a few beats)
   5 Sustained clonus

4. **Frontal release signs**
   These primitive reflexes are typically seen with dementia or frontal lobe disease, but they may also occur in normal individuals.
   a. **Snout, suck, and root reflexes**
      These reflexes are elicited by lightly tapping the upper lip or the side of the mouth.
   b. **Palmomental reflex**
      Lightly stroking the palm results in ipsilateral contraction of the mentalis muscle. A unilateral palmomental contraction implies contralateral frontal lobe disease.
   c. **Grasp reflex**
      Placing two fingers in the palm results in involuntary grasping.
   d. **Glabellar reflex**
      Obligatory blinking occurs each time the glabellar area between the eyes is tapped.

Sensory

Sensory testing, because of its subjectivity, is the most difficult and least reliable part of the neurologic examination. In patients with depressed level of consciousness or severe inattention, sensory testing usually provides little useful information and should be omitted. In most cases, testing for signs of sensory loss is unnecessary unless the patient has symptoms of sensory loss. **The key to a successful and efficient sensory examination is to know what you're looking for.** Sensory loss typically occurs in specific patterns, which you should try to rule in or rule out (Box 2–4).

A few simple rules can help make the sensory examination easier and are noted in Box 2–5.

1. **Primary sensory modalities**
   Sensation is mediated by two pathways: the dorsal columns,

---

Box 2–4. PATTERNS OF SENSORY LOSS

Hemisensory loss (cortical lesions)
Stocking-glove sensory loss (neuropathy)
Spinal level and Brown-Séquard's syndrome (spinal cord lesions)
Dermatomal sensory loss (nerve root lesions)
Peripheral nerve sensory loss (mononeuropathy)
Saddle anesthesia (lesion in cauda equina or conus medullaris)

> **Box 2–5. RULES FOR SENSORY EXAMINATION**
>
> 1. *Don't ask leading questions.*
>   When testing for hemisensory loss, ask "Does this feel the same on both sides?" If you ask "Which side feels sharper?", you are likely to get inconsistent (and insignificant) lateralizing responses.
> 2. *When mapping a region of sensory loss, move from the affected into the normal region.*
>   Patients are better able to detect when a pinprick turns sharp than when it becomes dull.
> 3. *Beware of fatigue.*
>   Cooperation in the sensory examination takes concentration, and patients may become fatigued. Rather than taking a thorough, top-to-bottom approach, start your sensory examination by getting right to the point.

which mediate vibration and joint position, and the spinothalamic tracts, which mediate pain and temperature. Touch is mediated by both sensory pathways and is thus usually the last modality to be affected.

  a. **Light touch**

    Test by lightly touching with fingertips or cotton wool. *Allodynia* refers to pain in response to a normally nonpainful stimulus (e.g., light touch).

  b. **Pinprick**

    Use a clean safety pin. *Hyperalgesia* refers to an exaggerated painful sensation; *hyperpathia* refers to an abnormal painful sensation (e.g., burning, tingling).

  c. **Temperature**

    Test with the handle of a reflex hammer or tuning fork submerged under cold tap water.

  d. **Vibration**

    Apply a 128-Hz tuning fork to the toes, medial malleolus, patella, fingers, wrist, and elbow, and ask when the sensation stops. In the elderly, vibration is commonly absent or reduced in the feet.

  e. **Joint position (proprioception)**

    Grasp the sides of the digit and ask the patient to identify small (5 to 10 degrees), random, up or down movements. Remember that even with complete proprioceptive loss, 50% of responses will be correct!

2. **Cortical sensory modalities**

    If the primary sensory modalities are intact, disturbances of these modalities imply dysfunction of the contralateral parietal

Table 2-4 □ SOME ABNORMALITIES OF GAIT

Gait	Features
Hemiparetic	Patient drags or circumducts the affected leg (moves stiffly in a circular motion outward and forward) and has a reduced ipsilateral arm swing
Ataxic	Patient has a wide-based stance with a veering and staggering gait; patient may consistently fall to the same side as the affected cerebellum
Parkinsonian	Patient has a stooped posture, takes small steps (festination), hesitates and freezes, and turns "en bloc"
Steppage	Patient lifts the knee high off the ground because of inability to dorsiflex at the ankle; patient has foot slap (results from peripheral neuropathy)
Waddling	Patient's pelvis drops on non–weight-bearing side with each step (results from myopathy with hip girdle weakness)
Scissor	Patient's gait is stiff, with short steps that cross forward on each other (results from spastic paraparesis)
Apraxic	Patient's gait is slow and unsteady; patient has trouble initiating steps, and the feet barely elevate off the floor (i.e., "magnetic gait") (results from hydrocephalus or frontal lobe disease)
Hysterical	Patient has a bizarre, wild, careening gait but never falls; patient shows excellent balance

lobe. *The main utility of cortical sensory testing is for the detection of subtle hemisensory neglect.*

a. **Double simultaneous stimulation (face-hand test)**

Have the patient close the eyes; quickly touch one cheek and the contralateral hand at the same time. *Extinction* refers to consistent neglect of the hand stimulus on one side and implies a lesion of the contralateral parietal lobe. *Caudal neglect* refers to the tendency to consistently neglect the hand stimulus on either side; it occurs with dementia and frontal lobe disease.

b. **Graphesthesia**

Have the patient close the eyes and identify a number traced on the palm.

c. **Stereognosis**

Ask the patient to close the eyes and identify a key, coin, paperclip, or similar object placed in the palm.

Gait and Station

Disturbances of gait can result from dysfunction in one of many neurologic subsystems, including the motor cortex, corticospinal tracts, basal ganglia, cerebellum, vestibular system, peripheral nerves, muscles, and visual and proprioceptive afferent tracts. **Hence, gait testing is an excellent screening procedure, and many practitioners make it the first part of the neurologic examination.**

Specific components of gait analysis include *posture, width of stance, length of stride, arm swing,* and *balance*. Specific types of gait disturbance are listed in Table 2–4. Test the following:

- **Natural gait**
- **Tandem gait**
  Have the patient walk a straight line, touching toe to heel.
- **Toe walking**
- **Heel walking**
- **Sitting to standing**
  To assess proximal leg strength, have the patient stand up from a chair with the arms folded.
- **Romberg's test**
  Have the patient stand with eyes open and feet together. If the patient cannot do so, suspect a severe cerebellar or vestibular disturbance. *If substantial instability or falling occurs only after the patient closes the eyes, Romberg's test is positive.* A positive test indicates either *proprioceptive* (i.e., neuropathy or dorsal column disease) or *vestibular* dysfunction.
- **Pull test**
  Stand behind the patient and pull back on the shoulders. Normally, the patient should be able to regain balance after one step. Falling or retropulsion (many backward steps) suggests *impaired postural reflexes,* as occurs with parkinsonism.

chapter 3 | Diagnostic Studies

A thorough history and examination should enable you to localize the disease process and generate a differential diagnosis. Confirmation of the diagnosis will usually require neurodiagnostic testing. When any of the tests described here is performed, it is essential to know what you are looking for and to understand the sensitivity (likelihood of a true positive result if the disease is present) and specificity (likelihood of a true negative result if the disease is absent) of each test for diagnosing the disease in question. Risks, benefits, and cost must also be considered.

■ LUMBAR PUNCTURE

Examination of the cerebrospinal fluid (CSF) by lumbar puncture (LP) is essential for diagnosing meningitis and subarachnoid hemorrhage when computed tomography (CT) is negative. It can also be helpful in evaluating peripheral neuropathy, carcinomatous meningitis, pseudotumor cerebri, multiple sclerosis (MS), and a variety of other inflammatory disorders.

- **Technique of LP**

    Proper positioning is the key to success (Fig. 3–1). Position the patient's back at the edge of the bed, with the head flexed, and the legs curled up in the fetal position. Place a pillow under the head; it may be helpful to place another pillow between the legs. *Ensure that the shoulders and hips are*

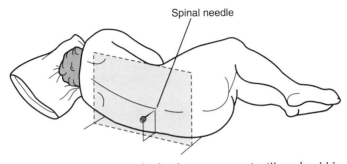

Figure 3–1 □ Positioning for lumbar puncture. A pillow should be placed beneath the head. Hips and shoulders should be parallel to each other and perpendicular to the bed. The spinal needle should be parallel to the bed.

parallel to each other and perpendicular to the bed (i.e., not tilted forward). Locate the interspace between L4 and L5, which lies at the intercristal line (across the tops of the iliac crests), and insert the needle one level above, between L3 and L4. After sterilizing the area and locally injecting 2% lidocaine, insert a 20- or 22-gauge needle, parallel to the bed and tilted slightly cephalad. As you enter the subarachnoid space, you will feel a slight "pop." Measure the opening pressure and collect the CSF.

- **Examination of the CSF**

    This examination should always include a cell count (2 ml), protein and glucose analysis (2 ml), a Gram stain and culture (2 ml), and a CSF Venereal Disease Research Laboratory (VDRL) test (1 ml). Additional CSF tests are listed in Table 3–1. If red blood cells (RBCs) are encountered, check for xanthochromia, a yellowish tinge that differentiates true subarachnoid hemorrhage (>12 hours old) from a traumatic tap. To evaluate the significance of white blood cells (WBCs) in a traumatic tap, recall that the normal ratio of WBCs to RBCs in peripheral blood is 1:700.

- **Complications of LP**

    The most frequent complication (in approximately 5% of patients) of LP is *spinal headache*, which results from persistent leakage of CSF from the entry site, leading to low intracranial

Table 3–1 □ CSF TESTS

- Cell count
- Protein and glucose levels
- Gram stain and culture
- VDRL test
- India ink test (for *Cryptococcus neoformans*)
- Wet smear (for fungi and amebae)
- Stain and culture for AFB (for tuberculosis)
- Cryptococcal antigen titers
- pH and lactate levels (abnormal in MELAS)
- Oligoclonal bands (abnormal in multiple sclerosis)
- IgG index (intrathecal IgG production)
- Latex agglutination bacterial antigen tests (for pneumococcus, meningococcus, and *Haemophilus influenzae*)
- Viral isolation studies
- Cytology (requires fixation in formalin)
- Lyme disease antibody titers (compare with serum titers) and Western blot
- Polymerase chain reaction for Lyme disease, tuberculosis, HSV-1 infection, cytomegalovirus infection, and others
- CSF ACE activity (abnormal with tuberculosis or sarcoidosis)

ACE = angiotensin-converting enzyme; AFB = acid-fast bacteria; CSF = cerebrospinal fluid; HSV-1 = herpes simplex virus 1; IgG = immunoglobulin G; MELAS = mitochondrial encephalomyopathy, lactic acidosis, and stroke; VDRL = Venereal Disease Research Laboratory.

pressure (ICP) and traction on the pain-sensitive intracranial dura when the patient is upright. The risk is minimized by keeping the patient supine for 3 to 6 hours after the procedure. Other complications are rare and occur only in patients with predisposing conditions: (1) *meningitis* can result if the needle is passed through infected tissue (e.g., cellulitis) before penetrating the dura, (2) *epidural hematoma* with compression of the cauda equina can result in patients with coagulopathy, (3) *tentorial herniation* can result in patients who have space-occupying lesions or severe basilar meningitis, and (4) *complete spinal block* and cord compression can result in patients who have a partial spinal block. These predisposing conditions are relative (not absolute) contraindications to LP, and the risk/benefit ratio of performing or not performing the procedure must be considered in each case.

■ COMPUTED TOMOGRAPHY

CT provides "slice" images of the brain by sending axial x-ray beams through the head. The amount of radiation involved is essentially harmless. Tissues are differentiated by the degree to which they attenuate the x-ray beams:

Low attenuation (appears **black**)
- Air (darkest)
- Fat
- CSF and water

Medium attenuation (appears **gray**)
- Edematous or infarcted brain
- Normal brain
- Subacute hemorrhage (3 to 14 days old)

High attenuation (appears **white**)
- Acute hemorrhage
- Intravenous contrast material
- Bone or metal (brightest)

- **Intravenous contrast material**
    When injected, contrast material is normally confined to the cerebral vessels. Hence, *contrast enhancement detects the presence of a disrupted blood-brain barrier*. Contrast is useful in patients with suspected neoplasm, abscess, vascular malformation, or new-onset seizures.

■ MAGNETIC RESONANCE IMAGING

Magnetic resonance imaging (MRI) provides greater resolution and detail than does CT but takes longer to perform. MRI is superior to CT for evaluating the brain stem and posterior fossa and is superior to myelography for identifying intramedullary spinal cord lesions. Because it uses a powerful magnetic field, there is no exposure to radiation. However, MRI is contraindicated in patients with implanted ferromagnetic objects such as pacemakers, orthopedic pins, and older aneurysm clips.

- **T1 images**

    T1 images (TE <50, TR <100) are best for showing *anatomy*. CSF and bone appear black, normal brain appears gray, fat and subacute blood (>48 hours old) appear white. Most pathologic processes (e.g., infarction, tumor) are associated with increased water content and hence appear darker than normal brain.

- **T2 and FLAIR images**

    T2 (TE >80, TR >2000) and FLAIR (fluid attenuation inversion recovery) images are best for showing *pathology*. Most pathologic processes (e.g., infarction, tumor) lead to bright high-signal (white) changes, which reflect increased tissue water content. FLAIR is somewhat more sensitive than T2 in general; the CSF appears dark on FLAIR but bright on T2. Blood on T2 varies in signal intensity according to the age of the hemorrhage, as depicted in Table 3–2.

- **Diffusion-weighted imaging**

    Diffusion-weighted imaging (DWI) is useful for detecting *hyperacute ischemia* in patients with acute stroke. Severe cerebral ischemia produces an immediate reduction in the diffusion coefficient of water, resulting in high-intensity (bright) signal changes on these images within minutes. Over several hours, DWI lesions become associated with high-intensity lesions seen on T2 and FLAIR as the ischemic tissue progresses to infarction. "T2 shine-through" refers to the tendency for high-intensity T2 lesions to produce increased signal on DWI, falsely indicating reduced diffusion.

Table 3–2 □ EVOLUTION OF APPEARANCE OF HEMORRHAGE ON MRI

Feature	T1 Image	T2 Image	Metabolic Change
Blood			
4–6 hours	No change	○	Intact RBC with oxyhemoglobin
7–72 hours	No change	●	Intact RBC with deoxyhemoglobin
4–7 days	○	●	Intact RBC with methemoglobin
1–4 weeks	○	○	Free methemoglobin
Months	●	●	Hemosiderin with macrophages
Edema	●	○	Increased water content

● = low signal, appears dark; ○ = high signal, appears bright; MRI = magnetic resonance imaging; RBC = red blood cell.

- **Proton density images**
  Proton density images are partway between T1 and T2 images in signal density. Their main utility is for differentiating periventricular pathology (e.g., white matter demyelination) from CSF.
- **STIR sequences**
  STIR (short tau inversion recovery) sequences allow summation of T1 and T2 signals and drop-out of fat. They are useful for evaluating mesial temporal sclerosis in patients with epilepsy.
- **Flow voids**
  Flow voids appear black on both T1 and T2 images, and they represent high-velocity blood flow (e.g., normal cerebral vessels or arteriovenous malformation [AVM]).
- **MR angiography**
  MR angiography produces images of the extracranial and intracranial cerebral circulation with the brain and skull "subtracted out." The resolution is adequate for the evaluation of large-scale lesions (e.g., internal carotid artery stenosis and large aneurysms) but is inferior to standard angiography for evaluating smaller lesions (e.g., beading, distal spasm).
- **MR venography**
  MR venography provides subtraction images of the major venous sinuses. It can be useful for diagnosing dural sinus thrombosis but is less sensitive than angiography.

■ MYELOGRAPHY

Myelography consists of injecting radiopaque dye into the spinal canal via either a lumbar or a suboccipital approach. After the patient is tilted, x-rays and axial CT slices allow visualization of the spinal subarachnoid space and can reveal extradural compressive lesions, ruptured intervertebral disks, and vascular malformations on the surface of the cord. In recent years, this test has been largely supplanted by MRI; however, myelography can still be useful if MRI is equivocal, and it remains essential for ruling out cord compression if MRI is not available. Complications are generally the same as those associated with LP.

■ DOPPLER ULTRASONOGRAPHY

- **Carotid duplex Doppler ultrasonography**
  This imaging technique can provide an accurate and noninvasive estimate of the degree of stenosis of the extracranial internal carotid arteries. B-mode ultrasonography gives a graphic image of the arterial wall and can detect plaques, whereas pulsed Doppler ultrasonography analyzes velocity

and turbulence related to stenosis. Results are generally classified as (1) normal, (2) <40% stenosis, (3) 40 to 60% stenosis, (4) 60 to 80% stenosis, (5) 80 to 99% stenosis, and (6) occlusion. If carotid Doppler scans suggest occlusion, confirmation with angiography is required, because high-grade stenosis cannot be ruled out in all cases. Positioning of the transducer over the posterior neck can also differentiate normal, high-resistance, and absent flow in the proximal vertebral arteries.
- **Transcranial Doppler (TCD) ultrasonography**
  This technique measures the velocity of blood flow in the intracranial proximal cerebral arteries (internal carotid artery [ICA] siphon, middle cerebral artery [MCA], anterior cerebral artery [ACA], posterior cerebral artery [PCA], ophthalmic, basilar, and vertebral). The main parameters obtained by TCD ultrasonography are blood flow velocity and pulsatility. TCD ultrasonography can be useful for the following:
  1. Diagnosing intracranial stenosis or occlusion
  2. Evaluating the hemodynamic significance of carotid stenosis or occlusion (look for blunted poststenotic flow in the MCA and reversed collateral flow in the ACA or ophthalmic artery)
  3. Assessing vasospasm in patients with subarachnoid hemorrhage (high-velocity flow)
  4. Screening for arteriovenous malformations (high-velocity flow, very low pulsatility)
  5. Identifying severely increased ICP (low-velocity flow, high pulsatility)
  6. Diagnosing brain death (systolic spikes with absent diastolic flow)

■ ANGIOGRAPHY

Cerebral angiography provides high-resolution images of the extracranial and intracranial cerebral vasculature (Fig. 3–2). The procedure is performed by threading a small catheter into the cerebral vessels via the femoral artery. Angiography is useful for identifying the following:
1. Occluded or stenotic vessels
2. Arterial dissections
3. Aneurysms
4. Arteriovenous malformations
5. Vasculitic narrowing ("beading")
6. Dural venous sinus thrombosis
- **Complications**
  Although infection or bleeding at the puncture site can occur, the most important complication (in 1 to 2% of patients) is stroke, which results from emboli generated by the

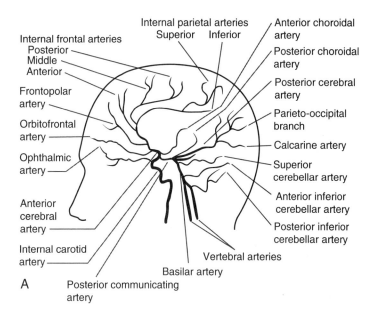
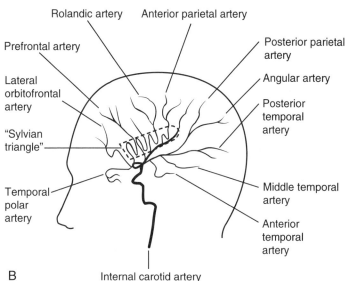

Figure 3–2 □ Diagram of a lateral cerebral angiogram. *A*, Anterior cerebral and posterior cerebral arteries. *B*, Middle cerebral artery.

catheter and which occurs most frequently in older patients with atherosclerotic disease.

■ ELECTROMYOGRAPHY AND NERVE CONDUCTION STUDIES

Electromyography (EMG) and nerve conduction studies assess the integrity and function of muscle and nerve, respectively, and essentially serve as extensions of the clinical examination.
- **EMG**

This test can help distinguish neuropathic from myopathic disease, define the precise distribution of muscle involvement, and aid in the diagnosis of specific muscle disorders with unique features (e.g., myotonia). The procedure is performed by inserting a needle electrode into a muscle and analyzing motor unit potentials, both at rest (spontaneous activity) and with varying degrees of muscle contraction. The following parameters are analyzed:
  1. **Insertional activity.** Excessive insertional activity is seen in both neuropathic and myopathic disease and hence is nonspecific.
  2. **Spontaneous activity.** Normal muscle is electrically silent. Spontaneous muscle fiber contractions *(fibrillation potentials* and *positive sharp waves)* and spontaneous motor unit discharges *(fasciculations)* usually signify muscle denervation. After an acute nerve injury (e.g., disk herniation and nerve root compression), spontaneous activity usually takes 2 weeks to appear. *Paraspinal muscle denervation* implies nerve root injury as opposed to more distal lesions of the plexus or peripheral nerve. *Myotonia* is a special form of continuous motor unit activity characterized by high-frequency waxing and waning discharges, producing a "dive bomber" sound.
  3. **Motor unit potential.** This parameter can differentiate myopathy from denervation. Neuropathic features reflect reinnervation of previously denervated motor units, resulting in *high-amplitude, polyphasic potentials*. Myopathic features reflect loss of muscle fiber mass, resulting in *low-amplitude, polyphasic potentials of short duration*.
  4. **Recruitment pattern.** Voluntary muscle contraction leads to progressive recruitment of motor units and to a dense interference pattern that completely obliterates the baseline. In neuropathic disease, there are fewer motor units in the affected muscle, resulting in a *reduced* or *discrete recruitment* of motor units. Myopathic disease, with random loss of muscle fibers, leads to *early recruitment* and a *low-amplitude interference pattern*.

5. **Single-fiber EMG (SFEMG).** This technique examines the temporal relationship between firing of single muscle fibers innervated by the same motor neuron. Impaired neuromuscular transmission (e.g., in myasthenia gravis) results in a varying interval, referred to as a "jitter."

- **Nerve conduction studies**

Nerve conduction studies can be performed on motor or sensory nerves. The procedure is performed by applying electrical stimulation to skin sites overlying a peripheral nerve and recording the speed of conduction and amplitude of the "downstream" action potential. The following parameters are analyzed:

1. **Conduction velocity.** Conduction velocity is generally reduced (<60% of normal) in demyelinating neuropathy. *Conduction block* reflects focal demyelination and is identified when nerve stimulation proximal to the block leads to a compound muscle action potential (CMAP) amplitude that is less than 50% of that obtained by stimulating distal to the block.
2. **Amplitude.** The amplitude of the CMAP correlates with the number of muscle fibers activated by stimulation of the peripheral nerve. In general, reduced CMAP amplitude with relatively preserved conduction velocity is characteristic of *axonal neuropathy*.
3. **Late responses.** *F waves* result from antidromic conduction followed by orthodromic conduction in the same nerve. Delayed or absent F waves, in combination with normal peripheral nerve conduction, implies disease of the proximal nerve (e.g., root compression, early Guillain-Barré syndrome). The *H reflex* is the electrical counterpart of the ankle jerk and can be performed to assess the integrity of the S1 root; the antidromic potential travels down a sensory nerve, synapses in the spinal cord, and then travels orthodromically down a motor nerve.
4. **Repetitive stimulation.** Muscle responses to repetitive stimulation are useful for assessing neuromuscular junction disease. In myasthenia gravis (see Chapter 15), repetitive stimulation at 2 to 3 Hz produces a characteristic *decremental response* (>10% drop in amplitude between the first and the fifth CMAP).

■ ELECTROENCEPHALOGRAPHY

Electroencephalography (EEG) provides a multichannel recording of the surface electrical activity of the brain. Background rhythms (Fig. 3–3) are analyzed with regard to amplitude and frequency (delta waves, <4 Hz; theta waves, 4 to 7 Hz; alpha waves, 8 to 13 Hz, and beta waves, >13 Hz). In the awake, normal adult, a posterior dominant alpha rhythm is detected when the eyes are closed and the patient is in a relaxed state. Sleep results in characteristic sequential changes (progressive slowing, vertex transients, sleep spindles, and K complexes) that reflect highly organized synchronous activity. The primary utility of EEG is for evaluating epileptiform disorders and causes of diffuse encephalopathy.

- **Seizure disorders**

  The main value of EEG in patients with seizures is for detecting *interictal epileptiform activity* (spikes and sharp waves). Focal epileptiform activity reflects a single irritative focus and corresponds with partial-onset seizures, whereas paroxysmal spike-and-wave discharges of diffuse origin correspond with generalized-onset seizures (Fig. 3–4). Occasionally an *electrographic seizure* will be recorded by chance during the examination. The absence of epileptiform discharges does not imply the absence of a seizure disorder, however, because 20 to 40% of EEG recordings in patients with epilepsy appear normal. *Sleep, sleep deprivation, hyperventilation,* and *photostimulation* can be used to elicit epileptiform activity or absence seizures, and they are collectively referred to as activation procedures. EEG can also be used to identify *nonconvulsive status epilepticus* (complex-partial or absence status) in patients with prolonged postictal or otherwise unexplained impairment of consciousness.

- **Diffuse encephalopathy**

  Diffuse background slowing (in the range of theta and delta waves) is an almost universal finding in patients with impaired level of consciousness of any cause. In patients with

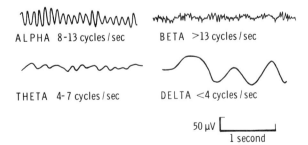

Figure 3–3 □ Basic EEG rhythms. (From Solomon GE, Kutt H, Plum F: Clinical Management of Seizures, 2nd ed. Philadelphia, WB Saunders Co, 1983.)

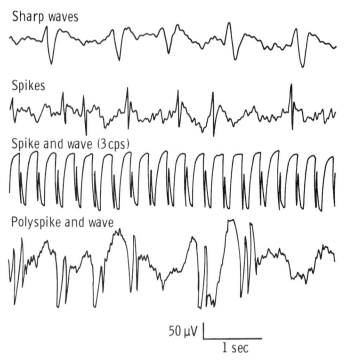

Figure 3-4 □ Paroxysmal EEG patterns seen in patients with epilepsy. (From Solomon GE, Kutt H, Plum F: Clinical Management of Seizures, 2nd ed. Philadelphia, WB Saunders Co, 1983.)

focal lesions (e.g., stroke or brain tumor), the slowing is usually more pronounced in the ipsilateral hemisphere. In most patients in whom the cause of encephalopathy is readily identified (e.g., drug overdose, head trauma), EEG is not helpful. However, in some instances, unique patterns that can point to a specific diagnosis are identified:

1. **Periodic lateralizing epileptiform discharges (PLEDs).** These discharges can occur with large destructive lesions of any type and do not always correspond with clinical seizure activity. In patients with encephalitis, bilateral PLEDs are highly suggestive of herpes simplex infection.
2. **Triphasic waves.** Triphasic waves are nonspecific but can occur with high frequency in patients with metabolic encephalopathy (e.g., in hepatic, renal, and pulmonary failure).
3. **Beta activity.** Beta activity combined with diffuse slow-

ing suggests intoxication with barbiturates, benzodiazepines, or other sedative-hypnotic drugs.
  4. **Periodic discharges.** Periodic discharges consisting of bisynchronous bursts of high-amplitude, sharp waves are characteristic of subacute sclerosing panencephalitis (SSPE) and Jakob-Creutzfeldt disease.
- **Prognosis in coma**
  In hypoxic-ischemic coma, prognosis for recovery of consciousness is related to the severity of slowing and attenuation of the background rhythm. A *burst-suppression pattern, diffuse low-amplitude attenuation,* and *lack of reactivity to external stimuli* imply a poor prognosis. Keep in mind, however, that prognosis is usually related more to the cause of coma than to the depth of coma. *Alpha coma* and *spindle coma patterns* tend to occur with brain stem coma, but they do not have important prognostic significance.
- **Brain death**
  Electrocerebral silence can be used as a confirmatory test for brain death (see Chapter 19).

■ EVOKED POTENTIALS

Evoked potentials provide a recording of electrical activity in central sensory pathways produced by visual, auditory, or sensory stimulation. Signals are recorded by placing electrodes over the scalp or the spine and using a computer to average and amplify the signal, which results in a characteristic pattern of waveform peaks that have approximate anatomic correlates. There are three types of evoked potential studies:
- **Visual evoked responses (VER)**
  The visual stimulus is delivered as an alternating checkerboard pattern or a stroboscopic flash; the waveform corresponds with stimulation of the occipital cortex.
- **Brain stem auditory evoked responses (BAER)**
  Auditory signals are delivered by clicks through earphones. The waveform corresponds with stimulation of CN 8, the cochlear nucleus, pons, and inferior colliculus.
- **Somatosensory evoked potentials (SSEP)**
  Electrical stimuli are delivered to peripheral nerves. The waveform corresponds with stimulation of the lumbosacral or the brachial plexus, the cervicomedullary dorsal column nuclei, and the sensory cortex.

The uses of evoked potentials in clinical practice are as follows:
  1. **Multiple sclerosis.** Evoked potentials can be used to support the diagnosis in a patient with a single symptom by identifying subclinical demyelination at a differ-

ent anatomic site (e.g., abnormal VERs in a patient with transverse myelitis).
2. **Brain stem lesions.** Brain stem lesions can be verified and localized with BAER.
3. **Acoustic neuroma.** BAER can be used to verify CN 8 injury.
4. **Spinal cord injury.** SSEP can be used for prognosis by differentiating complete from partial injury.
5. **Hypoxic-ischemic coma.** Absence of cortical potentials by SSEP on day 5 or later implies that consciousness will not be regained.

■ MUSCLE AND NERVE BIOPSY

Muscle and nerve biopsy specimens are extremely fragile, and the procedure should be performed only by an experienced surgeon with adequate neuropathology backup for processing and analysis. The sural nerve and gastrocnemius muscle are often examined together, although biopsy of almost any muscle can be performed. Muscle biopsy is essential for diagnosing causes of myopathy such as polymyositis, genetic biochemical deficiencies, mitochondrial disease, sarcoidosis, critical illness myopathy, and infection (e.g., trichinosis). The causes of neuropathy that can be diagnosed by nerve biopsy are listed in Table 20–4.

■ BRAIN BIOPSY

Brain biopsy can be performed either as an open procedure, usually of the anterior nondominant temporal lobe, or by using stereotactic needle localization. Although stereotactic biopsy is often necessary for deep lesions, the diagnostic yield is better with the open procedure because more tissue can be obtained. The main complication is hemorrhage (in approximately 1% of cases). Brain biopsy is of value for diagnosing brain tumors or abscess, central nervous system (CNS) vasculitis, neurosarcoidosis, encephalitis, and Jakob-Creutzfeldt disease.

PATIENT-RELATED PROBLEMS: THE COMMON CALLS

chapter 4

Seizures and Status Epilepticus

Seizures are dramatic and frightening for all who witness the event—patients, families, and staff—and tend to induce panic, rather than rational thought, even on a neurology service. It is your job to proceed in a logical and thorough manner to identify the cause of the seizure and to halt it if it persists.

Clinical seizures are caused by an excessive, synchronous, abnormal discharge of cortical neurons that produces a sudden change in neurologic function. Seizures are classified as *simple* if there is no impairment of consciousness or as *complex* if an alteration in consciousness occurs. Seizures may be *focal*, involving a single brain region and causing limited dysfunction, such as clonic movements of a single limb, paresthesias, or abnormal speech or behavior; or they may be *generalized*, involving the whole brain and producing loss of consciousness and convulsions. Most seizures last seconds to minutes. *Status epilepticus* is defined as continuous tonic-clonic seizure activity lasting 10 minutes or repetitive seizures over 30 minutes between which the patient does not return to a baseline neurologic level. *Epilepsy* is a chronic condition defined as recurrent, unprovoked seizures and is discussed in Chapter 26.

■ PHONE CALL

Questions

1. **Is the patient still seizing? If yes, how long has it been going on?**
    Any patient seizing on admission to the emergency room (ER) should be considered to be in status epilepticus until the course of the seizure is known.
2. **What is the patient's level of consciousness?**
    A patient may have a decreased level of consciousness if the seizure is still occurring (nonconvulsive status epilepticus) or if the patient is postictal. The two states can be difficult to differentiate without an electroencephalogram (EEG).
3. **Is this the first known seizure for this patient?**
    If the patient has a known history of epilepsy, there may be records available regarding anticonvulsants that have

worked or failed in the past. Other information regarding past seizures will be gained from taking the patient's history.

4. Is the patient on anticonvulsant medication?
Anticonvulsant levels need to be checked for any seizure patient on medication. Many anticonvulsants are epileptogenic at toxic levels.

5. Is the patient diabetic?
Focal or generalized seizures may be caused by hyper- or hypoglycemia.

6. Is the patient immunocompromised?
Additional elements in the differential diagnosis need to be considered in immunocompromised patients, particularly opportunistic infections such as toxoplasmosis, fungal meningitides, and tubercular meningitis.

Orders

If the patient is still seizing:
1. Have two intravenous (IV) setups ready at the bedside.
2. Have oral airway and Ambu bag available at the bedside.
3. Have lorazepam 8 mg ready at the bedside. Diazepam 10 mg is an alternative, but it has a shorter anticonvulsant activity (20 minutes versus 4 hours for lorazepam).
4. Clear any sharp or hard objects from the bed, put the side rails up, and pad the side rails.
5. Perform a finger stick glucose test.

If the patient has stopped seizing:
1. Have an oral airway ready at the bedside.
2. Perform a finger stick glucose test.

Inform RN

"Will arrive at the bedside in . . . minutes."

If the patient is still seizing, it must be considered a medical emergency. If the patient has stopped seizing, another seizure may occur within a few minutes.

■ ELEVATOR THOUGHTS

What is the differential diagnosis of seizures?

On your way to the bedside, you should generate a list of probable diagnoses based on the initial information you obtained from your telephone conversation with the nurse.

V (vascular): Intracranial hemorrhage, acute or chronic ischemic infarction, subarachnoid hemorrhage, arteriovenous malformation, venous sinus thrombosis, or amyloid angiopathy

I (infectious): meningitis (bacterial, viral, fungal), meningoencephalitis (herpes simplex encephalitis), or abscess (bacterial, fungal, or parasitic)

T (traumatic): new head injury (e.g., from a fall) or old head injury with subdural hematoma

A (autoimmune): systemic lupus erythematosus, central nervous system (CNS) vasculitis, or multiple sclerosis

M (metabolic/toxic): hypo- or hypernatremia, hypo- or hypercalcemia, hypo- or hyperglycemia, hypomagnesemia, hyperthyroidism, uremia, hyperammonemia, ethanol (EtOH) toxicity or EtOH withdrawal, other drugs including cocaine, phencyclidine, and amphetamines

I (idiopathic/iatrogenic): idiopathic epilepsy or medications (Table 4–1 lists common medications that can cause seizures)

N (neoplastic): brain metastasis or primary CNS tumor

S (structural): congenital structural defects (rare in adults)

Paroxysmal conditions that may mimic seizures: hypoglycemia, syncope, asterixis, stroke/transient ischemic attack, myoclonus, dystonia, tremor, narcolepsy, complicated migraine, panic attack, hyperventilation, malingering.

Table 4–1 □ COMMON MEDICATIONS THAT MAY CAUSE SEIZURES

Antidepressants
  Imipramine
  Amitriptyline
  Nortriptyline
  Bupropion
Antipsychotic agents
  Chlorpromazine
  Thioridazine
  Trifluoperazine
  Trifluoperazine
  Perphenazine
  Haloperidol
Analgesics
  Fentanyl
  Meperidine
  Pentazocine
  Propoxyphene
Local anesthetics
  Lidocaine
  Procaine
Sympathomimetics
  Terbutaline
  Ephedrine
  Phenylpropanolamine

Antimicrobial agents
  Penicillin, ampicillin
  Synthetic penicillins
  Cephalosporins
  Metronidazole
  Isoniazid
  Imipenem
  Pyrimethamine
Antineoplastic agents
  Vincristine
  Chlorambucil
  Methotrexate
  Carmustine (BCNU)
  Cytosine arabinoside
Bronchodilators
  Aminophylline
  Theophylline
Others
  Insulin
  Antihistamines
  Anticholinergics
  Atenolol
  Baclofen

■ MAJOR THREAT TO LIFE

- Aspiration of gastric contents if the airway is not protected
- Head injury
- Lactic acidosis, hypoxia, hyperthermia, rhabdomyolysis, cerebral edema, or hypotension from a prolonged seizure. These conditions may produce permanent brain injury.

Measures to prevent aspiration and subsequent injury to the patient are described in Management I. The patient should be positioned in the *lateral decubitus* position to prevent aspiration of gastric contents. All hard or sharp objects should be removed from the bed, the side rails should be up, and the side rails should be padded. Procedures for aborting an ongoing seizure are described below.

■ BEDSIDE

Quick Look Test

Is the patient still seizing?

Most seizures will have stopped by the time you arrive at the bedside. If there is still seizure activity, prepare to treat it.

If the patient has stopped seizing, assess the patient's level of consciousness.

Is the patient awake and alert? Is he or she interactive and conversing?

A period of lethargy or stupor may follow a generalized seizure. Focal deficits such as a hemiparesis may also be apparent from a quick look.

Does the patient look comfortable? Is there any sign of respiratory distress or agitation or any complaint of headache?

Management I

Treatment of an Ongoing Seizure

1. **Keep calm.** It is likely that others in the room are reacting with fear or panic. Ask family members to leave the room. Tell them you will speak with them as soon as the situation is evaluated and under control.
2. **Ensure that all measures have been taken to protect the patient from physical injury and aspiration of gastric contents.** Have one or two people maintain the patient in a lateral decubitus position (Table 4–2).
3. **Administer oxygen by nasal cannula or face mask,** particularly if the patient is older or has a history of cardiac disease.
4. **Watch and wait for 2 minutes.** A majority of seizures will

Table 4–2 □ SEIZURE PRECAUTIONS

Bed should be at the lowest position
Side rails should be up
Side rails should be padded
Patient should ambulate to bathroom only with supervision
Only axillary temperatures should be measured
Patient should be supervised when using sharp objects
Oral airway, oxygen, and suction should be at bedside

---

stop spontaneously within a short time. There is no immediate risk to the patient, provided the risks of aspiration and physical injury have been addressed. During the waiting period, do the following:

- Check the **finger stick glucose** level. If there is significant hypo- or hyperglycemia, this may be the first condition to treat.
- Make sure there are **two IV setups available,** at least one with 0.9% normal saline (NS). If the patient has no IV access, start an IV line. If the seizures stop within 3 minutes, however, IV insertion and blood drawing will be much easier.
- Draw **lorazepam 8 mg** in a 10-ml syringe.
- **Elicit any further history** not obtained in the initial phone call. Is this a first-ever seizure? Is the patient on anticonvulsants? What is the patient's admitting diagnosis? Is the patient diabetic? Is the patient immunocompromised? Has the patient been febrile in the last 24 hours? Ask for the chart to be brought to the bedside.
- **Observe the seizure type.** Generalized seizures, in which both sides of the body are involved and in which there is altered level of consciousness, are potentially the most dangerous if the seizures persist for longer than 30 minutes. A partial seizure, in which a single limb or side of the body is involved, may suggest a structural lesion.

5. **If the seizure has not remitted in 2 minutes,** ensure that an IV line is available. If the patient has no IV access, have one or two people hold the forearm while the most experienced person available inserts two IV lines and draws blood. Avoid the antecubital area because convulsions may cause flexion of the arm and block off the IV site.
6. Order the following **blood tests:** complete blood cell count (CBC), electrolytes, glucose, magnesium (Mg), calcium (Ca), ammonia, EtOH level, toxicology screen, and anticonvulsant level (if applicable).
7. If the patient is hypoglycemic, give **glucose (50 ml of D50W)** by slow, direct injection. If there is any history or suspicion

of alcoholism, administer **thiamine 100 mg by slow, direct injection over 3 to 5 minutes.** The administration of thiamine will prevent susceptible patients from developing Wernicke's encephalopathy. If hypoglycemia is the cause of the seizure, the seizure should stop, and the patient should wake up soon after the glucose administration.
8. If glucose levels are normal or after glucose has been given, administer **lorazepam 0.1 mg/kg in 2-mg increments by IV push over 2 to 3 minutes.**

    An Ambu bag with face mask should be at the bedside because benzodiazepines can cause respiratory depression. Alternatives to lorazepam include **diazepam 5 to 10 mg given by IV push in NS or rectally in gel form**, or **midazolam 0.2 mg/kg IV or sublingually.** Lorazepam may be given intramuscularly (IM) and may be helpful if no peripheral IV access can be achieved.

Treatment of Status Epilepticus

1. If the seizure has not stopped with a full dose of a benzodiazepine, administer **fosphenytoin** (the prodrug of phenytoin) **15 to 20 mg/kg as a slow IV push or IV infusion** (Fig. 4–1). (This loading dose corresponds to approximately 1500 mg in a 70-kg patient.) The rate of administration should not exceed 200 mg/min because fosphenytoin can cause cardiac arrhythmias, prolongation of the QT interval, and hypotension. The electrocardiogram (ECG) should be monitored continuously, and the blood pressure should be checked each minute during the infusion. The rate of administration should be slowed if ECG changes or hypotension occurs. The usual protocol is to give **500 mg with a slow IV push over 5 minutes, and then repeat twice.** If IV access is unavailable, fosphenytoin can also be given IM. If the patient is known to be on phenytoin already and is suspected of having subtherapeutic levels, **a load of 10 mg/kg bolus** may be given. Fosphenytoin, like most anticonvulsants, may be epileptogenic at high concentrations.
2. Approximately 70% of prolonged seizures will be brought

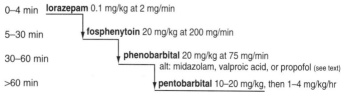

Figure 4–1 □ Standard medication protocol for status epilepticus.

under control with a combination of lorazepam and fosphenytoin, but if the seizure lasts longer than 30 minutes, transfer the patient to an intensive care unit (ICU) for probable intubation. Prolonged status epilepticus may require active treatment of hypoxia, hypotension, cardiac arrhythmias, cardiac failure, lactic acidosis, hyperpyrexia, electrolyte disturbances, or rhabdomyolysis.
3. Once the patient is in the ICU, if the patient is continuing to seize despite a full fosphenytoin load, the next step is to administer barbiturates. **Phenobarbital should be infused IV at a rate of 75 mg/min and should be stopped at a loading dose of 15 to 20 mg/kg.** Thereafter, give **10 to 15 mg/kg PO or IV every 12 hours.** Intubation, if not already done, is required at this point. Continue monitoring the blood pressure and ECG, along with continuous EEG monitoring, as a standard of care. Twenty to 30% of patients will continue to have electrographic seizure activity that is not clinically apparent. Alternatives to phenobarbital include **midazolam (Versed) 0.2 mg/kg bolus, followed by IV infusion of 0.1 to 2 mg/kg/hour, propofol** (a unique GABA agonist) **3 to 5 mg/kg loading dose, followed by IV infusion of 2 to 10 mg/kg/hour,** or **valproic acid (Depacon) IV 15 to 60 mg/kg IV bolus followed by 10 to 15 mg/kg IV every 6 hours** (see Table 4–3).
4. If there is no response to full doses of a benzodiazepine and two anticonvulsants, consider the seizure to be refractory status epilepticus. As the next step, administer **pentobarbital 5 to 20 mg/kg loading dose and then 1 to 4 mg/kg per hour as a maintenance infusion.** Monitor the EEG continuously to keep the patient in a burst suppression pattern. Hypotension is nearly always encountered with pentobarbital, and pressors may be required. General anesthesia with halothane and neuromuscular blockade has been used in some cases to avoid rhabdomyolysis, but this eliminates the ability to follow the neurologic examination.
5. Although nearly all seizures may be brought under control with anticonvulsant therapy (Table 4–3), continued control may be impossible until the underlying cause is identified and treated.

Evaluation and Initial Management If the Seizure Has Stopped

A single first seizure that has stopped often does not need to be treated. Anticonvulsant therapy should be reserved for patients who have had more than one seizure or who have risk factors that make another seizure more likely. The potential danger to the patient is not over, however. A patient who has had one seizure may have another seizure within a few minutes.

Table 4-3 □ DRUGS USED FOR THE TREATMENT OF STATUS EPILEPTICUS

Drug	Loading Dose	Maximum Loading Rate	Continuous Infusion Dose
Lorazepam	0.1 mg/kg IV	2 mg/min to max 8 mg	N/A
Fosphenytoin or phenytoin	20 mg/kg IV	200 mg/min or 50 mg/min for phenytoin	N/A
Phenobarbital	20 mg/kg IV	75 mg/min	N/A
Valproic acid	15-60 mg/kg	20 mg/min	N/A
Midazolam	0.2 mg/kg IV	N/A	0.1-0.4 mg/kg/hour
Propofol	1-2 mg/kg IV	N/A	2-10 mg/kg/hour
Pentobarbital	5-20 mg/kg IV	N/A	1-4 mg/kg/hour

Order "seizure precautions" for the patient (see Table 4-2). Remember also that a seizure is a symptom, not a disease. Your primary job now should be to identify the cause of the seizure and to treat the underlying condition.

1. **Draw blood and order the following tests:** CBC, electrolytes, glucose, Mg, Ca, ammonia, EtOH level, toxicology screen, and anticonvulsant levels.
2. **Ensure that there is intravenous access.** Start an IV running to keep the vein open with 0.9% NS.
3. **Ask for the chart** to be brought to the bedside while you perform a selective physical examination.

Selective Physical Examination

Initial physical examination of a patient who has had a seizure should take no more than 5 minutes. Important clues to the etiology of the seizure may emerge. Pay particular attention to unilateral focal deficits that could indicate a structural lesion.

General Physical Examination

Vital signs Fever could be a clue to an infectious cause, although a prolonged seizure may cause hyperpyrexia. Dyspnea may suggest hypoxia. Cardiac arrhythmia or tachycardia could suggest a cardioembolic or syncopal event. Hypertensive encephalopathy may present with seizures.

HEENT Look for evidence of bites on the tongue, lips, or buccal mucosa. Look for any evidence of

	new or old head injury. Check the fundi for papilledema.
Neck	Look for neck stiffness (meningismus).
Skin	Look for cafe au lait spots or port-wine stains as a sign of neurocutaneous disorders (e.g., neurofibromatosis or Sturge-Weber syndrome). Hematomas, lacerations, or even fractures may have been produced as a consequence of the seizure.
Chest	Focal decreased breath sounds or rales may be a clue to aspiration. Cardiac murmur or arrhythmia may suggest a cardioembolic event.
GU	Incontinence, particularly urinary, may accompany a generalized seizure.

Neurological Examination

Assess for new or residual focal deficits:

The *level of consciousness* may be decreased after a seizure. A period of lethargy, stupor, or inattentiveness may follow a generalized seizure. If the patient is awake, have him or her count backward from 20 to 1 as a screening test for attentiveness.

Aphasia has been partially screened for by asking the patient to count backward from 20 to 1. If the patient is unable to do this task, he or she may be either too inattentive, in which case aphasia testing will be futile, or aphasic. Ask the patient to show two fingers, then to repeat an unfamiliar phrase (e.g., "The spy fled to Greece").

Hemiparesis may be obvious, as evidenced by an inability to lift an arm or leg, or it may be subtle, as detected by a widened palpebral fissure, a flattened nasolabial fold, or a pronator drift when arms are extended with palms up.

Reflex asymmetry or a unilateral Babinski's sign may be indicative of a focal lesion.

Selective History and Chart Review

Reassess the timing, circumstances, and duration of the seizure. Try to establish with the patient or with witnesses whether this was indeed a seizure. An aura is often present at the onset of a seizure, which is thought to represent the beginning of the abnormal epileptic discharges. Auras are most commonly olfactory, gustatory, or other visceral sensations that precede motor or sensory activity. Were there rhythmic, synchronous movements of more than one body part? Identify a "focal signature" if present; that is, did the seizure begin in one part of the body and then progress or become generalized? Were there head and eye deviations at the beginning? A seizure that begins focally can aid in the localization of the underlying pathology. If both sides of the body were involved, did the patient lose consciousness, become incontinent, or bite the tongue or mouth?

From the chart, look for clues to the underlying cause. Check for the following:

1. Medications the patient is on that are potentially epileptogenic (see Table 4–1).
2. History of alcohol or drug use.
3. Underlying medical problems that could cause seizures, including hepatic or renal disease, prior head injury, cerebrovascular disease, connective tissue diseases, porphyria, or carcinoma (lung, breast, and colon cancer are the most common tumors that metastasize to the brain).
4. HIV infection. Patients who are immunocompromised, particularly patients with acquired immunodeficiency syndrome (AIDS), are predisposed to opportunistic infections such as toxoplasmosis, tubercular meningitis, and cryptococcal meningitis and to CNS lymphoma.
5. Recent laboratory results: electrolyte, glucose, Ca and Mg levels, thyroid and liver function tests, toxicology screen, EtOH levels, and anticonvulsant levels.

■ MANAGEMENT II

Having accumulated information from the history, the physical examination, and the laboratory, a working differential diagnosis should be generated. As always, in an acute situation, the differential diagnosis should include the most dangerous diagnosis as well as the most likely. Management should proceed from the differential diagnosis.

1. If a **metabolic cause** is identified or suspected, the underlying cause should be treated appropriately.
2. If the examination reveals a focal deficit, if the onset of the seizure appeared to be focal, or if the patient has new-onset seizures, a **computed tomography (CT) or magnetic resonance imaging (MRI) scan** should be obtained. If there is no renal insufficiency, contrast should be administered. Keep in mind that a cerebral infarction may not be detectable by CT within the first 6 hours.
3. If no immediately treatable metabolic cause is identified or if a structural lesion is suspected, a loading dose of **fosphenytoin 15 to 20 mg/kg** should be given. If there is little concern of another seizure's occurring within a short period of time (as opposed to a patient with suspected alcohol or sedative withdrawal, HIV positivity, or a structural lesion, for example), the loading dose may be given orally as phenytoin.

4. If there is no evidence of a major mass effect or increased intracranial pressure on imaging and an infectious etiology is suspected, a **lumbar puncture** may be performed so that antibiotic therapy, if warranted, may be targeted as specifically as possible. If infection is suspected, other supportive evidence should be sought as well, such as blood cultures, urine cultures, and chest x-ray.
5. If treatment was given to correct abnormal laboratory results, those tests should be repeated, including electrolytes, Mg, Ca, and glucose. If fosphenytoin was administered, a blood level should be ordered for the next morning.
6. An **EEG** should be obtained if the diagnosis of seizure is at all uncertain; it also serves the purpose of guiding long-term management. In most cases, an EEG is not helpful in the acute situation, except when treating prolonged status epilepticus.
7. If **no underlying cause** for seizures is determined, idiopathic epilepsy may be the diagnosis. An EEG is often helpful in differentiating specific epileptic syndromes. Treatment with an appropriate anticonvulsant would then be indicated. See Chapter 26 for treatment of epilepsy.

chapter 5 | Stupor and Coma

Stupor and coma refer, respectively, to moderate and severe depression of the level of consciousness. The acute onset of stupor or coma is a medical emergency. A wide variety of metabolic and structural disorders can produce this state. Management should focus on stabilizing the patient, establishing a diagnosis, and treating the underlying cause.

■ PHONE CALL

Questions

1. **What are the vital signs?**
2. **Is the airway protected?**
    Stuporous and comatose patients are at high risk for *aspiration*, because of impaired cough and gag reflexes, and *hypoxia*, which results from diminished respiratory drive. Endotracheal intubation is the most effective method for securing the airway and ensuring adequate oxygenation.
3. **Is there any history of trauma, drug use, or toxin exposure?**
    Obtain a quick description of recent events and pre-existing medical or neurologic conditions. Check the Emergency Medical Service sheet.
4. **Is someone available to provide further history?**
    Relatives, friends, ambulance personnel, or anyone else who has had recent contact with the patient should be identified and instructed to wait for further questioning.

Orders

1. **Call the anesthesiology service for intubation if the patient is deeply comatose or exhibiting signs of respiratory compromise.**
    In stuporous patients with normal respirations, give 100% oxygen via face mask until hypoxemia is ruled out.
2. **Order an intravenous line.**
3. **Order a finger stick glucose measurement.**
    This should always be checked immediately, because hypoglycemia is a rapidly treatable cause of stupor or coma that can coexist with other diagnoses (e.g., sepsis, cardiac arrest, or trauma).

4. **Order diagnostic blood tests.**
   - Serum chemistries (glucose, electrolytes, blood urea nitrogen [BUN], creatinine)
   - Complete blood cell count (CBC)
   - Arterial blood gas
   - Calcium, magnesium
   - Prothrombin time (PT)/partial thromboplastin time (PTT)
5. **If the etiology of coma is unclear** order toxicology screen, thyroid function tests, liver function tests, serum cortisol, and ammonia level.
6. **Insert a Foley catheter.**
7. **Order urinalysis, electrocardiogram (ECG), and chest x-ray.**
8. **Give emergency treatment.** These measures are often given "in the field," or whenever the cause of coma is unclear.
   - **Thiamine 100 mg intravenously (IV)**
     Thiamine reverses coma resulting from acute thiamine deficiency (Wernicke's encephalopathy). It must be given *before* dextrose because hyperglycemia can lead to consumption of thiamine and acute worsening of Wernicke's encephalopathy.
   - **50% dextrose 50 ml (1 ampule) IV**
   - **Naloxone (Narcan) 0.4 to 0.8 mg IV**
     Naloxone reverses coma caused by opiate intoxication. Up to 10 mg may be required to reverse severe intoxication.
   - **Flumazenil (Romazicon) 0.2 to 1.0 mg IV**
     Flumazenil reverses coma caused by benzodiazepine intoxication. Up to 3 mg may be required. *Do not give flumazenil if seizures have occurred, because flumazenil may precipitate further seizures.*

■ ELEVATOR THOUGHTS

What causes stupor or coma?
The causes of stupor and coma (Table 5–1) can be broadly grouped into three categories:
1. **Structural intracranial disorders (33%)**
   In most cases, these disorders are diagnosed by positive brain imaging (computed tomography [CT] or magnetic resonance imaging [MRI]) or by lumbar puncture (LP).
2. **Toxic or metabolic disorders (66%)**
   Abnormal blood tests usually, but not always, confirm these disorders.
3. **Psychiatric disorders (1%)**

Stupor and coma result from diseases affecting either both of the cerebral hemispheres or the brain stem. As a rule, *unilateral hemispheric lesions* do not produce stupor or coma unless they are of a mass sufficient to compress either the

Table 5–1 □ CAUSES OF STUPOR AND COMA

1. **Structural intracranial disorders**
   a. Trauma
      (1) Epidural, subdural, intracerebral, or subarachnoid hemorrhage
      (2) Diffuse axonal injury
      (3) Concussion
   b. Cerebrovascular events
      (1) Intracerebral or subarachnoid hemorrhage
      (2) Hemispheric or brain stem infarction
      (3) Dural sinus thrombosis
      (4) Hypertensive encephalopathy
   c. Infection
      (1) Meningitis
      (2) Encephalitis
      (3) Abscess
   d. Inflammatory disorders
      (1) Autoimmune vasculitis or cerebritis
      (2) Demyelinating disease (e.g., multiple sclerosis)
   e. Neoplasm
   f. Hydrocephalus
2. **Toxic or metabolic disorders**
   a. Global hypoxia-ischemia
   b. Electrolyte or acid-base disorders
      (1) pH disturbances
      (2) Hyper- or hyponatremia
      (3) Hyper- or hypoglycemia
      (4) Hyper- or hypocalcemia
   c. Drug intoxication or withdrawal
   d. Temperature disorder (hyper- or hypothermia)
   e. Organ system dysfunction
      (1) Liver (hepatic encephalopathy)
      (2) Kidney (uremia)
      (3) Thyroid (myxedema, thyrotoxicosis)
      (4) Adrenal (hyper- or hypoadrenalism)
   f. Seizure and postictal states
   g. Thiamine or vitamin B_{12} deficiency
3. **Psychogenic coma**

contralateral hemisphere or the brain stem. *Focal brain stem lesions* produce coma by disrupting the reticular activating system. *Metabolic disorders* impair consciousness by diffuse effects on both the reticular formation and the cerebral cortex.

■ MAJOR THREAT TO LIFE

Three common and treatable causes of coma can rapidly lead to death:

- **Herniation and brain stem compression**
  Space-occupying mass lesions that produce coma are a neurosurgical emergency (Fig. 5–1).
- **Increased intracranial pressure (ICP)**
  Increased ICP can lead to impaired cerebral perfusion and global hypoxic-ischemic injury (see Chapter 12).
- **Meningitis or encephalitis**
  Death from bacterial meningitis or herpes encephalitis can be prevented with early treatment (see Chapter 22).

■ BEDSIDE

Selective History

The cause of coma can frequently be determined by the history. Ask family, friends, ambulance personnel, or others who have had recent contact with the patient about the following:

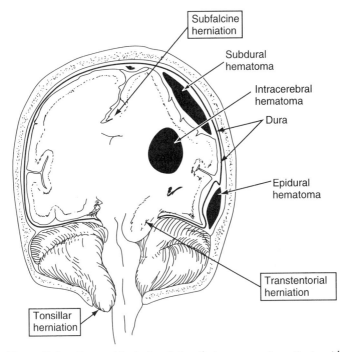

Figure 5–1 □ Types of brain herniation that can occur in patients with compartmentalized intracranial pressure.

1. Recent events
   When was the patient last seen? How was the patient discovered? Were there any preceding neurologic complaints? Was there any recent trauma or toxin exposure?
2. Medical history
3. Psychiatric history
4. Medications
5. Use of drugs or alcohol

Selective Physical Examination

With or without history, clues to the etiology of coma can be elicited from the physical examination.

General Physical Examination

Vital signs	*Severe hypertension* suggests a structural central nervous system (CNS) lesion with increased ICP or hypertensive encephalopathy.
Skin	Look for external signs of trauma, needle marks, rashes, cherry redness (suggests carbon monoxide poisoning), or jaundice.
Breath	Alcohol, acetone, or fetor hepaticus (from liver failure) can lead to a pungent or "fruity" smell.
Head	The skull should be inspected for fractures, hematomas, and lacerations.
Ear, nose, and throat	*Cerebrospinal fluid (CSF) otorrhea or rhinorrhea* results from skull fracture with disruption of the dura (a positive dextrose stick test, indicating a high level of glucose, differentiates CSF from mucus). *Hemotympanum* is also highly suggestive of skull fracture. *Tongue biting* suggests an unwitnessed seizure.
Neck (do not manipulate the neck if there is suspicion of cervical spine fracture)	Stiffness suggests meningitis or subarachnoid hemorrhage.

Neurologic Examination

The goals of the neurologic examination are (1) to determine the depth of coma and (2) to localize the process leading to coma.

1. **General appearance**
   Open eyelids and a slack jaw indicate deep coma. Head and gaze deviation suggest a large ipsilateral hemispheric lesion. Observe for *myoclonus* (which suggests a metabolic process), *rhythmic muscle twitching* (which is indicative of seizure activity), or *tetany* (spontaneous, prolonged muscle spasms).
2. **Level of consciousness**
   Many inexact terms are used to describe depressed level of consciousness (e.g., somnolent, clouded, drowsy, obtunded). Because of the lack of precision associated with these terms, it is much more useful to **document the response of the patient to a specific stimulus;** for example, "opens eyes temporarily and responds with brief phrases to repeated questioning," or "moans and localizes to sternal rub." Responses to verbal and noxious stimuli can be used to generate a **Glasgow Coma Scale score** (Table 5–2), a reproducible and widely used method for quantifying level of consciousness. For the sake of simplicity, we advocate describing nonalert patients as *lethargic, stuporous,* or *comatose.*
   a. **Lethargy**
      Lethargy resembles sleepiness, except that the patient is incapable of becoming fully alert. These patients are conversant but inattentive and slow to respond. They are unable to adequately perform simple concentration tasks, such as counting from 20 to 1 or reciting the months in reverse.

Table 5–2 □ GLASGOW COMA SCALE

Parameter	Patient Response	Score
Eye opening	Spontaneous	4
	To voice	3
	To pain	2
	None	1
Best motor response	Obeys commands	6
	Localizes to pain	5
	Withdraws to pain	4
	Flexor posturing	3
	Extensor posturing	2
	None	1
Best verbal response	Conversant and oriented	5
	Conversant and disoriented	4
	Uses inappropriate words	3
	Makes incomprehensible sounds	2
	None	1
Total score		3–15

b. **Stupor**

Stupor is characterized by incomplete arousal to painful stimuli. There is little or no response to verbal commands. Painful stimulation results in brief responses to questions, exclamations ("ouch"), or moaning. The patient may obey commands temporarily when aroused by noxious stimuli but more often only localizes to pain.

c. **Coma**

Coma is defined by the absence of verbal or complex motor responses to any stimulus. *A Glasgow Coma Scale score of 8 or lower is frequently used to define coma.*

3. **Respirations**

Abnormal respiratory patterns (Fig. 5–2) occur frequently with coma and can aid in localization. Respirations in intubated patients can be observed by briefly disconnecting the endotracheal tube from the ventilator.

a. **Patterns without localizing value**

(1) **Depressed respirations** can occur with severe coma of any cause.

(2) **Cheyne-Stokes respiration** is characterized by alternating periods of hyperventilation and apnea. It usually occurs with bihemispheric lesions or metabolic encephalopathy. Slow-cycling *Cheyne-Stokes respirations are considered to represent a "stable" breathing pattern that does not imply impending respiratory arrest.* Rapid-cycling Cheyne-Stokes respirations may be more ominous.

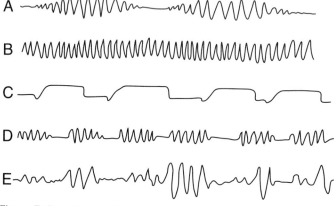

Figure 5–2 □ Abnormal respiratory patterns associated with coma. Tracings represent chest wall excursion; upward deflections represent inspiration. *A*, Cheyne-Stokes respiration. *B*, Central neurogenic hyperventilation. *C*, Apneustic breathing. *D*, Cluster breathing. *E*, Ataxic breathing.

(3) **Hyperventilation** in comatose patients is most often due to systemic disease. Hyperventilation associated with *metabolic acidosis* can result from lactic acidosis, ketoacidosis, uremia, or organic acid poisoning. An association with *respiratory alkalosis* can result from hypoxia or hepatic encephalopathy. **Central neurogenic hyperventilation** is sometimes associated with CNS lymphoma or brain stem damage from tentorial herniation.
- b. **Patterns with localizing value**
  - (1) **Apneustic breathing** is characterized by a prolonged inspiratory phase (the inspiratory cramp) followed by apnea. It implies pontine damage.
  - (2) **Cluster breathing** consists of brief cycles of shallow hyperventilation with periods of apnea. It has less of a crescendo-decrescendo quality than Cheyne-Stokes respiration and is often a sign of pontine or cerebellar damage.
  - (3) **Ataxic (Biot's) breathing,** an irregular, chaotic breathing pattern, implies damage to the medullary respiratory centers and is usually seen in association with posterior fossa lesions. *Progression to apnea occurs frequently.*
4. **Visual fields**
   Visual fields should be tested with threatening movements, which normally evoke a blink. Asymmetry of this response implies hemianopia.
5. **Fundoscopy**
   Papilledema occurs after prolonged (>12 hours) elevation of ICP, and only rarely does it develop acutely. Thus, the absence of papilledema does not rule out increased ICP. *Spontaneous venous pulsations* are difficult to identify, but their presence implies normal ICP. *Subhyaloid hemorrhages* appear as globules of blood on the retinal surface and are commonly associated with subarachnoid hemorrhage.
6. **Pupils**
   The shape, size, and reactivity to light of the pupils should be noted.
   - a. **Symmetry and normal reactivity to light** implies structural integrity of the midbrain. *Reactive pupils in conjunction with absent corneal and oculocephalic responses are highly suggestive of metabolic coma.*
   - b. **Midposition (2 to 5 mm) fixed or irregular pupils** imply a focal midbrain lesion.
   - c. **Pinpoint reactive pupils** occur with pontine damage. Opiates and cholinergic intoxication (e.g., with pilocarpine) also produce small reactive pupils.
   - d. **A unilateral dilated and fixed pupil** usually occurs with

CN 3 compression in the setting of uncal herniation. Ptosis and exodeviation of the eye are also seen. *An acutely "blown" pupil represents an immediate threat to life and requires urgent intervention.*
   e. **Bilateral fixed and dilated pupils** can reflect central herniation, global hypoxia-ischemia, or poisoning with barbiturates, scopolamine, atropine, or glutethimide.
7. **Ocular movements**

   Horizontal conjugate gaze is mediated by the *frontal eye fields* and the *pontine gaze centers*. The frontal eye fields, when activated, drive gaze to the opposite side. The pontine gaze centers, when activated, drive gaze to the same side. Vertical conjugate gaze is mediated by centers in the *midbrain tegmentum and lower diencephalon*. In unresponsive patients, conjugate eye movements can be actively elicited by testing the **oculocephalic and oculovestibular reflexes** (Fig. 5–3). Both reflexes are mediated by stimulating the semicircular canals, with CN 8 input to the vestibular nuclei and bilateral connections to the third, fourth, and sixth nuclei. *Thus, intact eye movements indicate brain stem integrity from the level of CN 3 to CN 8 (midbrain and pons).*
   a. **The position of the eyes at rest** should be noted.
      (1) **Gaze deviation away from the hemiparesis** results from hemispheric lesions contralateral to the hemiparesis.
      (2) **Gaze deviation toward the hemiparesis** can result from the following:
         (a) Pontine lesions contralateral to the hemiparesis
         (b) "Wrong-way gaze" from thalamic lesions contralateral to the hemiparesis
         (c) Seizure activity in the hemisphere contralateral to the hemiparesis
      (3) **Forced downward eye deviation** results from lesions of the midbrain tectum. Association with impaired pupillary reactivity and refractory nystagmus is known as *Parinaud's syndrome.*
      (4) **Slow roving eye movements** may be conjugate or dysconjugate and are not of localizing value. They are most frequently associated with bilateral hemispheric dysfunction and active oculocephalic reflexes.
      (5) **Ocular bobbing** consists of fast downward "bobbing" with slow return to the primary position. It results from bilateral damage to the pontine horizontal gaze centers.
      (6) **Saccadic (fast) eye movements** are not seen in coma and imply psychogenic unresponsiveness.
   b. **The oculocephalic (doll's eye) reflex** should be noted.

      This reflex is elicited by briskly turning the head side to

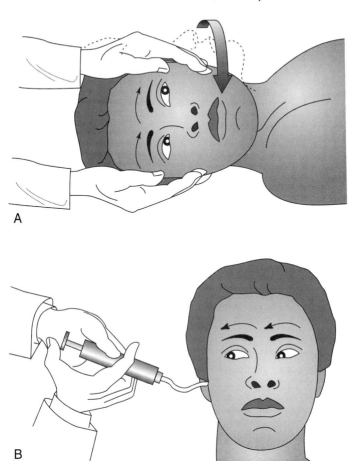

Figure 5–3 □ *A,* "Doll's eye" maneuver (oculocephalic reflex): with an intact brain stem (cranial nerves 3 through 8), the eyes move opposite to the direction of head turning. *B,* Cold caloric test (oculovestibular reflex): with an intact brain stem, injecting cold water in the auditory canal results in tonic conjugate eye deviation toward the cold ear.

side. In alert patients, supranuclear cortical inputs to the oculomotor nuclei control eye movement, and the response cannot be elicited. *An intact response consists of full conjugate eye movement opposite to the direction of head movement.*

A full and easy-to-elicit reflex ("ball-bearing eyes")

implies bilateral cerebral hemisphere dysfunction and structural integrity of the brain stem, as seen with metabolic coma.
  c. **The oculovestibular (cold caloric) reflex** should be tested.
    This reflex is a more potent method for eliciting conjugate eye movements. The head is tilted 30 degrees above horizontal, and the ear is lavaged with 30 to 60 ml of ice water using butterfly tubing attached to a syringe. *A normal response consists of tonic eye deviation toward the cold ear and fast nystagmus away from the cold ear (mediated by the frontal lobe contralateral to the direction of the fast component).*
    (1) **Tonic phase bilaterally intact, with absent fast responses** suggests coma from bihemispheric dysfunction.
    (2) **Conjugate gaze paresis** can result from unilateral hemispheric or pontine lesions.
    (3) **Asymmetric eye weakness** implies a brain stem lesion. CN 3 paresis, CN 6 paresis, and internuclear ophthalmoplegia are the most commonly identified abnormalities.
    (4) **Absent oculovestibular responses** are seen with deep coma of any cause and imply severe depression of brain stem function.
8. **Corneal reflex**
   Stroking the cornea with sterile gauze or cotton normally results in bilateral eye closure. The afferent limb of the reflex is mediated by CN 5, and the efferent limb by CN 7.
9. **Gag reflex**
   In intubated patients, this reflex can be tested by gently manipulating the endotracheal tube.
10. **Motor responses**
    Motor responses are the single best indicator of the depth and severity of coma.
    a. **Spontaneous movements** should be observed for symmetry and purpose. Preferential movement on one side indicates weakness of the unused limbs.
    b. **Limb tone** should be tested for symmetry.
       Tone in the upper extremities is tested by passive motion at the elbow and wrist. Lower extremity tone is tested by a quick lifting motion under the thigh; if the heel elevates off the bed, tone is abnormally increased. *Bilaterally increased lower extremity tone is an important sign of herniation.*
    c. **Induced movements** should be tested systematically by observing responses to stimuli of increasing intensity, in the following order:
       (1) **Verbal command.** Ask the patient to open the eyes, protrude the tongue, raise one arm, and show two fingers. *Hand squeezing often occurs as an automatic re-*

sponse and, in isolation, should not be taken as evidence of the patient's following commands.
  (2) **Sternal rub.** Apply gentle pressure with fingertips. Proceed to deep knuckle pressure if there is no response.
      (a) **Purposeful localizing responses** consist of precise hand movements and active attempts to ward off the examiner.
      (b) **Gross localizing responses** are slower and less accurate. They occur with deepening coma or with nondominant hemispheric lesions causing impaired spatial discrimination.
  (3) **Nailbed pressure.** Use the handle of the reflex hammer and gradually increase the pressure on each extremity.
      (a) **Withdrawal** is mediated by the motor cortex. The movements are sudden, nonstereotyped, and variable in intensity.
      (b) **Flexor (decorticate) posturing** (Fig. 5–4) results from damage to the corticospinal tracts at the level of the *deep hemisphere or upper midbrain*. The full response consists of flexion with adduction of the arms and extension of the legs.
      (c) **Extensor (decerebrate) posturing** (see Fig. 5–4) consists of extension, adduction, and internal rotation of the arms and extension of the legs. It results from corticospinal tract damage at the level of the *pons or upper medulla*.
11. **Sensory responses**
    Asymmetry of response to noxious stimulation suggests a lateralizing sensory deficit.
12. **Reflexes**
    a. **Deep tendon reflexes**
       Asymmetry indicates a lateralizing motor deficit caused by a structural lesion.
    b. **Plantar reflexes**
       Bilateral Babinski's responses can occur with structural or metabolic coma.

■ DIAGNOSTIC TESTING

Once the history and neurologic examination are completed, a differential diagnosis should be generated. Most patients in stupor or coma can be placed into one of three categories on the basis of neurologic findings:
1. **Nonfocal examination with brain stem intact**
   This category is characterized by reactive pupils, full eye

70 Patient-Related Problems: The Common Calls

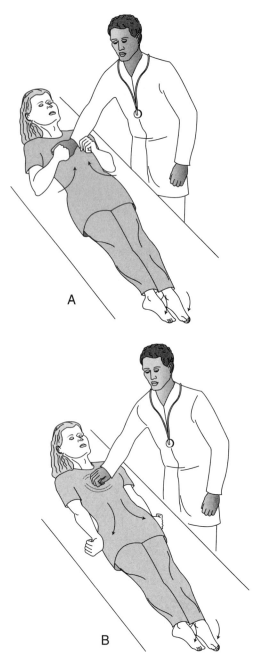

Figure 6–4 □ *A,* Decorticate (flexor) posturing. *B,* Decerebrate (extensor) posturing.

movements, and symmetric motor responses and suggests a toxic-metabolic etiology, CNS infection, or hydrocephalus.
2. **Focal hemispheric signs**
These signs are characterized by contralateral hemiparesis and gaze paresis and suggest a structural CNS lesion such as stroke, subdural hematoma, or neoplasm.
3. **Focal brain stem signs**
These signs are characterized by abnormal pupil reactivity, cranial nerve signs, and motor posturing and suggest a brain stem lesion or a space-occupying lesion associated with herniation.

Because it is important to quickly rule out life-threatening conditions in patients with coma, diagnostic testing should generally proceed in the following order in all patients until a diagnosis is established:
1. **Head CT (or MRI) scan**
Intravenous contrast material should be given if a tumor or an abscess is suspected. Order bone windows if there is a history of trauma.
2. **Lumbar puncture**
LP should be performed to rule out meningitis, encephalitis, or subarachnoid hemorrhage if the diagnosis is not established by CT or MRI. *Never postpone treatment for meningitis or encephalitis if there is a delay in obtaining the CSF.*
3. **Electroencephalogram (EEG)**
An EEG may be necessary to rule out *nonconvulsive status epilepticus,* a postictal state, or metabolic coma if the diagnosis is not established by CT and LP.

Pseudocoma states should be considered if the cause of coma remains unclear after diagnostic testing.
- **Psychogenic coma**
Psychogenic coma occurs in patients who are physiologically awake but unresponsive. Clues to the diagnosis include negativistic behavior (active resistance to eye-opening or passive limb movement), avoidance behavior (the hand avoids the face when dropped from above the head), intact saccadic eye movements and nystagmus on cold caloric testing, and recovery of alertness in response to very painful stimuli.
- **Locked-in syndrome**
Locked-in syndrome refers to bilateral pontine damage (usually from infarction) that renders the patient awake but completely paralyzed except for vertical eye movements. *Ocular bobbing* is a common finding.
- **Akinetic mutism**
Akinetic mutism refers to states of extreme psychomotor retardation (abulia) resulting from extensive thalamic or frontal lobe damage. These patients appear awake but demon-

strate reduced spontaneity and exhibit only limited responses after extremely long delays.

■ MANAGEMENT

Emergency Treatments for Patients in Coma

1. **Space-occupying lesions** require prompt neurosurgical evaluation because emergent decompression may be lifesaving.
2. **Increased intracranial pressure,** if suspected, should be treated immediately. Stepwise treatment includes
   a. *Head elevation*
   b. Intubation and *hyperventilation*
   c. *Sedation* if severe agitation is present (**midazolam 1 to 2 mg IV** is an effective, short-acting agent)
   d. *Osmotic diuresis* with **20% mannitol 1 g/kg via rapid IV infusion**
      These therapies can be used to "buy time" before definitive neurosurgical intervention. **Dexamethasone 10 mg IV every 6 hours** may also be of benefit for reducing edema associated with tumor or abscess. After these emergency treatments, an ICP monitor should be inserted to further guide management (see Chapter 12).
3. **Encephalitis** from herpesvirus infection, if suspected, should be treated empirically with **acyclovir 10 mg/kg IV every 8 hours.** Further diagnostic testing should proceed as outlined in Chapter 22.
4. **Meningitis,** if suspected, should be treated empirically. Cover with **ceftriaxone 1 g IV every 12 hours** and **ampicillin 1 g IV every 6 hours** pending CSF culture results.

General Care of the Comatose Patient

1. **Airway protection**
   Adequate oxygenation and ventilation and prevention of aspiration are the goals. Most patients will require endotracheal intubation and frequent orotracheal suctioning. *Nonintubated stuporous patients should always be designated to receive nothing by mouth (NPO).*
2. **Intravenous hydration**
   Use only isotonic fluids (e.g., normal saline) in patients with cerebral edema or increased ICP.
3. **Nutrition**
   Administer enteral feeds via a small-bore nasoduodenal tube. Nasogastric tubes impair the integrity of the upper and lower esophageal sphincters and increase the risk of gastroesophageal reflux and aspiration.

4. **Skin**
   Order that the patient be turned every 1 to 2 hours to prevent pressure sores. An inflatable or foam mattress and protective heel pads may also be beneficial.
5. **Eyes**
   Prevent corneal abrasion by taping the eyelids shut or by applying a lubricant.
6. **Bowel care**
   Constipation can be avoided by giving a stool softener **(docusate sodium 100 mg three times a day).** Intubation and steroids may predispose to gastric stress ulceration, and this should be prevented by giving an H_2 blocker **(ranitidine 50 mg IV every 8 hours).**
7. **Bladder care**
   Indwelling urinary catheters are a common source of infection and should be used judiciously. Use intermittent catheterization every 6 hours when possible.
8. **Joint mobility**
   Order daily passive range-of-motion exercises to prevent contractures.
9. **Deep vein thrombosis (DVT) prophylaxis**
   Immobility is a major risk factor for DVT and subsequent pulmonary embolism. Order heparin **5000 U subcutaneously (SC) every 12 hours,** external pneumatic compression stockings, or both.

■ PROGNOSIS

The prognosis for recovery from coma depends primarily on the cause, rather than on the depth, of coma. Coma from drug intoxication and metabolic causes carries the best prognosis; patients with coma from traumatic head injury fare better than those with coma from other structural causes; and coma from global hypoxia-ischemia carries the least favorable prognosis. Simple bedside testing can be used to prognosticate outcome as early as 3 days after hypoxic-ischemic coma (Fig. 5–5). Confirmation of a hopeless situation in patients with hypoxic-ischemic coma can be attained with somatosensory evoked potential testing. Absent cortical responses with medial nerve stimulation 5 days or more after the onset of coma implies a 100% likelihood of a vegetative outcome. This information may be useful for helping families to decide whether to withdraw life support.

Persistent vegetative state (PVS) refers to a state of "eyes-open unresponsiveness" that is applied to patients in coma for 30 days or more. These patients assume normal sleep-wake cycles and display primitive responses to stimuli, such as chewing, sucking, and grasping, but demonstrate no evidence of conscious aware-

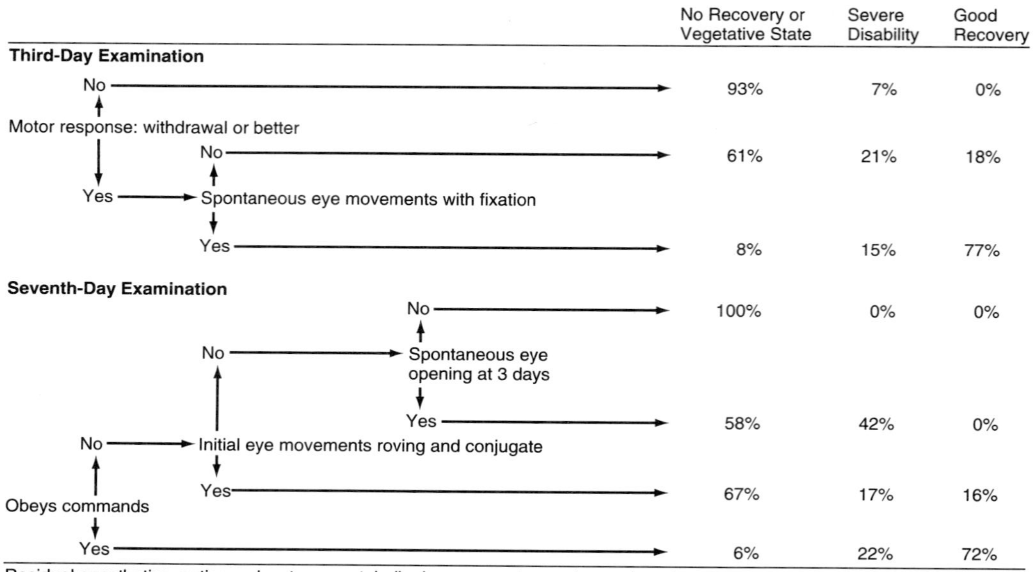

	No Recovery or Vegetative State	Severe Disability	Good Recovery
Third-Day Examination			
No → Motor response: withdrawal or better	93%	7%	0%
No → Spontaneous eye movements with fixation	61%	21%	18%
Yes	8%	15%	77%
Seventh-Day Examination			
No → Spontaneous eye opening at 3 days	100%	0%	0%
Yes → Initial eye movements roving and conjugate	58%	42%	0%
No → Obeys commands	67%	17%	16%
Yes	6%	22%	72%

Residual anesthetics, anticonvulsants, or metabolic derangements may be confounding.

Figure 5–5 □ Features predictive of recovery from hypoxic-ischemic coma. Outcomes refer to best functional state attained within the first year. (Modified from Levy DE, Caronna JJ, Singer BH, et al: Predicting outcome from hypoxic-ischemic coma. JAMA 1985;253:1420. Copyright © 1985, American Medical Association.)

ness. Prognostication is important, because this information may influence decisions to withhold life-sustaining measures such as cardiopulmonary resuscitation (CPR) or intensive care unit (ICU) care. Recovery of consciousness from PVS is generally defined as return of the ability to communicate or follow commands. By this criterion, 15% of adult patients with nontraumatic injury and 50% of patients with traumatic injury who are still in a vegetative state after 1 month will recover consciousness by 12 months. Recovery of consciousness after 12 months in a PVS is exceedingly rare.

chapter 6

Acute Stroke

Stroke should be suspected whenever a patient presents with the characteristic sudden onset of focal neurologic signs, such as hemiparesis, hemisensory loss, hemianopia, aphasia, or ataxia (Table 6–1). Time is of the essence for treating stroke, because the "therapeutic window" is only 3 to 6 hours. Because of the importance of early intervention in acute stroke, the emphasis of emergency room (ER) management should not be on identifying subtle, unusual, or interesting neurologic signs but on

1. **Stabilizing the patient**
2. **Obtaining blood tests, an electrocardiogram (ECG), and a chest radiograph**
3. **Establishing the diagnosis by history and physical examination**
4. **Obtaining a head computed tomography (CT) or magnetic resonance imaging (MRI) scan as soon as possible**

Further management of the patient, once the diagnosis has been established and the patient has left the ER, is discussed in Chapter 24.

■ PHONE CALL

Questions

1. What were the presenting symptoms?
2. Exactly when did the symptoms begin?
3. What are the vital signs?

Table 6–1 □ PRESENTATIONS OF ACUTE STROKE

- Abrupt onset of facial or limb weakness (usually hemiparesis)
- Sensory loss in one or more extremities
- Sudden change in mental status (confusion, delirium, lethargy, stupor, or coma)
- Aphasia (incoherent speech, lack of speech output, or difficulty understanding speech)
- Dysarthria (slurred speech)
- Loss of vision (hemianopic or monocular) or diplopia
- Ataxia (truncal or limb)
- Vertigo, nausea and vomiting, or headache

4. Does the patient have a history of hypertension, diabetes, or cardiac disease?
5. Is the patient taking aspirin or warfarin?

It is particularly important to perform an urgent CT scan in patients taking warfarin, in order to rule out intracerebral hemorrhage, because early treatment with fresh frozen plasma (FFP) can be lifesaving.

Orders

1. Establish an intravenous line with **0.9% normal saline (NS) at 20 ml/hour.** Hypotonic fluids such as D5W and half-normal saline aggravate cerebral edema.
2. Provide oxygen via a nasal cannula (if patient is tachypneic).
3. Keep the patient NPO (nothing by mouth).
4. Obtain an ECG.
5. Obtain a chest radiograph.
6. Obtain a stat noncontrast head CT scan.
7. Perform the following diagnostic blood tests:
   - Complete blood cell count (CBC) and platelet count
   - Serum chemistries (glucose, electrolytes, blood urea nitrogen [BUN], creatinine)
   - Prothrombin time (PT)/partial thromboplastin time (PTT)
8. If indicated, perform the following tests:
   - Alcohol level
   - Liver function tests
   - Arterial blood gases
   - Toxicology screen

■ ELEVATOR THOUGHTS

What are the causes of stroke?
1. **Infarction: causes 80% of all strokes**
   a. Embolic
      (1) Cardiogenic embolism
         (a) Atrial fibrillation or other arrhythmia
         (b) Left ventricular mural thrombus
         (c) Mitral or aortic valve disease
         (d) Endocarditis (infectious or noninfectious)
      (2) Paradoxical embolism (patent foramen ovale)
      (3) Aortic arch embolism
   b. Atherothrombotic (large- or medium-vessel disease)
      (1) Extracranial disease
         (a) Internal carotid artery
         (b) Vertebral artery
      (2) Intracranial disease
         (a) Internal carotid artery

(b) Middle cerebral artery
(c) Basilar artery
  c. Lacunar (small penetrating artery occlusion)
2. **Intracerebral hemorrhage (ICH): causes 15% of all strokes**
   a. Hypertensive
   b. Arteriovenous malformation
   c. Amyloid angiopathy
3. **Subarachnoid hemorrhage (SAH): causes 5% of all strokes**
4. **Miscellaneous causes (can lead to infarction or hemorrhage)**
   a. Dural sinus thrombosis
   b. Carotid or vertebral artery dissection
   c. Central nervous system (CNS) vasculitis
   d. Moyamoya disease (progressive intracranial large artery occlusion)
   e. Migraine
   f. Hypercoagulable state
   g. Drug abuse (cocaine or amphetamines)
   h. Hematologic disorders (sickle cell anemia, polycythemia, or leukemia)
   i. MELAS (mitochondrial encephalopathy, lactic acidosis, and stroke)
   j. Atrial myxoma

■ MAJOR THREAT TO LIFE

- **Transtentorial herniation**
    Occurs primarily in the following presentations:
    1. Massive hemispheric infarction or hemorrhage
    2. Intraventricular extension of ICH or SAH
- **Cerebellar infarction or hemorrhage**
    All patients with large cerebellar lesions require neurosurgical evaluation because emergent decompression can be lifesaving.
- **Aspiration**
    Aspiration pneumonia is a common cause of death in stroke patients. All patients should be considered to have impaired swallowing until proven otherwise.
- **Myocardial infarction (MI)**
    Acute MI complicates approximately 3% of acute ischemic strokes.

■ BEDSIDE

Quick Look Test

What is the patient's level of consciousness?
   The urgency of the situation can be assessed immediately by

evaluating the level of consciousness. *Patients in stupor or coma are at the highest risk for further deterioration and are most likely to benefit from urgent intervention.*

Airway and Vital Signs

Is the patient in respiratory distress?
If the patient's breathing appears labored, check arterial blood gas levels and start oxygen. **Patients with severe dyspnea or depressed level of consciousness (stupor or coma) should be intubated prior to CT scanning.** Failure to control the airway in either setting can lead to massive aspiration or to respiratory arrest.

What is the blood pressure?
Hypertension occurs frequently after stroke as a nonspecific response to cerebral injury. In ischemic stroke, this response may be advantageous, because increased cerebral perfusion pressure improves blood flow in regions of marginally perfused brain (the ischemic penumbra) that have lost the capacity to autoregulate. As a result, *overly aggressive blood pressure (BP) reduction in acute ischemic stroke patients can lead to increased infarction and neurologic deterioration.* For this reason, only severe hypertension should be treated prior to CT scanning unless there is a nonneurologic indication (Box 6–1).

Box 6–1. GUIDELINES FOR ER TREATMENT OF HYPERTENSION IN ACUTE STROKE

Treat hypertension if a nonneurologic hypertensive emergency exists:
1. Acute myocardial ischemia
2. Cardiogenic pulmonary edema
3. Malignant hypertension (retinopathy)
4. Hypertensive nephropathy
5. Aortic dissection

Also treat hypertension if the BP is highly elevated on three repeated measurements 15 minutes apart:
1. Systolic BP >220 mm Hg
2. Diastolic BP >120 mm Hg

Otherwise, systolic BPs of 160 to 220 mm Hg should *not* be treated prior to CT scanning. If hemorrhage is identified by CT, reduction of the systolic BP to 150 to 180 mm Hg should be considered.

If the patient meets one of the criteria listed in Box 6–1 and needs urgent BP control, start with IV labetalol.
1. Order **100 mg of IV labetalol in a 20-ml syringe (5 mg/ml)** to the bedside.
2. Order a labetalol drip to the bedside **(200 mg in 200 ml NS)**.
3. **IV push 20 mg of labetalol over 2 minutes; repeat 40 to 80 mg at 10-minute intervals** until the desired BP is attained.
4. Once the desired BP is attained, start infusion of **2 mg/min (120 ml/hour)** and titrate.

If labetalol fails to control hypertension and increased intracranial pressure (ICP) is not a concern, start **nitroprusside IV 50 mg/250 ml D5W (200 µg/ml) at 3 ml/hour (10 µg/min)** and titrate.

Low BP in acute stroke is unusual. Hypotension that is severe enough to precipitate cerebral infarction is rare but can occur in patients with severe carotid artery or intracranial artery stenosis.

What is the heart rate?
Rapid atrial fibrillation may require treatment with **digoxin 0.125 to 0.5 mg IV** or **verapamil 5 to 10 mg IV** for rate control prior to CT scanning.

What is the temperature?
The most common cause of fever in a stroke patient is aspiration pneumonia. If fever is present, order blood and urine cultures and consider administering antibiotics empirically **(cefoxitin 1 g IV every 6 hours** or **cefuroxime 750 mg IV every 8 hours).**

Selective History

If possible, obtain an eyewitness to corroborate the patient's account. Be sure to check the following:
1. **What time did the stroke begin?**
   Approximately 30% of strokes occur at night and present upon awakening.
2. **What were the initial symptoms?**
   A maximal deficit at onset in a fully alert patient supports cerebral infarction and suggests embolism in particular. Loss of consciousness, headache, or vomiting supports intracerebral hemorrhage. Inquire specifically about the following:
   - Headache or neck pain (hemorrhage or dissection)
   - Loss of consciousness
   - Confused or slurred speech
   - Visual disturbances
   - Dizziness or vertigo (brain stem ischemia)

- Weakness or clumsiness
- Numbness or paresthesias
- Gait instability
3. Were there any antecedent attacks consistent with transient ischemic attack (TIA)?
4. Was any seizure activity observed?
5. What is the patient's medical history?
6. Has the patient used drugs or alcohol recently?
    Cocaine can precipitate infarction or hemorrhage.
7. What medications is the patient taking?

Selective Physical Examination

General Physical Examination

Neck	Auscultate for carotid bruits. Neck stiffness suggests subarachnoid hemorrhage.
Lungs	Check for aspiration pneumonia or congestive heart failure.
Heart	Murmurs suggest valvular heart disease and a possible source of embolism.

Neurologic Examination

Because time is of the essence, the initial neurologic examination needs to be systematic and efficient. The goal is to simply localize and characterize the severity of the deficit. An experienced examiner can accomplish this in 10 to 15 minutes; a more detailed examination should be carried out later.

- **Mental status**
  1. **Level of consciousness and attentiveness**
  2. **Concentration.** Ask the patient to count from 20 to 1 or to recite the months in reverse.
  3. **Orientation**
  4. **Aphasia.** Check the fluency of spontaneous speech, naming, repetition, and paraphasic errors (word or syllable substitutions).
  5. **Hemispatial neglect.** Forced head and gaze deviation implies a large hemispheric lesion.
- **Cranial nerves**
  1. **Fundus.** Check for papilledema.
  2. **Visual fields.** Ask the patient to count fingers in all four quadrants. Check the patient's blink-to-threat if the patient is inattentive.
  3. **Pupils**
  4. **Extraocular movements**
  5. **Face.** A widened palpebral fissure and flattened nasolabial fold are indicative of facial weakness.
  6. **Palate and tongue.** Check for symmetry and adequacy of the gag reflex.

- **Motor**
  1. **Spontaneous movements.** Preferential movement of the limbs on one side indicates paresis of the unused limbs. If the patient is unresponsive, check for a preferential localizing response to sternal rub.
  2. **Limb tone.** Increased tone occurs with deep lesions in the internal capsule or brain stem.
  3. **Arm (pronator) drift.** If the patient is unable to follow commands, passively elevate both arms and check whether one falls preferentially.
  4. **Power.** Check strength against active resistance at the shoulders, wrists, hips, and ankles.
- **Reflexes**
  1. **Deep tendon reflex**
  2. **Plantar reflex**

Proceed with the neurologic examination if the patient's level of consciousness allows:

- **Sensory**
  1. **Pinprick or pinch test** identifies a lateralizing deficit.
- **Coordination**
  1. **Finger-to-nose test** identifies intention tremor and past pointing.
  2. **Gait and station.** Check for reduced arm swing on the paretic side. A wide base is indicative of truncal ataxia.

■ MANAGEMENT I: ACUTE MANAGEMENT

Once the history and examination are completed, you should be able to localize the lesion clinically. **The main differential diagnoses are infarction and hemorrhage, which can be accurately diagnosed only by CT.** Hence, all further management decisions (anticoagulation, BP management, or further workup) will depend on the results of the head CT.

Hemorrhage

Radiographic Assessment

Blood is readily identified by the presence of a high-density (bright) signal (Fig. 6–1*A*). If ICH is present, be sure to check for the following radiographic findings:

- *Subarachnoid hemorrhage* (Fig. 6–1*B*) in association with intraparenchymal hemorrhage suggests a ruptured aneurysm and requires angiography.
- *Intraventricular hemorrhage* (Fig. 6–1*C*) in association with ventricular enlargement requires neurosurgical evaluation for possible emergent ventriculostomy.

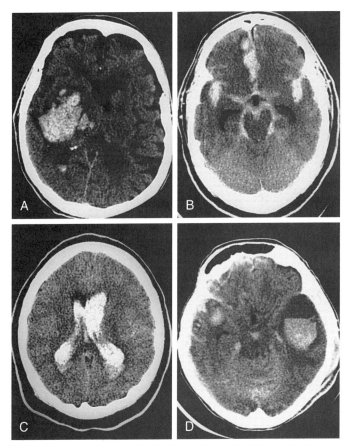

Figure 6–1 □ CT scans of brain hemorrhage. *A,* Intracerebral hemorrhage. *B,* Subarachnoid hemorrhage. *C,* Intraventricular hemorrhage. *D,* Acute hemorrhage with fluid/fluid level, indicative of a clotting disturbance.

- *Fluid/fluid levels* within a hematoma (Fig. 6–1D) result from separation of red blood cells and plasma and are indicative of a coagulopathy.
- *Edema and mass effect* usually lead to delayed neurologic deterioration when associated with a large hemorrhage (>30 ml). An abnormally large or an irregular amount of edema associated with hemorrhage suggests (1) hemorrhagic infarction, (2) bleeding associated with neoplasm, or (3) venous infarction from dural sinus thrombosis.

Checklist for Acute Management of Intracerebral Hemorrhage

1. **Rule out coagulopathy.**
   Confirm that the PT and PTT are normal. If the PT is elevated, give **FFP 4 to 8 U IV every 4 hours** and **vitamin K 15 mg IV push, then subcutaneously (SC) three times a day** until the PT is normalized. Reverse heparin anticoagulation with **protamine sulfate 10 to 50 mg slow IV push** (1 mg reverses approximately 100 units of heparin).
2. **Control severe hypertension.**
   In contrast to the approach taken with acute cerebral infarction, a somewhat more aggressive approach to BP control is suggested for patients with acute ICH, because high levels may lead to worsening of perilesional edema. Although the optimal management has yet to be established, we advocate reduction of systolic BPs that are higher than 180 mm Hg to levels between 150 and 180 mm Hg using a labetalol drip (see Airway and Vital Signs).
3. **Obtain a neurosurgical evaluation.**
   The criteria for emergent evacuation of intracerebral hemorrhage are controversial. Surgery can be lifesaving if the patient is deteriorating and signs of herniation appear. Consideration should also be given to inserting a *ventricular drain* in stuporous or comatose patients with intraventricular hemorrhage or a *parenchymal ICP monitor* in patients with large, deep hemorrhages who are not candidates for surgery.
4. **Consider angiography** to rule out an aneurysm or arteriovenous malformation (AVM). This is particularly important in young (less than 50 years of age), nonhypertensive patients.
5. **Consider mannitol (1 g/kg IV)** for deepening coma or if clinical signs of brain stem compression are evident (see Chapter 12 for further details). **Steroids such as dexamethasone have not been shown to be effective in patients with ICH.**
6. **Consider phenytoin loading (10 to 20 mg/kg IV or by mouth [PO])** in patients with large hemorrhages and depressed level of consciousness.
   In general, anticonvulsants can be withheld unless there

is evidence of seizure activity. However, prophylactic treatment is reasonable if the patient's condition is critical enough to require intubation, treatment of increased ICP, or surgery.

Additional guidelines for the management of ICH or SAH are included in Chapter 24 and under Management II: General Care in this chapter.

Infarction

Radiographic Assessment

Infarction appears as a lucent (dark) signal on a CT scan but may not be apparent until 12 to 24 hours after onset. Early signs of infarction (Fig. 6–2) are important to recognize and include (1) loss of definition of the gray-white junction, (2) mild sulcal effacement, and (3) subtle, hazy lucency. The CT scan is frequently negative in patients with lacunar or brain stem infarction, and in these cases, MRI will frequently delineate the lesion. Newer MRI techniques such as diffusion-weighted imaging (DWI) may reveal ischemia or early infarction in the first few hours after stroke onset.

Affected Vascular Territory

Identification of the affected vascular territory can provide important information regarding the mechanism of the infarction. The topography of the major arterial territories of the brain are shown in Figure 6–3. Examples of the three main patterns of infarction, described below, are shown in Figure 6–4.

1. **Territorial infarction** respects the margins of an entire vascular territory or one of its branches. The cause is usually

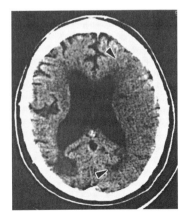

Figure 6–2 □ Early cerebral infarction, with loss of gray-white definition and sulcal effacement. (*Arrowheads* indicate anterior and posterior borders of the territory of the middle cerebral artery.)

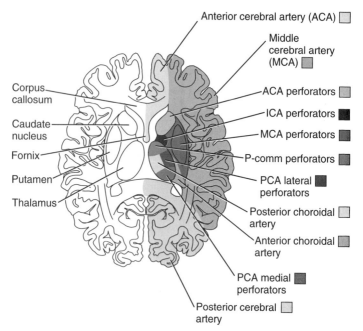

Figure 6–3 □ Axial section at the level of the thalamus showing the anatomic distribution of the major cerebral vascular territories. P-comm, posterior communicating artery. (Redrawn from Tatu L, et al: Arterial territories of the human brain: Cerebral hemispheres. Neurology 1998;50:1699–1708.)

embolism, with infarction occurring in brain regions immediately distal to the site of occlusion.

2. **Border-zone infarction** may occur either (1) along the boundaries between different vascular territories (watershed infarction) or (2) in the deepest and least well-collateralized regions of a vascular territory (internal border-zone infarction). In either case, the cause is usually distal hemodynamic perfusion failure related to a more proximal stenosis or occlusion.
3. **Lacunar infarction** appears as a small, deep infarction within the territory of a single, small penetrating artery. The mechanism is usually related to occlusion within the course of the small vessel (microatheroma or lipohyalinosis).

Goals of Management

1. **Limiting or reversing ongoing acute ischemia (3-hour window)**

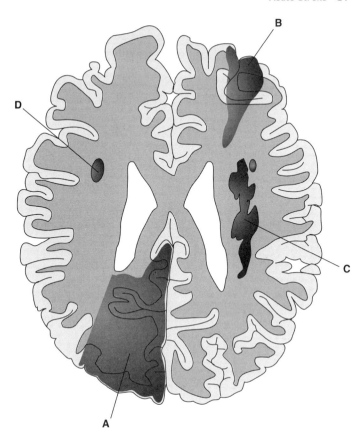

Figure 6–4 □ Schematic representation of different topographic patterns of cerebral infarction. *A*, territorial infarction (from posterior cerebral artery occlusion); *B*, watershed border-zone infarction (between the territories of the anterior cerebral artery and the middle cerebral artery); *C*, internal border-zone infarction (deep middle cerebral artery territory); *D*, lacunar infarction (lenticulostriate-penetrating artery occlusion).

Thrombolysis with **tissue plasminogen activator (t-PA)** is the only currently approved treatment for reversing ischemia in acute stroke. It carries a 6% risk of significant bleeding and should be given only within 3 hours of onset and only if the head CT scan is normal. It should be administered by experienced clinicians only.

2. **Preventing neurologic deterioration related to an evolving stroke (72-hour window)**

Stroke progression occurs in 20 to 40% of hospitalized patients with ischemic stroke, with the risk being highest in the first 24 hours. Clinical deterioration can result from one of three mechanisms:

- **Extension of ischemic territory.** This may result from either *progressive thrombosis within an occluded vessel* (e.g., progressive brain stem infarction in a patient with basilar artery thrombosis) or *distal perfusion failure related to a more proximal stenosis or occlusion* (e.g., enlargement of internal border-zone infarction in a patient with internal carotid artery [ICA] occlusion).

    Approach: Heparin may prevent progressive thrombosis, and optimization of volume status and blood pressure may mitigate perfusion failure.

- **Hemorrhagic conversion.** This problem is frequently identified radiographically but rarely results in clinical symptoms. The three main risk factors are increased patient age, large infarct size, and acute hypertension.

    Approach: Defer anticoagulation of high-risk patients for 48 to 72 hours; treat severe hypertension.

- **Progressive edema and infarct swelling.** This problem is generally limited to large infarcts. Brain edema generally peaks 3 to 5 days after onset and is rarely a problem within the first 24 hours.

    Approach: Treatment with mannitol is beneficial. Avoid hypotonic fluids. *Steroids are not effective.*

3. **Preventing early recurrent stroke (30-day window)**

Approximately 5% of patients hospitalized for ischemic stroke experience a second stroke within 30 days. This risk is highest (greater than 10%) in patients with severe carotid stenosis and cardioembolism and lowest (1%) in patients with lacunar infarction.

Approach: Early treatment with heparin may reduce the risk of early recurrent stroke in patients with cardioembolism or large-artery stenosis but has not been proved to do so.

Checklist for Acute Management of Ischemic Stroke

1. **IV t-PA (0.9 mg/kg IV over 1 hour with 10% of the dose given as an initial bolus; maximum of 90 mg)** if onset is definitely within 3 hours and CT shows no signs of widespread early infarction.
2. **Consider angiography** for local intra-arterial thrombolysis with **t-PA (5 to 25 mg) between 3 and 6 hours after onset** if the patient has not received IV t-PA, a major hemispheric or basilar artery syndrome is present, and an experienced interventional neuroradiologist is available.

3. **Consider cardiac rhythm monitoring** for patients with evidence of arrhythmia or myocardial ischemia.
4. **Consider intensive care unit (ICU) observation** in patients with clinical or radiographic signs of massive hemispheric or cerebellar infarction, depressed level of consciousness, respiratory distress, or stroke-in-evolution.
5. **Obtain a neurosurgical evaluation** for possible decompressive surgery in patients with large cerebellar infarction or complete middle cerebral artery territory infarction with midline shift and deteriorating level of consciousness.
6. **Consider MRI** in patients with posterior circulation strokes or if the infarction is not well delineated by CT.
7. **Consider IV heparin** (start at **800 U/hour, 20,000 U in 500 ml NS at 20 ml/hour**) in the following situations:
   - Suspected cardioembolic stroke
   - TIAs or infarction related to carotid artery stenosis
   - Stroke-in-evolution
   - Arterial dissection
   - Dural sinus thrombosis

   Keep in mind that heparin is relatively contraindicated in patients with large infarcts associated with mass effect or hemorrhagic conversion.
8. **Order a noninvasive neurovascular workup.**

   Proper decisions regarding the treatment of cerebral infarction are based on elucidation of the mechanism of the stroke.

   The following tests should be performed in every patient:
   - *Echocardiography* is an important technique for identifying cardiac sources of emboli. In many patients, transthoracic echocardiography is adequate. *Transesophageal echocardiography* provides more-detailed views of the left atrium and aortic arch and is a more sensitive test for detecting mural thrombi and valvular vegetations. An *agitated saline study* ("bubble study") is highly sensitive for detecting right-to-left atrial shunts, consistent with a patent foramen ovale.
   - *Carotid Doppler ultrasonography* is needed to rule out carotid stenosis that is symptomatic and greater than 70%, which is an indication for carotid endarterectomy.

   The following tests should be performed in selected patients:
   - *Transcranial Doppler ultrasonography* can be used to diagnose occlusion or stenosis of the major intracranial arteries. Abnormal intracranial waveforms and collateral flow patterns can also be used to determine whether a stenosis found in the neck is hemodynamically significant.

- *Magnetic resonance angiography* can be used to diagnose extracranial or intracranial stenosis or occlusion.
- *Holter monitoring* may be useful for detecting intermittent atrial fibrillation.
9. **Consider blood testing** to identify unusual causes of stroke, particularly in young patients.
    - *Blood cultures* if endocarditis is suspected.
    - *Procoagulant workup:* protein C activity, protein S activity, antithrombin III activity, lupus anticoagulant, anticardiolipin antibodies, Factor V Leiden mutation, prothrombin gene mutation. *Note:* These tests should be obtained before anticoagulation is started.
    - *Vasculitis workup:* antinuclear antibody (ANA), rheumatoid factor (RF), rapid plasma reagin (RPR), hepatitis virus serologies, erythrocyte sedimentation rate (ESR), serum protein electrophoresis (SPEP), cryoglobulins, and herpes simplex virus (HSV) serologies.
    - *Coagulation profile* to rule out disseminated intravascular coagulation (DIC).
    - *Beta-human chorionic gonadotropin (β-hCG)* testing to rule out pregnancy in young women with stroke.

Refer to Chapter 24 for further discussion of specific ischemic stroke syndromes, evaluation of TIAs, and the secondary prevention of ischemic stroke.

■ MANAGEMENT II: GENERAL CARE

Much of the morbidity and mortality associated with stroke is related to nonneurologic complications, which can be minimized by adherence to these guidelines:

1. **Fever**

    Fever exacerbates ischemic brain injury and should be treated aggressively with antipyretics (acetaminophen) or a cooling blanket, if necessary.

2. **Nutrition**

    Stroke patients are at high risk for aspiration. Patients with depressed level of consciousness, brain stem strokes, bilateral strokes, and large hemispheric strokes carry the highest risk. Formal assessment of swallowing ability by a speech pathologist should be completed before patients at risk are fed. Start enteral feeding via a nasoduodenal tube within 24 hours after the stroke if the patient cannot swallow safely.

3. **Intravenous hydration**

    Hypovolemia is common among stroke patients and should be corrected with isotonic crystalloid. Avoiding volume depletion may be particularly important in patients with intracardiac thrombi (dehydration has been linked to progressive thrombus formation) or hemodynamic stroke. Hypotonic fluids (e.g., D5W and 0.45% saline) can aggravate cerebral edema and should be avoided.

4. **Glucose**

    Hyperglycemia and hypoglycemia can lead to exacerbation of ischemic injury. Although the clinical relevance of these effects in humans is unclear, it seems prudent to prevent hyperglycemia (glucose level higher than 240 mg/dl) by avoiding administration of IV dextrose solutions and by treating with insulin, if needed.

5. **Pulmonary care**

    Chest physical therapy (every 4 hours) should be ordered to prevent atelectasis in immobilized patients.

6. **Activity**

    Patients with stroke should be mobilized and engaged in physical therapy as soon as possible. For immobilized patients, order patient turning every 2 hours (to prevent pressure sores) and joint range-of-motion exercises four times a day to prevent contractures. Heel splints to maintain the ankle in dorsiflexion can also prevent shortening of the Achilles tendon. Have the patient taken out of bed to a chair every day as soon as feasible.

7. **Prophylaxis for deep vein thrombosis (DVT)**

    Ischemic stroke patients with significant immobility who are not on IV heparin should be treated with **heparin 5000 U every 12 hours** to prevent formation of DVT. This treatment can be started safely in patients with ICH after 48 hours.

8. **Bladder care**

    Indwelling urinary catheters should be used judiciously; order intermittent catheterization every 6 hours when possible.

chapter 7

Spinal Cord Compression

Spinal cord compression is one of the few true neurologic emergencies. The more severe the syndrome, the more acute the injury is likely to have been. Unlike the brain, which may have remarkable functional recovery, the spinal cord, once damaged, rarely recovers function. Patients with cord compression resulting from neoplastic disease of the spine who cannot walk before the onset of treatment will rarely walk again. Diagnosis of spinal cord injury depends on a clear understanding of the anatomy of the cord and the supportive structures.

■ PHONE CALL

This chapter will be most useful for patients in whom spinal cord compression is known or suspected. The response to such a call should focus on establishing the diagnosis and assessing the acuteness of the injury.

Questions

1. What is the patient's general condition?
2. What are the vital signs? Is the patient in any respiratory distress?
3. Does the patient have back pain?
4. Is there history of trauma to the neck or back?
5. Does the patient have any known cancer or infection?
    Back pain in a cancer patient is considered to result from a vertebral metastasis until it is proved otherwise.
6. How long has the problem been going on?

Orders

If trauma or an unstable spine is suspected, give the following orders:
1. **Immobilize the neck (back).**
    A Philadelphia collar or a backboard should be used to ensure adequate stability (Fig. 7–1). If such equipment is unavailable immediately, the cervical spine can be immobilized by holding the head firmly in a neutral position, using both hands.
2. **Check vital signs.**
    Injury above the C5 level may compromise respiratory

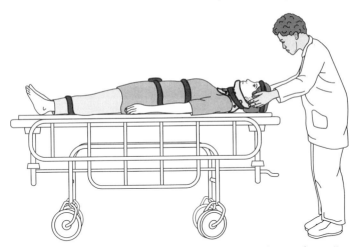

Figure 7-1 □ Stabilizing the neck and back with a Philadelphia collar and a backboard.

function. Cervical spinal injury, particularly with complete transection, may result in loss of sympathetic control, causing hypotension and bradycardia. Fever may point to an infectious process.

3. **Obtain plain x-rays of the neck (back) (anteroposterior and lateral).**

   Flexion and extension views, if done carefully by an experienced staff, may be helpful. Even if there is no suspicion of trauma, the pattern of bony abnormality may suggest subluxation, unsuspected pathologic fracture from neoplasm, osteomyelitis, or other infection. In most circumstances, plain x-rays can provide quick information that can then be followed up by computed tomography (CT) or magnetic resonance imaging (MRI) once an initial assessment is done.

4. **Notify the neurosurgical team or specialized spinal unit, if available.**

   Direct trauma to the spinal cord can produce a myelopathy, but it is the secondary effects from bleeding, dislocation, or osseous or articular instability that can be devastating; these secondary effects are preventable if properly identified and addressed.

Inform RN

"Will arrive at the bedside in . . . minutes."

Spinal cord compression is a medical emergency. Delay may cause irreversible neurologic dysfunction.

■ ELEVATOR THOUGHTS

What is the differential diagnosis of spinal cord compression?
Physical examination and often radiographic evaluation are needed to confirm a compressive myelopathy. You should be thinking first of the three categories of disease that are the most likely to cause spinal cord compression: trauma, infection, and neoplasm. Four other categories complete the differential diagnosis list.

1. **Trauma**

    Trauma is the most acute form of spinal cord compression. A history of a motor vehicle accident or sports-related accident is commonly elicited. Flexion, extension, compression, or rotation injuries in addition to direct blunt or penetrating trauma may produce a compressive myelopathy. Cervical disks tend to herniate centrally, producing an anterior cord syndrome.

2. **Infection**

    Infections of the spine most often occur in the thoracic or lumbar spine. Infections can take the following forms:
    - Epidural abscesses. Seen commonly in intravenous (IV) drug users, these are most often bacterial (e.g., *Staphylococcus aureus, Escherichia coli*).
    - Spinal tuberculosis (Pott's disease). This occurs in debilitated or immunocompromised patients or in those known to have pulmonary tuberculosis.
    - Vertebral osteomyelitis. *Staphylococcus* species, *Streptococcus* species, *E. coli,* or *Brucella* species may cause pathologic fractures or produce epidural abscesses.

3. **Neoplasm**

    Metastases are the most common neoplasm seen in bony disease of the spine (Fig. 7–2). The thoracic spine is most often affected because of venous drainage of visceral organs through spinal extradural venous plexuses. Meningiomas may appear as extradural tumors, with a predominance in the thoracic region. The female/male ratio is 9:1. Neurofibromas or schwannomas may arise on spinal roots and cause cord compression as they expand. Ependymomas are intrinsic cord tumors that could mimic extra-axial compressive lesions.

4. **Degenerative disease**

    Cervical disks herniate centrally, in contrast to lumbar disks, which herniate laterally and cause radicular symptoms. Thoracic disk protrusions are rare. An acute cauda equina syndrome may be produced by herniation at L1–L2.

5. **Congenital disease**

    Arnold-Chiari malformation, with or without syringomyelia, may produce cervical myelopathy. Congenital defects

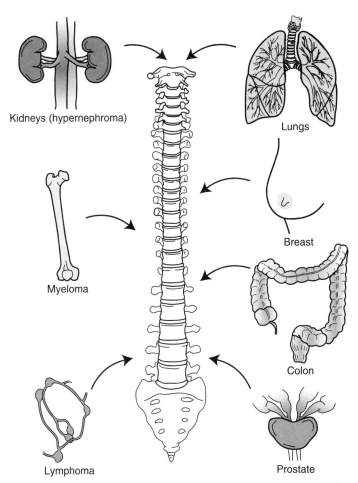

Figure 7–2 □ Neoplasms that commonly metastasize to or involve the spine: carcinoma of the lung, breast, colon, and prostate; hypernephroma; myeloma; and lymphoma.

of the atlantoaxial joint may predispose to subluxation or dislocation. A tethered cord produces a spastic diplegia of the legs. Relatively minor trauma may bring an occult malformation to clinical prominence.

6. **Inflammatory disease**

    Rheumatoid arthritis is the most common disease affecting the stability of the upper cervical spine and may allow atlantoaxial translocations.

7. Vascular disease

Epidural and subdural hematomas of the spine are very rare. They may be seen in patients taking anticoagulant medication. Arteriovenous malformations of the spine are rare.

■ MAJOR THREAT TO LIFE

- **Respiratory compromise** (cervical lesions) may require immediate intubation. Diaphragm weakness may result in hypoventilation and respiratory acidosis.
- **Autonomic dysregulation may produce hypotension** that does not respond to volume challenge. This phenomenon may be part of spinal shock. The hypotension may respond to pressors (e.g., dopamine).

■ BEDSIDE

Quick Look Test

What is the general condition of the patient?
Respiratory distress may necessitate immediate intubation. Look for retraction of the supraclavicular muscles as a sign of accessory respiratory muscle use because of diaphragmatic weakness.

Does the patient look cachectic or ill, suggesting cancer or general debilitation?

Is there urinary or bowel incontinence, suggesting sacral cord involvement?

Is there flushing or diaphoresis, suggesting autonomic dysregulation?

Management

If, after a quick look, the patient appears unstable, notify the surgical team, the anesthesiology service, and/or the neurosurgery service and address cardiopulmonary dysfunction. Stability of the neck should be ensured.

1. **Anti-inflammatory treatment**
   a. **Trauma**
      For **acute traumatic spinal cord injury,** the following protocol for methylprednisolone administration should be initiated:
      (1) **Methylprednisolone 30 mg/kg IV bolus over 15 minutes**

(2) 45-minute pause
(3) **Methylprednisolone 5.4 mg/kg/hr continuous IV infusion over the next 23 hours**
b. **Tumor**
For known or suspected **spinal neoplasm,** administer **dexamethasone 100 mg IV bolus** immediately.
2. **Blood tests**
In any patient with suspected spinal cord compression, routine blood tests should be performed in preparation for possible surgical decompression: complete blood cell count (CBC), chemistry panel, coagulation profile, and blood type and hold.
3. **Imaging**
If the patient is hemodynamically stable and not in respiratory distress, notify the appropriate radiologic personnel. Your patient will require an MRI scan as soon as your examination can provide anatomic localization and a working differential diagnosis. Myelography in combination with CT has nearly uniformly been replaced by MRI. CT may be superior to MRI only in spinal trauma to define subtle bony abnormalities or fractures.

Selective Physical Examination

Do not move the patient with a suspected spine injury until adequate immobilization of the neck or back has been ensured (e.g., with a Philadelphia collar).

The anatomy of the white matter tracts and cell groups in the spinal cord is consistent from patient to patient. Precise localization of the involved level and structure of the cord will, therefore, provide valuable early information about the likely pathogenesis of the injury. An anterior cord syndrome localized to the cervical region, for example, suggests cervical disk herniation. A posterior cord syndrome at the thoracic level suggests bony metastasis. Figure 7–3 shows a representative cross section of the spinal cord. Table 7–1 outlines the features of the main spinal cord syndromes. Note that at each level, lower motor neuron signs result from cell groups exiting the cord at that level, and upper motor neuron signs are present below the level of injury.

General Physical Examination

Vital signs	Evaluate as described earlier; look for any signs of autonomic instability.
HEENT	Trauma to the neck should be suspected when there is trauma to the face and body. Battle's sign (ecchymosis over the mastoid process), raccoon sign (periorbital ecchymosis), hemotympanum, and

Patient-Related Problems: The Common Calls

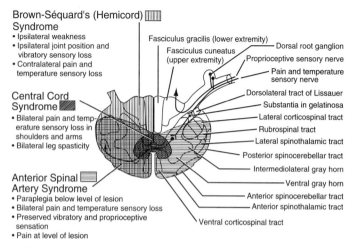

Brown-Séquard's (Hemicord) Syndrome
- Ipsilateral weakness
- Ipsilateral joint position and vibratory sensory loss
- Contralateral pain and temperature sensory loss

Central Cord Syndrome
- Bilateral pain and temperature sensory loss in shoulders and arms
- Bilateral leg spasticity

Anterior Spinal Artery Syndrome
- Paraplegia below level of lesion
- Bilateral pain and temperature sensory loss
- Preserved vibratory and proprioceptive sensation
- Pain at level of lesion

Labels: Fasciculus gracilis (lower extremity); Fasciculus cuneatus (upper extremity); Dorsal root ganglion; Proprioceptive sensory nerve; Pain and temperature sensory nerve; Dorsolateral tract of Lissauer; Substantia in gelatinosa; Lateral corticospinal tract; Rubrospinal tract; Lateral spinothalamic tract; Posterior spinocerebellar tract; Intermediolateral gray horn; Ventral gray horn; Anterior spinocerebellar tract; Anterior spinothalamic tract; Ventral corticospinal tract

Figure 7–3 □ Cross section of the spinal cord at the cervical level.

	cerebrospinal fluid (CSF) otorrhea suggest basilar skull fracture.
Spine	Percuss the spine with a fist or lightly with a tendon hammer. Tenderness to percussion suggests bony disease and will help localize the lesion for the rest of the examination and for a focal radiographic evaluation. Remember that the spinal cord comes down only to L1 in adults, unless there is a tethered cord. Tenderness in the lower lumbar or sacral spine may cause radicular symptoms but does not suggest cord compression.
Musculo-skeletal	Look for signs of rheumatoid arthritis, which can be associated with atlanto-occipital dislocation.

Neurologic Examination

- **Motor**

  Test strength in the legs and the arms. Symmetric loss of lower extremity power with preserved strength in the arms may be the first clue to thoracic cord involvement. If there is bilateral weakness in both the arms and the legs, suggesting cervical involvement, there should be upper motor neuron signs in the legs. Note that if the spinal injury is acute, muscle tone may be decreased below the level of the injury.

Table 7-1 □ MAJOR SPINAL CORD SYNDROMES

Syndrome	Common Causes	Features
Hemicord syndrome (Brown-Séquard's paralysis)	Penetrating injury Extrinsic compression	Contralateral spinothalamic loss Ipsilateral paresis Ipsilateral dorsal column loss Preserved light touch *Note:* deficits appear 1 to 2 levels below injury
Anterior cord syndrome	Anterior spinal artery infarct "Watershed" (T4–T6) ischemia Acute cervical disk herniation	Bilateral spinothalamic loss Preserved dorsal column sensation Upper motor neuron paralysis below lesion Lower motor neuron paralysis at lesion Sphincter dysfunction
Central cord syndrome	Syringomyelia Hypotensive spinal cord ischemia Spinal trauma (flexion-extension injury) Spinal cord neoplasm	Lower motor neuron weakness in arms Variable leg weakness and spasticity Severe pain and hyperpathia Spinothalamic loss in arms Sphincter dysfunction or urinary retention
Posterior cord syndrome	Trauma Posterior spinal artery infarct	Dorsal column sensory loss Pain and paresthesias in neck, back, or trunk Mild paresis

- **Sensory**

    Look for a sensory level. Bilateral weakness with a concordant sensory level is pathognomonic for spinal cord injury. Vibratory sense may be the first to go, particularly with a posterior cord syndrome, but the pinprick test (with a previously unused safety pin) is the most precise and reproducible. Remember, pain and temperature sensory neurons entering the cord ascend ipsilaterally for two to three spinal segments in the dorsolateral tract of Lissauer before crossing just anterior to the central canal to join the contralateral spinothalamic tract located in the lateral cord. Therefore, loss of pinprick or temperature sensation at a given level may indicate pathology two to three segments above the level detected on examination. A dermatome chart can be found in Appendix A–5.

    Perineal sensory loss (saddle anesthesia) suggests injury to the conus medullaris. Patchy sensory loss in the lower extremities with radicular-type pain and bilateral weakness may suggest involvement of the cauda equina, rather than of the spinal cord.

    Mark the borders of a sensory disturbance with a pen for comparison with future examinations.

- **Reflexes**

    Hyporeflexia is often present at the level of the spinal cord injury, with hyperreflexia below the level of injury. If the injury is acute, the only upper motor neuron sign may be a Babinski sign. Loss of the "anal wink" (contraction of the anal sphincter in response to pinprick in the perineum) indicates possible conus medullaris involvement.

- **Cranial nerves and mental status examination**

    These may be done briefly to rule out involvement of central nervous system (CNS) structures above the spinal cord. A perisagittal mass lesion, such as a falx meningioma or a CNS lymphoma, may produce bilateral leg weakness and urinary incontinence, mimicking a thoracic cord lesion. Other mental status signs, such as personality change, lethargy, or disinhibition, may be a clue to CNS pathology. Lower brain stem signs may accompany high cervical cord injury, particularly if there is a congenital deformity of the brain or atlantoaxial joint.

Selective History and Chart Review

1. *Reassess the timing, duration, and course of the symptoms.*

    Development over minutes to hours suggests trauma or infarction. Progression over hours to days suggests an infectious etiology. An epidural abscess may be present even in the absence of fever or an elevated white blood cell count.

Development of weakness or sensory loss over days to weeks suggests a neoplasm.
2. *Review the presence and character of pain.*
   Radicular pain will help localize and confirm extramedullary spinal involvement. Abrupt onset of radicular or diffuse pain, flaccid weakness, sphincter dysfunction, and a thoracic sensory level suggest spinal cord infarction. Bilateral radicular pain in an unusual distribution (e.g., L2 or L3) may indicate a cauda equina syndrome. Rectal pain may be the first sign of a conus medullaris lesion.
3. *Review the chart for history of illicit drug use* (this predisposes to epidural abscess and osteomyelitis), tuberculosis, or cancer.
4. *Check recent laboratory values* to assess for possible infection or chronic disease.

Surgical Intervention

Fractures, subluxations, and dislocations require reduction into normal alignment. Cervical traction may succeed in reducing a displacement, but it should be performed only by experienced personnel, usually under radiographic guidance. Open reductions may be required for more complex fractures or dislocations.

Neurosurgical decompressive laminectomy is the operation of choice for epidural abscess. Investigations should proceed without delay when an epidural abscess is suspected to avoid its progression to irreversible spinal cord injury. Patients who are paraplegic at the start of the operation rarely regain function. For pyogenic osteomyelitis, direct ventral spinal canal decompression is often necessary. A second, reconstructive operation may be required after the infection is brought under control with appropriate antibiotics. Decompressive laminectomy may also be needed for acute myelopathy or cauda equina syndrome resulting from disk herniation in the lumbar region. An anterior approach may be necessary to remove a herniated cervical disk. Finally, in the rare case of epidural or subdural hematoma, decompressive laminectomy is again the treatment of choice.

For **neoplastic spinal cord compression,** the first step after administration of high-dose steroids and accurate localization by examination and MRI is surgical decompression. Once the pressure has been relieved, further treatment usually requires tissue biopsy. Many tumors may be radiosensitive, but most radiotherapy units require a definite tissue diagnosis. If the surgeons have performed a decompression procedure, open biopsy may be possible. An alternative procedure is CT-guided needle biopsy.

chapter 8 | Delirium

The term *delirium* is synonymous with the term *acute confusional state*. Delirium is common in hospitalized patients, particularly in the elderly, and refers to an acute, global disorder of thinking and perception, characterized by impaired consciousness and inattention. Restlessness, agitation, and combativeness may be seen, as well as bizarre behavior and delusions. A call to evaluate delirium may therefore be one for "agitation" or "confusion." Delirium may be distinguished from dementia by the fact that with dementia alone, the sensorium remains clear, despite the occurrence of confusion and disorientation. Furthermore, it should be emphasized that although delirium is often defined as a transient condition, it may take days to weeks to clear, and if delirium is left untreated, the mortality rate may be as high as 25% in elderly inpatients. As with other mental status alterations discussed in this book, delirium is a symptom, not a disease. Successful management depends on accurate diagnosis of the underlying condition.

■ PHONE CALL

Questions

1. **Is the patient fully awake and alert? In what way is the patient confused? When did the change occur?**
   Clarify the acuteness and nature of the mental status change. It is important to distinguish between acute and chronic changes and also to distinguish delirium from dementia (see Chapter 18) and stupor (see Chapter 5).
2. **What are the vital signs?**
   Fever suggests infection; tachypnea may suggest hypoxia, metabolic acidosis, or hyperglycemia (Kussmaul's respiration); and irregular heart rhythm may suggest cardioembolic stroke.
3. **Was there any head injury?**
4. **What is the patient's underlying medical condition?**
   Diseases that are likely to cause metabolic disarray, such as renal or liver disease, endocrinopathies, diarrheal illnesses, or malignancy, may alter electrolytes. Human immunodeficiency virus (HIV) infection or acquired immune deficiency syndrome (AIDS) opens a wider array of differential diagnoses.

5. **Is the patient diabetic?**
   Both hypoglycemia and hyperglycemia can cause altered mental status.
6. **Is the patient known to be a user of alcohol, nicotine, or other nonprescription drugs?**

Orders

1. Order a finger stick glucose level.
2. If the patient is tachypneic or drowsy, obtain arterial blood gas measurements. A pulse oximeter may be useful for monitoring oxygen saturation.
3. Provide orientation and reassurance to the patient. Make sure the room is well lit. The treatment of the behavioral and emotional manifestations of delirium, to the extent possible, will make the subsequent etiologic evaluation easier.
4. Restrain the patient with a Posey chest restraint if necessary. Significant agitation or combativeness may put the patient or those nearby at risk for physical injury.
5. If possible, do not medicate. Perform the evaluation first. If sedation is given before a good neurologic examination can be obtained, the opportunity for making a diagnosis may be lost.

Inform RN

"Will arrive at the bedside in . . . minutes."

■ ELEVATOR THOUGHTS

What are the causes of delirium?
V (vascular): stroke (infarct or hemorrhage causing a sensory aphasia), subarachnoid hemorrhage, hypertensive encephalopathy, cholesterol emboli syndrome
I (infectious): herpes simplex encephalitis or other viral encephalitis; bacterial, fungal, or rickettsial meningoencephalitis; neurosyphilis; Lyme disease; parasitic abscess (e.g., toxoplasmosis, cysticercosis), bacterial abscess; HIV encephalitis; systemic infection such as urosepsis or pneumonia
T (traumatic): open or closed head trauma, acute or chronic subdural hematoma
A (autoimmune): systemic lupus erythematosus (SLE), multiple sclerosis
M (metabolic/toxic): hypoglycemia or hyperglycemia, hyponatremia, hypercalcemia, hepatic encephalopathy, uremia, porphyria; drug or alcohol ingestion or withdrawal
I (iatrogenic): drug toxicity (particularly in the elderly)—psy-

chotropic drugs, steroids, digoxin, cimetidine, anticonvulsants, anticholinergics, dopaminergics (see Table 8–1 for common medications with central nervous system [CNS] side effects); rare—heavy metal poisoning, pellagra, vitamin B_{12} or folate deficiency, Wilson's disease

N (neoplastic): primary brain tumor, metastatic brain disease, paraneoplastic syndrome (limbic encephalitis with small-cell lung cancer)

S (seizure): postictal state, nonconvulsive status epilepticus (rare)

Other (psychiatric): bipolar disorder/mania, psychosis

■ MAJOR THREAT TO LIFE

- **Expanding mass lesion with impending herniation**
  Although it is rare for a mass lesion to progress to impending herniation without focal neurologic signs, the first changes may be confusion or altered state of consciousness. Progression can be rapid if there is an expanding subdural hematoma or edema from subarachnoid hemorrhage.
- **Bacterial meningitis or encephalitis**
  Bacterial meningitis is a major treatable illness that can be fatal if missed. Other meningitides are likely to be less fulminant yet can also be fatal if left untreated. Herpes simplex encephalitis is the most common sporadic encephalitis. Aside from direct brain damage from infection, encephalitides can produce edema and subsequent herniation.
- **Delirium tremens**
  Usually occurring more than 48 hours after cessation of alcohol consumption, the autonomic instability of delirium tremens may produce high fevers, tachycardia, and severe fluctuations in blood pressure (Fig. 8–1). Mortality rate is about 15%.

■ BEDSIDE

Quick Look Test

Does the patient look ill or well?

Is the patient in respiratory distress?

What are the vital signs?
If there is a fever, meningitis must be ruled out. An irregular heart rhythm may suggest atrial fibrillation. Markedly elevated blood pressure, particularly diastolic blood pressure greater than 120 mm Hg, may produce hypertensive encephalopathy,

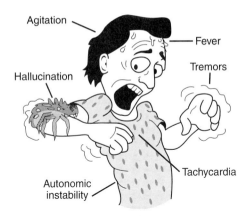

Figure 8–1 □ Delirium tremens.

which is characterized by headache, confusion, and irritability, with lethargy developing over hours to days.

Selective Physical Examination I

General Physical Examination

Breath	• The odor of alcohol or fetor hepaticus may suggest the etiology.
HEENT	• Look for external signs of head trauma—scalp lacerations or bruises, Battle's sign, raccoon eyes, papilledema.
Neck	• Nuchal rigidity, Kernig's sign, Brudzinski's sign
Cardiopulmonary	• Tachypnea can indicate hypoxia or metabolic acidosis. Rales or decreased breath sounds may help diagnose a pneumonia. Listen for irregular heart rhythm and for murmurs to suggest valvular heart disease.
Abdomen	• Percuss the liver. Hepatomegaly may be the physical manifestation of hepatic encephalopathy or may direct your management to consideration of alcohol withdrawal. Look for ascites.
Extremities	• Look for clubbing as a sign of chronic pulmonary disease, peripheral edema as a sign of cardiac or renal failure, and splinter hemorrhages as a sign of

emboli. **Asterixis** is a sign of metabolic disarray, for example, from renal or hepatic failure.

Neurologic Examination
- **Mental status**
  1. Assess the patient's **alertness:** Is the patient fully awake and alert? Assess the patient's **attentiveness**. Does the patient maintain eye contact? Does he or she glance about the room as if having hallucinations? One simple test of sustained attention is to ask the patient to recite the days of the week backward or to count backward from 20 to 1.
  2. Listen for **paraphasias** in spontaneous speech to suggest a sensory aphasia. Test **comprehension**. Ask the patient to follow progressively complex commands (e.g., "Show two fingers," "Point to the ceiling and then to the floor," and "Tap each shoulder twice with your eyes closed").
  3. Assess **thought content**. Tangential or pressured speech, delusions, flight of ideas, hallucinations, perceptual illusions, and disorientation may be seen with psychiatric disease or acute encephalopathies.
- **Cranial nerves**
  1. **Pupils.** Pinpoint pupils may result from opiate overdose. Widely dilated pupils could be a sign of cholinergic overdose (e.g., organophosphate poisoning). Asymmetric pupils can indicate uncal herniation from intracranial mass effect. Argyll Robertson pupils are seen with CNS syphilis (periaqueductal midbrain lesion [see Chapter 22]).
  2. **Facial asymmetry** in the form of a flattened nasolabial fold or a wider palpebral fissure may be a subtle sign of an intraparenchymal mass or stroke.
  3. Assess swallowing capacity and gag reflex.
- **Motor**

  Depending on how cooperative your patient is, you may be able to test strength by confrontation. In an inattentive patient, observe limb movements for asymmetry. Lateralizing weakness suggests an intracranial lesion. Tremor may indicate alcohol withdrawal or intoxication.
- **Sensory**

  A detailed sensory examination requires sustained cooperation that an inattentive patient often cannot give. Response to a brief noxious stimulus (e.g., a pinch or pulling hair on the arm) is a quick way to assess gross sensory function. If the limb is paretic, the response may be a facial grimace.
- **Gait**

  Ataxia may suggest intoxication.

- Reflexes
  Babinski's response or reflex asymmetry suggests lateralized intracranial pathology.

Selective History and Chart Review

1. **Review medications**
   Have any new medications been started recently? Particularly in the elderly, drug toxicity is a common cause of change in mental status. Table 8–1 lists common medications that can cause delirium.
2. **Review medical or psychiatric history**
   Known metabolic disorders such as renal or hepatic disease or past episodes of psychosis would be crucial to make a diagnosis.

Table 8–1 □ COMMON MEDICATIONS THAT CAN CAUSE DELIRIUM

Anticholinergics
  Trihexyphenidyl HCl (Artane)
  Benztropine mesylate (Cogentin)
Anticonvulsants
  Phenytoin (Dilantin)
  Phenobarbital
  Valproic acid (Depakene/Depakote)
Antihistamines
  Diphenhydramine (Benadryl)
  Dextromethorphan hydrobromide + promethazine (Phenergan)
  Cimetidine (Tagamet)
Benzodiazepines
  Diazepam (Valium)
  Temazepam (Restoril)
  Triazolam (Halcion)
Corticosteroids
  Prednisone
  Dexamethasone (Decadron)
Dopaminergic drugs
  L-dopa (Sinemet)
  Pergolide (Permax)
  Bromocriptine (Parlodel)
Digoxin
Disulfiram
Indomethacin
Lithium
Opiates

■ MANAGEMENT I: CONTROL OF DELIRIUM

1. **Treatment of agitation**

   Treatment of delirium depends on the correct identification of the underlying condition. If agitation or combativeness is likely to interfere with the investigation or if there is physical threat to the patient or to the staff, the best medications to use are butyrophenones (e.g., haloperidol [Haldol]), group 3 phenothiazines (e.g., trifluoperazine), or benzodiazepines. See Table 8–2 for drugs used to control agitation and delirium. **Haldol 2 to 10 mg intramuscularly (IM)** may be expected to reach peak serum levels in 20 to 40 minutes. Repeating the dose up to 20 mg may be necessary in severe cases. For mild agitation or in the elderly, an initial dose of 1 to 2 mg may be sufficient. For moderate agitation, use 4 mg initially. For violent, combative patients, 6 to 10 mg can be used as an initial dose. If an acute dystonic reaction occurs with Haldol, **diphenhydramine 25 to 50 mg IM** may be given, even though the anticholinergic effect may worsen the delirium. Haloperidol should be avoided in alcohol withdrawal, benzodiazepine withdrawal, and hepatic encephalopathy. For acute agitation in these settings, a benzodiazepine such as **lorazepam 1 to 2 mg IM** may be given. (Higher doses may be required if tolerance has developed in the setting of chronic alcohol or benzodiazepine abuse.) **Naloxone (Narcan) 1 to 2 ampules, given intravenously (IV), IM, or subcutaneously (SC) every 5 minutes**, should be reserved for the lethargy of suspected opiate intoxication.

2. **The following blood tests should be ordered immediately:**

Table 8–2 □ DRUGS USED IN THE TREATMENT OF ACUTE AGITATION AND DELIRIUM

Drug	Starting Dose
Antipsychotics	
Haloperidol (Haldol)	0.5–5 mg PO/IM
Risperidone (Risperdal)	1–2 mg PO
Clozapine (Clozaril)	25 mg PO
Olanzapine (Zyprexa)	5–10 mg PO
Trifluoperazine (Stelazine)	1–2 mg IM; 2–5 mg PO
Benzodiazepines	
Lorazepam (Ativan)	0.5–2 mg IV/IM/PO
Alprazolam (Xanax)	0.25–0.5 mg PO
Diazepam (Valium)	2.5–5 mg IV; 2–10 mg PO

- Complete blood cell count (CBC) with differential
- Electrolyte panel, including stat glucose
- Full chemistry panel, including liver function tests
- Urine toxicology screen (if drug intoxication is suspected)
- Urine and blood cultures (if fever is present)
- Arterial blood gases
- Calcium, phosphate
- Erythrocyte sedimentation rate may be measured, but its specificity is low.

3. A chest x-ray should be obtained if fever or dyspnea is present.

■ MANAGEMENT II: TREATMENT OF LIFE-THREATENING DISORDERS

1. **Bacterial meningitis**

    Delirium with fever should be treated as bacterial meningitis until proved otherwise. As a rule, a head computed tomography (CT) scan should be ordered before a lumbar puncture is performed. If there is no papilledema on examination, no coagulopathy, and no focal deficit (including gait ataxia), and a head CT is not readily available, a lumbar puncture may almost always be done without risk of herniation. (See Chapter 3 for a discussion of lumbar puncture.) Cerebrospinal fluid (CSF) should be sent for cell count, protein and glucose determinations, microbial cultures (bacterial, fungal, mycobacterial), and Venereal Disease Research Laboratory (VDRL) test, and for Gram, acid-fast bacillus, and India ink stains. CSF findings in bacterial meningitis are cloudy fluid with 50 to 20,000 white blood cells, predominantly leukocytes, elevated protein level, and decreased glucose level (see Table 22–1). The causative organism may be identified and antibiotic sensitivity may be obtained in more than 80% of the cases. Empirical treatment of bacterial meningitis prior to definitive identification in adults should be **ampicillin 1 g IV every 6 hours** and a third-generation cephalosporin (e.g., **ceftriaxone 2 g IV every 12 hours**). See Chapter 22 for details.

2. **Delirium tremens**

    The autonomic instability of delirium tremens is treated supportively, with acetaminophen (Tylenol) or a cooling blanket for fevers. Continuous cardiac monitoring may be necessary if arrhythmias develop. **Valium 5 to 10 mg IV load**, with **subsequent doses of 2 to 5 mg IV every 30 to 60 minutes**, should be used. Sedation should be titrated to minimize agitation. Tremulousness may be used as a clinical monitor of the effectiveness of the benzodiazepine. An alternative is **chlordiazepoxide (Librium) 25 to 100 mg every 6 hours by mouth (PO)**. The dose should be tapered as the symptoms subside. **Thiamine 100 mg IV, IM, or PO** should be given daily for 3 days to prevent the development of Wernicke's encephalopathy.

3. **Suspected mass lesion**
   If there is papilledema or a focality on examination, an emergent head CT or magnetic resonance imaging (MRI) scan should be obtained. For mass lesions, refer to the appropriate chapter for treatment of acute stroke (Chapter 6), increased intracranial pressure (Chapter 12), or brain tumor (Chapter 23).

Selective History and Chart Review

Once it is clear that the patient does not have a mass lesion, bacterial meningitis, or delirium tremens, you have time to make a more complete assessment of the situation. If family members are available, try to sort out the acuteness of the change. A chronic or fluctuating course in an elderly person may suggest that the apparent delirium is really a component of dementia. Alzheimer's disease and vascular dementia are the most common causes (see Chapter 18). A subacute course over days, with intermittent fevers, suggests a subacute or chronic encephalomeningitis, such as herpes simplex encephalitis, tubercular meningitis, or cryptococcal meningitis.

Review the chart. What are the patient's medical conditions? What medications is he or she on? Were any medications recently added that are known to have CNS effects (see Table 8–1)? The offending agent should be stopped or substituted. Do the most recent laboratory values suggest metabolic abnormalities? Renal and hepatic failure are the most common sources of metabolic encephalopathy (Box 8–1). Is the patient HIV positive? Acute HIV infection may cause a meningoencephalitis. Immunocompromised patients are at risk for a variety of opportunistic infections that can cause encephalopathy, particularly cryptococcal and tuberculous meningitis, toxoplasmosis, and CNS syphilis. Malignancy, most notably small-cell lung carcinoma, can cause a paraneoplastic "limbic encephalitis," in addition to altering electrolytes with syndrome of inappropriate antidiuretic hormone (SIADH).

■ MANAGEMENT III: TREATMENT OF OTHER DISORDERS

1. **Hypoglycemia and hyperglycemia**
   Hypoglycemia may be rapidly corrected with a bolus of

> **Box 8–1. HEPATIC ENCEPHALOPATHY**
>
> Hepatic encephalopathy usually appears in a patient with liver function already compromised from alcoholic cirrhosis, chronic hepatitis, or malignancy. An increased protein load, such as from a gastrointestinal bleed, causes ammonia to accumulate in the brain. Whether the high level of ammonia itself or the increase in concentration of its metabolites produces the alterations in consciousness is not known. Examination may reveal abdominal ascites, an enlarged (or shrunken) liver, and asterixis, in addition to changes in mental status, namely inattention, disorientation, and confusion. In the later stages, focal signs such as hemiparesis or dysconjugate gaze may appear. Management is directed at reducing the protein load with dietary protein restrictions and **neomycin 2 to 4 g per day PO,** which reduces the population of ammonia-producing bacteria in the bowel. **Lactulose 15 to 45 ml two to four times per day** to induce diarrhea may also help reduce intestinal bacteria. Ammonia levels should be followed as an indication of the effectiveness of therapy. If acute agitation requires treatment, use benzodiazepines such as **diazepam 5 to 10 mg every 8 hours. Haloperidol should be avoided.** When hepatic encephalopathy is suspected, be sure to obtain a stool guaiac test and a hematocrit.

50 ml D50W IV by direct injection. Do not forget that **thiamine (100 mg PO or IM)** must be given first to prevent possible induction of Wernicke's encephalopathy. Maintenance with D5W may be necessary if the hypoglycemia is prolonged. Hyperglycemia (diabetic ketoacidosis) requires administration of insulin, repletion of intravascular volume, and often, management of acidosis and potassium. The level of monitoring required is best handled in an intensive care unit (ICU).

2. **Hyponatremia and hypernatremia**

    Management of hyponatremia and hypernatremia usually involves treating the underlying cause (e.g., renal disease, vomiting and diarrhea, hypothalamic or adrenal dysfunction, or SIADH from malignancy or medications). Treatment with IV fluids and electrolytes differs depending on volume status (see Table 21–3). Too rapid a correction of hyponatremia may precipitate central pontine myelinolysis, an acute demyelinating syndrome occurring mostly in patients with poor nutritional status, causing quadriplegia, dysarthria, and pseudobulbar palsy.

3. **Hypocalcemia**
   Severe hypocalcemia (<7.0 mg/dl) may be treated with **10 to 20 ml (1 to 2 g) of 10% calcium gluconate IV in 100 ml D5W over 30 minutes**. If the patient is hyperphosphatemic, correction with glucose and insulin is required before giving calcium IV. Patients on digoxin should have continuous cardiac monitoring, as calcium potentiates digoxin's action.
4. **Uremia with renal failure**
   Symptomatic uremia with renal failure causing delirium may necessitate urgent hemodialysis.
5. **Sepsis**
   Delirium caused by sepsis should clear spontaneously with appropriate treatment of the infection.
6. **Psychiatric causes**
   Psychiatric causes of delirium may generally be treated acutely with **haloperidol 1 to 5 mg PO or IM**. Psychiatric consultation should be obtained for definitive treatment.
7. **Seizures**
   Delirium from a **postictal state** should clear progressively over minutes to hours. An electroencephalogram (EEG) should be ordered within the next few days. **Nonconvulsive status epilepticus** is a neurologic emergency that requires EEG for definitive diagnosis. (See Chapter 4 for further discussion of seizure management.)
8. **Nicotine withdrawal**
   In rare instances, delirium can occur in heavy smokers due to nicotine withdrawal. Application of a **transdermal 21-mg nicotine patch** can result in dramatic improvement in some cases.

chapter 9 | Head Injury

The initial assessment of head injury in the emergency room (ER) can be frantic, with resuscitation measures, history taking, and examination occurring simultaneously. An organized approach is essential to ensure that vital components of the evaluation are not omitted. **The immediate goal is to judge the severity of the injury as minimal, moderate, or high.** This aspect of the injury can be quickly assessed at the time of arrival.

■ PHONE CALL

Questions

1. **What are the vital signs?**
   If the patient is in respiratory distress, the spine should be immobilized (this should have been done already) and nasotracheal intubation should be performed.
2. **What were the circumstances and the mode of injury?**
   The force and location of head impact should be determined as precisely as possible.
3. **Did the patient experience loss of consciousness?**
   Concussion refers to temporary loss of consciousness that occurs at the time of impact. Because patients are amnestic following concussion, only an eyewitness can accurately gauge the duration of loss of consciousness.
4. **Has the patient's neurologic status deteriorated since the time of impact?**
   Progressive decline in level of consciousness after an injury suggests an expanding *subdural or epidural hematoma.*
5. **What is the patient's level of consciousness now?**
   This should be assessed using the Glasgow Coma Scale (see Table 5–2).
6. **Has the patient recently ingested drugs or alcohol?**
   Intoxication can confound assessments of mental status and may lead to withdrawal symptoms.
7. **Is there significant extracranial trauma?**
   The patient should be quickly examined for external signs of trauma to the neck, chest, abdomen, and limbs.

Determination of the Severity of Injury

At this juncture, you should have enough information to classify the injury severity as **minimal, moderate,** or **high.** Subse-

quent diagnostic testing and management should proceed according to the algorithm in Figure 9–1.
1. **Minimal-risk group**
    - Glasgow Coma Scale score of 15 (alert, attentive, and oriented) and normal neurologic findings on examination
    - No concussion, or concussion in the absence of moderate-risk group criteria
2. **Moderate-risk group**
    - Glasgow Coma Scale score of 9 to 14 (confused, lethargic, or stuporous) or minor focal neurologic deficit (i.e., nystagmus, facial droop)
    - Concussion if age > 60 years, headache, or minor external signs of trauma are present
    - Posttraumatic amnesia
    - Vomiting
    - Seizure
    - Major external trauma (Battle's sign, raccoon eyes, etc.)
3. **High-risk group**
    - Glasgow Coma Scale score of 3 to 8 (comatose)
    - Progressive decline in level of consciousness
    - Major focal neurologic deficit (i.e., hemiparesis, aphasia)
    - Penetrating skull injury or palpably depressed skull fracture

Orders

1. For *all patients*, **order cervical spine radiographs (anteroposterior, lateral, and odontoid views).**
    All patients with traumatic injury above the level of the clavicles should have cervical spine films to rule out a fracture. Before a cervical collar can be removed, the cervical spine must be cleared completely from C1 to C7.
2. **For all patients with *moderate or severe injury*, give the following orders:**
    a. **Start an intravenous (IV) line with normal (0.9%) saline or lactated Ringer's solution.**
       Isotonic fluids replace intravascular volume more effectively than do hypotonic fluids, and they do not aggravate cerebral edema.
    b. **Order diagnostic blood tests.**
       (1) Spun hematocrit
       (2) Complete blood cell count (CBC) and platelet count
       (3) Serum chemistries (glucose, electrolytes, blood urea nitrogen [BUN], creatinine)
       (4) Prothrombin time (PT)/partial thromboplastin time (PTT)
       (5) Toxicology screen and serum alcohol level
       (6) Type and hold

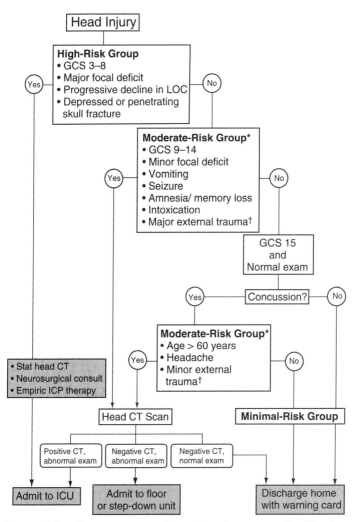

Figure 9–1 □ Emergency room diagnostic and treatment algorithm for head injury. (Refer to text for details.) CT, computed tomography; GCS, Glasgow Coma Scale score; ICP, intracranial pressure; ICU, intensive care unit; LOC, level of consciousness.
*One or more criteria may be present.
†Above the level of the clavicles.

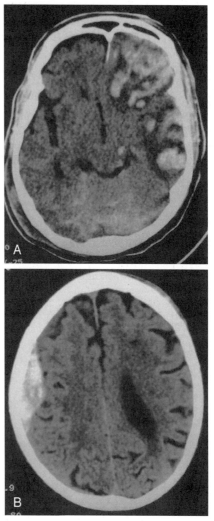

Figure 9–2 □ *A*, Left frontal and temporal cerebral contusions with surrounding edema. *B*, Small right parietal epidural hematoma *(convex shape)*.

c. **Obtain a head computed tomography (CT) scan with bone windows.**

Skull radiographs are not necessary if a head CT scan is performed, because CT is more sensitive for detecting fractures. Intracranial hemorrhage will be detected in approximately 90 to 100% of high-risk patients, 5 to 10% of

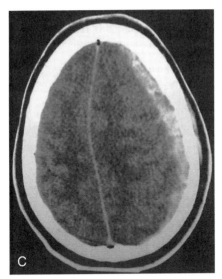

Figure 9-2 *Continued* □ C, Thin left subdural hematoma *(crescentic, convex shape)*. (Images courtesy of Dr. Robert De La Paz.)

moderate-risk patients, and 0% of minimal-risk patients. CT scans should be assessed for the following (Fig. 9-2):
  (1) Epidural and subdural hematoma
  (2) Subarachnoid and intraventricular blood
  (3) Parenchymal contusions and hemorrhages
  (4) Cerebral edema
  (5) Effacement of perimesencephalic cisterns
  (6) Midline shift
  (7) Skull fractures, sinus opacification (air-fluid levels), and pneumocephalus
3. **For *comatose patients* (Glasgow Coma Scale score ≤8) or in patients with signs of herniation, give the following orders:**
  a. **Elevate head of the bed 30 degrees.**
  b. **Hyperventilate the patient.**
    Intubate the patient. Use intermittent mandatory ventilation (IMV) at a rate of 16 to 20 cycles per minute with tidal volumes set at 10 to 15 ml/kg. Adjust settings to attain a P_{CO_2} of 28 to 32 mm Hg. Severe hypocapnia (<25 mm Hg) may lead to excessive vasoconstriction and cerebral ischemia and should be avoided.
  c. **Administer mannitol 20% 1.0 to 1.5 g/kg IV.**
    Mannitol should be given "wide open." The patient should be re-examined 30 minutes after mannitol is given

to assess for signs of improvement. Additional doses should be guided by an intracranial pressure (ICP) monitor (see Chapter 13).
d. **Insert a Foley catheter.**
e. **Obtain a neurosurgical consultation.**

■ ELEVATOR THOUGHTS

What are the most important sequelae of traumatic head injury?
1. **Concussion**
   Concussion refers to temporary loss of consciousness that occurs at the time of impact. It is usually associated with a short period of amnesia. The majority of patients with concussion have normal CT or magnetic resonance imaging (MRI) scans, reflecting the fact that concussion results from physiologic (rather than structural) injury to the brain. *Approximately 5% of patients who have sustained concussion will have an intracranial hemorrhage.*
2. **Epidural hematoma**
   Epidural bleeding usually results from a tear in the middle meningeal artery. Approximately 75% of such cases are associated with a skull fracture. The classic clinical course (seen in only one third of patients) proceeds from immediate loss of consciousness (concussion) to a lucid interval, which is followed by a secondary depression of consciousness as the epidural hematoma expands. Epidural blood takes on a bulging convex pattern on the CT scan (see Fig. 9–2) because the collection is limited by firm attachments of the dura to the cranial sutures. Progression to herniation and death can occur rapidly because the bleeding is from an artery.
3. **Subdural hematoma**
   Subdural bleeding usually arises from a venous source, with blood filling the potential space between the dural and arachnoid membranes. CT usually reveals a crescentic collection of blood across the entire hemispheric convexity (see Fig. 9–2). *Elderly and alcoholic patients are particularly prone to subdural bleeding;* in these patients, large hematomas can result from trivial impact or from acceleration/deceleration injuries (e.g., whiplash injury).
4. **Parenchymal contusion and hematoma**
   Cerebral contusions result from "scraping" and "bruising" of the brain as it moves across the inner surface of the skull. The inferior frontal and temporal lobes are the common sites of traumatic contusion (see Fig. 9–2). With lateral forces, contusions can occur just deep to the site of impact (coup lesions) or at the opposite pole as the brain impacts on

the inner table of the skull (contrecoup lesions). Contusions frequently evolve into larger lesions over 12 to 24 hours, and in rare instances, contusions can develop de novo 1 or more days after injury ("spät hematoma").
5. **Axonal shearing injury**
   Persistent coma occurs frequently in patients with severe head injury with normal CT scans and normal ICP. In these cases, coma results from widespread stretching, shearing, and disruption of axons as a result of rotational forces. Bilateral motor posturing, hyperreflexia, and dysautonomia are common and result from injury to the corticospinal tracts and autonomic centers in the brain stem. Diffuse axonal injury is thought to be the single most important cause of persistent disability in patients with traumatic brain damage.
6. **Skull fracture**
   Skull fractures are important markers of potentially serious intracranial injury, but they rarely cause symptoms themselves. If the scalp is lacerated over the fracture, it is considered an open, or compound, fracture. *Linear fractures* account for 80% of all skull fractures and can usually be managed conservatively. *Basilar skull fractures* occur with more serious trauma and are frequently missed on routine skull x-ray films. These fractures may be associated with cranial nerve injury or cerebrospinal fluid (CSF) leakage from the nose or ear. *Comminuted and depressed fractures* are often associated with contusions of the underlying brain and usually require surgical debridement.

■ MAJOR THREAT TO LIFE

- Epidural hematoma
- Subdural hematoma
- Increased ICP

■ BEDSIDE

Quick Look Test

What is the level of consciousness?
   Almost all patients with potentially life-threatening lesions will have depressed level of consciousness (lethargy, stupor, or coma).

Airway and Vital Signs

Is the airway protected? What is the respiratory rate?
   Indications for intubation include depressed level of con-

sciousness, respiratory distress (rapid, shallow breathing), or respiratory depression.

What is the heart rate and blood pressure?

If the patient is *hypotensive,* bleeding into the abdomen, thorax, retroperitoneal space, or tissues surrounding a long-bone fracture should be excluded. *Spinal shock* can occur with cord injury and results from acute loss of sympathetic outflow. *Hypertension* associated with a wide pulse pressure and bradycardia (Cushing's reflex) may reflect increased ICP.

Selective Physical Examination

General Physical Examination

Head	• The skull should be palpated for fractures, hematomas, and lacerations. *Battle's sign* (ecchymosis over the mastoid process) and *raccoon sign* (periorbital ecchymosis) suggest, but do not confirm, basilar skull fracture.
Ear, nose, and throat	• *CSF otorrhea* and *CSF rhinorrhea* result from skull fracture with disruption of the dura. CSF can be differentiated from mucus by its high glucose content on dipstick testing; bloody CSF can be differentiated from frank blood by a positive *halo test* (a "halo" of CSF forms around the blood when CSF is dropped on a cloth sheet). *Hemotympanum* is also highly suggestive of skull fracture. *Tongue biting* suggests an unwitnessed seizure.
Neck	• Do not manipulate the neck until a cervical fracture has been ruled out.
Chest, abdomen, back, pelvis, and extremities	• It is essential to rule out important coexisting injuries in patients with head injury. The patient should be thoroughly examined, and x-rays, diagnostic peritoneal lavage, and other interventions should be performed prior to CT scanning as clinically indicated.

Neurologic Examination

Rapid neurologic examination of the patient with head injury should focus on the following:

- **Mental status**
  1. **Level of consciousness**
     Level of consciousness is best documented by using the Glasgow Coma Scale (see Table 5–2) and by describing specific stimuli and responses (e.g., "answers with brief confused responses to repeated questioning" or "moans and vocalizes in response to sternal rub").
  2. **Attention and concentration**
     Ask the patient to count from 20 to 1 or recite the months in reverse.
  3. **Orientation**
     Check for orientation to time, place, and situation.
  4. **Memory**
     Document *retrograde amnesia* by asking the patient to recall the last thing he or she remembers prior to the injury. Check for *anterograde amnesia* by asking about the first thing remembered after the injury. Check recall for three objects at 5 minutes.
- **Cranial nerves**
  1. **Pupils**
  2. **Extraocular movements**
     Nystagmus may be found in alert patients with dizziness or vertigo following concussion. An *exodeviated eye with a large pupil* suggests CN 3 compression from uncal herniation.
  3. **Facial nerve**
     The facial nerve is the most commonly injured cranial nerve in patients with closed head injury.
- **Motor**
  1. **Spontaneous movements**
     Preferential movement of the limbs on one side indicates paresis of the unused limbs. If the patient is unresponsive, check for a lateralized localizing response to sternal rub.
  2. **Limb tone**
     Increased tone may reflect an early stage of decortication (flexor posturing) or decerebration (extensor posturing).
  3. **Arm (pronator) drift**
     If the patient is unable to follow commands, passively elevate both arms and check to see whether one falls preferentially.
  4. **Power**
     Check strength against active resistance at the shoulders, wrists, hips, and ankles.
  5. **Reflexes**
- **Gait**
  1. **Normal gait**
  2. **Tandem (heel-to-toe) gait**
     It is particularly important to check gait in patients with

"mild injury" who are treated and released without a CT scan.

■ MANAGEMENT

Minimal-Risk Group

Patients in this group (see Fig. 9–1) can generally be discharged from the ER **without a head CT scan** as long as the following criteria are met:
- Neurologic examination (especially mental status and gait) is normal.
- Cervical spine radiograph is cleared.
- A responsible person is available to observe the patient over 24 hours, with instructions to return the patient to the ER if late symptoms (listed on a head injury warning card) develop.

Moderate-Risk Group

In patients who have suffered concussion, normal findings on neurologic examination and CT scan eliminate the need for hospital admission. These patients can be discharged home for observation, even in the presence of headache, nausea, vomiting, dizziness, or amnesia, because the risk of development of a significant intracranial lesion thereafter is minimal. Criteria for hospital admission after head injury are shown in Box 9–1.

Severe Head Injury

Following initial assessment and stabilization, **the immediate consideration in the patient with severe head injury is whether there is an indication for emergent neurosurgical intervention.** If the decision is made to operate, surgery should proceed imme-

---

Box 9–1. CRITERIA FOR HOSPITAL ADMISSION FOLLOWING HEAD INJURY

- Intracranial blood or fracture identified on head CT scan
- Confusion, agitation, or depressed level of consciousness
- Focal neurologic signs or symptoms
- Alcohol or drug intoxication
- Significant comorbid medical illness
- Lack of a reliable environment for subsequent observation

diately, because delays can only increase the likelihood of further brain damage during the waiting period.

The medical management of patients with severe injury should be carried out in an intensive care unit (ICU). Although little can be done about brain damage that occurs on impact, ICU care can play a major role in reducing secondary brain injury from hypoxia, hypotension, or increased ICP.

Checklist for Management of Severe Head Injury in the Intensive Care Unit

1. **Reassess airway and ventilation**
    In general, patients in stupor or coma (those unable to follow commands because of a depressed level of consciousness) should be intubated for airway protection. If there is no evidence of increased ICP, ventilatory parameters should be set to maintain P_{CO_2} at 40 mm Hg and P_{O_2} at 90 to 100 mm Hg.

2. **Monitor blood pressure (BP)**
    If the patient shows signs of hemodynamic instability (hypo- or hypertension), monitoring is best accomplished with an arterial catheter. Because autoregulation is frequently impaired with acute head injury, mean BP must be carefully maintained to avoid hypotension (mean BP $<$ 70 mm Hg), which can lead to cerebral ischemia, or hypertension (mean BP $>$ 130 mm Hg), which can exacerbate cerebral edema.

3. **Consult neurosurgery to insert an ICP monitor in patients with a Glasgow Coma Scale score of 8 or less**
    Because severe ICP elevations (Lundberg A waves or plateau waves) occur suddenly and without warning, a monitor should be inserted even if the patient does not currently show signs of increased ICP. Ventricular catheters are advisable if significant intraventricular hemorrhage with hydrocephalus is present. Otherwise, a parenchymal or epidural monitor should be used, because the associated risk of infection is significantly lower (see Chapter 12).

4. **Fluid management**
    Only isotonic fluids (normal saline or lactated Ringer's solution) should be administered to patients with head injury because the extra free water in half-normal saline or D5W can exacerbate cerebral edema.

5. **Nutrition**
    Severe head injury leads to a generalized hypermetabolic and catabolic response, with caloric requirements that are 50 to 100% higher than normal. Enteral feedings via a nasogastric or a nasoduodenal tube should be instituted as soon as possible (usually by hospital day 2).

6. **Temperature management**
   Fever (temperature >101°F) exacerbates cerebral injury and should be aggressively treated with acetaminophen or cooling blankets.
7. **Anticonvulsants**
   Fosphenytoin (15 to 20 mg/kg IV loading dose, then 300 mg/day IV) reduces the frequency of early (i.e., first week) posttraumatic seizures from 14% to 4% in patients with intracranial hemorrhage but does not prevent later seizures. If the patient has not experienced a seizure, phenytoin should be discontinued after 7 to 10 days. Levels should be monitored closely, because subtherapeutic levels frequently result from hypermetabolism of phenytoin.
8. **Steroids**
   Steroids have not been shown to favorably alter outcome in patients with head injury and may lead to increased risk of infection, hyperglycemia, and other complications. For this reason, *steroids such as dexamethasone have no role in the treatment of traumatic brain injury.*
9. **Prophylaxis for deep vein thrombosis (DVT)**
   Pneumatic compression boots are routinely used in immobilized patients to protect against lower-extremity DVT and the associated risk of pulmonary thromboembolism. **Heparin 5000 U subcutaneously (SC) every 12 hours** should be started 48 hours after injury even in the presence of intracranial hemorrhage.
10. **Prophylaxis for gastric ulcer**
    Patients on mechanical ventilation or with coagulopathy are at increased risk of gastric stress ulceration and should receive **ranitidine 50 mg IV every 8 hours** or **sucralfate 1 g by mouth (PO) every 6 hours**.
11. **Antibiotics**
    The routine use of prophylactic antibiotics in patients with open skull injuries is controversial. Penicillin may reduce the risk of pneumococcal meningitis in patients with CSF otorrhea, rhinorrhea, or intracranial air but may increase the risk of infection with more virulent organisms.
12. **Follow-up CT scan**
    In general, a follow-up head CT scan should be obtained 24 hours after the initial injury in patients with intracranial hemorrhage to assess for delayed or progressive bleeding.

Selected Complications of Severe Head Injury

1. **CSF leaks**
   CSF leaks result from disruption of the leptomeninges and occur in 2 to 6% of patients with closed head injury. CSF leakage ceases spontaneously with head elevation alone after a few days in 85% of patients; a lumbar drain may speed

this process in persistent cases. Although patients with CSF leaks are at increased risk for meningitis (usually from pneumococci), administration of prophylactic antibiotics is controversial. Persistent CSF otorrhea or rhinorrhea or recurrent meningitis is an indication for operative repair.
2. **Carotid cavernous fistulae**
   Carotid cavernous fistulae, characterized by the triad of *pulsating exophthalmos, chemosis, and orbital bruit,* may develop immediately or several days after injury. Angiography is required to confirm the diagnosis. Endovascular balloon occlusion is the most effective means of repair and can prevent permanent visual loss.
3. **Diabetes insipidus**
   Diabetes insipidus may result from traumatic damage to the pituitary stalk, resulting in cessation of antidiuretic hormone secretion. Patients excrete large volumes of dilute urine, resulting in hypernatremia and volume depletion. **Arginine vasopressin (Pitressin) 5 to 10 U IV, IM, or SC every 4 to 6 hours or desmopressin acetate (DDAVP) SC or IV 2 to 4 µg every 12 hours** is given to control urine output to less than 200 ml/hour, and volume is replaced with hypotonic fluids (D5W or 0.45% saline) depending on the severity of hypernatremia.
4. **Posttraumatic seizures**
   Posttraumatic seizures may be **immediate** (occurring within 24 hours), **early** (occurring within the first week), or **late** (occurring after the first week). Immediate seizures do not predispose to late seizures; early seizures, however, indicate an increased risk of late seizures, and these patients should be maintained on anticonvulsants. The overall incidence of late posttraumatic epilepsy (recurrent, unprovoked seizures) after closed head injury is 5%; the risk is approximately 20% in patients with intracranial hemorrhage or depressed skull fractures.

■ PROGNOSIS

The outcome after head injury is often a matter of great concern, particularly in patients with serious injuries. The admission Glasgow Coma Scale score has substantial prognostic value: patients scoring 3 or 4 have an 85% chance of dying or remaining in a vegetative state, whereas these outcomes occur in only 5 to 10% of patients with a score of 12 or higher. *Postconcussion syndrome* refers to a chronic profile of headache, fatigue, dizziness, inability to concentrate, irritability, and personality changes that develops in many patients following head injury. Often, there is overlap with symptoms of depression.

chapter 10 | Ataxia and Gait Failure

True ataxia implies a decomposition of coordinated posture and movement that is normally integrated by the cerebellum. Because almost every component of the nervous system contributes to maintenance of normal movement, gait, and posture, a call for a patient with gait failure requires consideration of a broad differential diagnosis. Successful evaluation begins with assessing the acuteness of the syndrome. Associated signs on examination will help with anatomic localization. Your management may range from emergent neurosurgical decompression of a cerebellar hematoma to a thorough laboratory evaluation to seek a cause for a chronic degenerative disease.

■ PHONE CALL

Questions

1. **When did the patient last walk normally?**
   This is the key question from which your route of investigation and management will spring. **If the patient was known to have been walking normally within the past 24 hours, you must rule out stroke, spinal cord compression** (see Chapter 7), **or a mass lesion in the posterior fossa.** These are medical emergencies. A subacute course (days to weeks) suggests an infectious, inflammatory, or neoplastic process. If the gait deterioration has occurred over weeks to months, your differential diagnosis will be weighted toward degenerative processes, either inherited or acquired.
2. **Has there been any trauma to the head, neck, or back?**
   A traumatic subdural hematoma or injury to the spinal cord or peripheral nerves may alter gait.
3. **What is the patient's level of consciousness?**
   Is the patient alert and awake, agitated, or confused? If a patient has an abnormal mental status in combination with ataxia or gait failure, acute intoxication or significant brain injury is likely.
4. **What are the vital signs?**
   Irregular heart rhythm may suggest cardioembolic stroke; fever may suggest an infectious process.

Orders

1. Maintain the patient at bed rest.

2. Use a chest restraint, if necessary, to prevent the patient from injuring himself or herself.
3. If there has been trauma to the head or neck, stabilize the cervical spine with a cervical collar (see Chapter 7).

■ ELEVATOR THOUGHTS

What is the differential diagnosis of gait failure?
Gait failure may occur as a result of damage to almost any part of the neural axis. Your initial examination of the patient will help establish whether you are dealing with disturbance of motor, sensory, or cerebellar function. Table 10–1 is an outline of the categories of diseases that cause gait dysfunction and the characteristic features of the gait disturbance. Table 10–2 provides a more detailed differential diagnosis of ataxia.

■ MAJOR THREAT TO LIFE

- **Cerebellar hemorrhage or infarction**
  Hematoma or infarction in the posterior fossa may progress to herniation and death if the lesion is large. It may require emergent neurosurgical evacuation.
- **Acute intoxication**
  Intoxication with sedatives such as barbiturate or alcohol may present initially as ataxia and may lead to respiratory failure.

■ BEDSIDE

Quick Look Test

Is the patient awake and alert?
A decreased level of consciousness in the presence of ataxia is more serious than ataxia alone.

Is there any evidence of head or neck trauma?
Head trauma rarely presents as ataxia alone but may require more immediate management. Vertebral artery dissection may result from trauma to the neck.

Has the patient been vomiting?
Nausea, vertigo, and vomiting are common symptoms that accompany posterior fossa disease.

Table 10–1 ◻ CLINICAL FEATURES OF GAIT DISTURBANCES

Disease Category	Features of Gait Failure
Focal brain injury (hemiparesis)	Spastically extended leg Spastically flexed arm Circumduction of paretic foot
Spinal cord injury (paraparesis)	Stiff, effortful movements at knees and hips Bilateral circumduction Toe-walking or scissoring gait
Peripheral or central deafferentation (sensory ataxia)	Wide-based stance and gait High-stepping gait Positive Romberg's sign
Cerebellar disease	Titubation (unsteady, oscillating posture) on sitting or standing Wide-based stance and gait Ataxia: staggering or lurching may be unilateral or bilateral
Normal-pressure hydrocephalus	"Magnetic," shuffling gait Many steps taken to turn 180 degrees
Lower motor neuron disease	Distal weakness (e.g., footdrop) High-stepping gait
Myopathy	Proximal leg weakness Difficulty arising from seated position Difficulty climbing stairs
Parkinsonism	Stooped posture Shuffling gait Retropulsion Difficulty initiating and terminating ambulation ("festinating gait")
Congenital/perinatal injury (cerebral palsy)	Spastically extended legs Spastically flexed arms Scissoring gait Adventitial movements (abnormal posturing or movements of one or more limbs)
Movement disorders (chorea, athetosis, or dystonia)	Adventitial movements may be present at rest Lurching gait

Table 10-2 □ DIFFERENTIAL DIAGNOSIS OF ATAXIA BY MODE OF ONSET

Mode of Onset	Disease Process
Acute (minutes to hours)	Cerebellar hemorrhage Cerebellar infarction Acute intoxication Head trauma Basilar migraine Dominant periodic ataxia (in children)
Subacute (hours to days)	Posterior fossa tumor Posterior fossa abscess Multiple sclerosis Toxins/intoxications Hydrocephalus Miller-Fisher variant of Guillain-Barré syndrome Viral cerebellitis (mostly in children)
Chronic (days to weeks)	Alcoholic cerebellar degeneration Paraneoplastic cerebellar syndrome Foramen magnum compression Chronic infection (e.g., Jakob-Creutzfeldt disease, rubella, panencephalitis) Hydrocephalus Vitamin E deficiency Hypothyroidism Inherited ataxias (autosomal recessive or dominant) Idiopathic degenerative ataxias
Episodic	Recurrent intoxications Multiple sclerosis Transient ischemic attacks Dominant periodic ataxia (children)

Modified from Harding AE: Ataxic disorders. *In* Bradley WG, Daroff RB, Fenichel GM, Marsden CD (eds): Neurology in Clinical Practice. Boston, Butterworth-Heinemann, 1991.

Selective History and Chart Review

The diagnosis for the etiology of gait failure can often be made on the history alone. If the patient is unable to give a history, get the history from a relative, nurse, or other witness. In the absence of a witness on hand, review the chart.

1. **When did the gait disturbance begin?**
2. **Was the onset sudden or gradual?**
3. **Why was the patient unable to walk? Was it because of weakness, imbalance, pain, or numbness?**
4. **Were there any accompanying symptoms?**

Diplopia, dysarthria, vertigo, or nausea suggests posterior fossa involvement. Unilateral weakness or numbness implies focal hemispheric brain injury (e.g., stroke). Urinary or fecal incontinence suggests spinal cord involvement. Pain radiating into the legs implies nerve root disease.

5. **Is the patient taking any medications that might cause ataxia?**

Most of the effects of medications are dose dependent (Table 10–3).

Selective Physical Examination I

General Physical Examination

Vital signs	• Fever may suggest an infectious etiology, such as **abscess, viral cerebellitis, or fungal infection.** Fever may also occur in some of the inherited metabolic ataxias (mostly in children). Irregular heart rhythm may suggest cardioembolic stroke.
HEENT	• Look for signs of head trauma. **Subdural or epidural hematoma** may produce hemiparesis.
Abdomen	• Look for signs of **chronic alcohol use,** such as hepatomegaly, caput medusae, or ascites. Hepatosplenomegaly may also appear in **Wilson's disease** and in some **inherited metabolic ataxias.**

Neurologic Examination

- **Mental status:** Establish level of alertness and attentiveness by asking the patient to count backward from 20 to 1 or to recite the months of the year backward.

Table 10–3 □ MEDICATIONS KNOWN TO CAUSE ATAXIA

Anticonvulsants	Immunosuppressants
Phenytoin	Cyclosporine A
Carbamazepine	Cytosine arabinoside
Primidone	Fluorouracil
Ethosuximide	Other medications (rarely cause ataxia)
Methosuximide	Phenothiazines
Sedatives	Monoamine oxidase inhibitors
Barbiturates	Reserpine
Benzodiazepines	Thiothixene
Chloral hydrate	Lithium salts
Paraldehyde	Nitrofurantoin

- Cranial nerves: Gait failure with almost any cranial nerve finding means there is brain stem or cerebellar involvement.
  1. **Pupils:** Pinpoint pupils may suggest **opiate intoxication**; asymmetric pupils may be a part of Horner's syndrome (miosis, ptosis, and anhidrosis), which, in combination with ataxia and contralateral pain and temperature sensory loss, makes up Wallenberg's (lateral medullary) syndrome. Small, irregular pupils that react to accommodation but not to light (Argyll Robertson pupils) may be a sign of **central nervous system syphilis, brain stem encephalitis, or mass effect on the midbrain.**
  2. **Extraocular movements: Nystagmus, particularly if vertical or dysconjugate, is a sign of injury to the brain stem or cerebellum.** Vertical (upbeat or downbeat) nystagmus is a reliable indicator of cerebellar or brain stem damage (see Chapter 13 for a more detailed discussion of nystagmus). Horizontal gaze palsies localize disease to a large hemispheric or small pontine lesion. Impaired upgaze, particularly in combination with retraction nystagmus and loss of pupillary accommodation, implies pressure on or damage to the tectum of the midbrain and can be seen in pineal region tumors or in hydrocephalus (Parinaud's phenomenon). CN 6 palsies may be a nonspecific sign of increased intracranial pressure. Oculoparesis, in combination with ataxia and areflexia, makes the diagnosis of the **Miller-Fisher variant of Guillain-Barré syndrome.**
  3. **CN 7:** Upper motor neuron facial paresis may be part of a hemiparesis or may indicate brain stem involvement if CN 6 is affected on the same side.
  4. **CN 8:** Tinnitus or hearing loss with ataxia suggests a **peripheral vestibular neuropathy or labyrinthitis,** particularly if there is a rotational component to the nystagmus.
  5. **CN 9 to CN 12:** Dysphagia, nasal speech, dysarthria, or tongue deviation may suggest a **brain stem stroke or mass lesion at the skull base,** producing spastic paraparesis and gait failure in addition to the lower cranial nerve findings.
- Cerebellar testing: Rapid, repetitive finger-thumb opposition (rapid alternating movements [RAM]) and finger-nose-finger (FNF) movements are two sensitive screening tests for cerebellar function. Irregular rhythm (dysdiadochokinesis) on finger tapping or ataxia of movements as the finger approaches the target on the FNF test suggests cerebellar dysfunction. The heel-knee-shin (HKS) test is the equivalent of the FNF test for the lower extremities. Figure 10–1 illustrates three common cerebellar tests (the FNF, RAM, and HKS tests). **Unilateral limb ataxia implies ipsilateral cerebellar hemisphere damage** because the cerebellar circuits that coor-

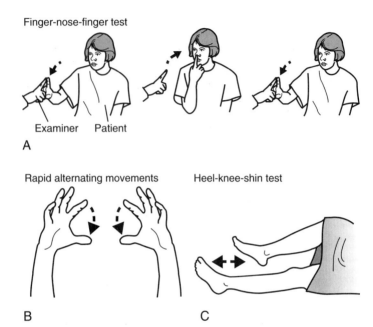

Figure 10–1 □ Cerebellar function tests. *A*, Finger-nose-finger test. Patient touches the finger of the examiner and his or her own nose sequentially. *B*, Rapid alternating movements. Patient taps the forefinger and thumb together as rapidly as possible. *C*, Heel-knee-shin test. Patient runs the heel up and down the opposite shin as accurately and rapidly as possible.

dinate movement cross twice, once while descending in the frontopontocerebellar pathway and a second time while ascending in the dentatothalamic, dentatorubral, and dentatocortical pathways. **Titubation (truncal ataxia) on sitting or standing or gait ataxia in the absence of limb ataxia suggests midline cerebellar damage.**

If the patient is able to stand, the gait evaluation is a crucial part of the examination for anatomic localization and determination of the underlying pathophysiology. Table 10–1 reviews the features of gait dysfunction that characterize different disease processes. The gait should be tested with the patient walking normally, walking on the toes, walking on the heels, and doing a tandem walk. Observe for symmetry of balance, stride, and arm swing.

- **Motor:** Test for strength by confrontation and look for pronator drift with the arms extended and palms up. (Pronator drift may be the only sign of a subtle hemiparesis.)
- **Sensory:** Temperature and vibration are the most sensitive parameters for testing sensory loss. Proprioceptive loss may indicate damaged posterior columns, as occurs in **vitamin B_{12} deficiency** (subacute combined degeneration) or **tabes dorsalis** (a now rare, late complication of syphilis).
- **Reflexes:** Unilateral hyperreflexia usually accompanies hemiparesis; bilateral hyperreflexia may indicate myelopathy; and areflexia is seen in peripheral neuropathy and in the **Guillain-Barré syndrome.**

■ MANAGEMENT I

Acute ataxia, particularly with any accompanying signs or symptoms of posterior fossa disease or increased intracranial pressure, must be treated with utmost urgency.

1. **Obtain a noncontrast head computed tomography (CT) or magnetic resonance imaging (MRI) scan.**
   If cerebellar hematoma or infarction is identified, proceed with the next steps.
2. **Admit the patient to an intensive care unit.**
3. **Consult with the neurosurgery service.** If there is hematoma near the brain stem or if the hematoma is large, rapid, and irreversible, neurologic deterioration may occur. Delayed deterioration may be the result of a rebleed or reactive edema formation. **Surgical evacuation of cerebellar hematoma greater than 3 cm in diameter has been shown to reduce morbidity and mortality rates for these patients.** Consideration for surgical evacuation is warranted, particularly if the patient is relatively young and is following a deteriorating course. **It may be necessary to place an intraventricular drain if hydrocephalus develops.**
4. **Cerebellar hematomas smaller than 3 cm may be managed medically with reasonably good results.** Therapy is largely supportive, with blood pressure control to a target maximum systolic blood pressure (SBP) of 160 to 180 mm Hg and control of coagulopathy with fresh frozen plasma if necessary. Hydrocephalus can develop even with smaller hematomas, necessitating neurosurgical placement of an intraventricular drain.
5. **Cerebellar infarction, if large, may produce the same syndrome of rapid progression to coma as does cerebellar hematoma.** As the infarcted territory becomes edematous, compression of the fourth ventricle may produce **obstructive hydrocephalus,** leading to further increase in intracranial

pressure. Cerebellar infarction in the posterior inferior cerebellar artery territory carries a worse prognosis than infarction in the anterior inferior cerebellar artery or superior cerebellar artery territories. **Surgical evacuation of a large cerebellar infarction may be lifesaving.** As noted in item 3, placement of an intraventricular drain may become necessary with cerebellar infarction if hydrocephalus develops.

Other causes of gait failure that require immediate management include cord compression or acute myelopathy (see Chapter 7), **subdural or epidural hematoma from head trauma** (see Chapter 9), **acute cerebral infarction** (see Chapter 6), **and acute intoxication** (see Chapter 5).

Selective Physical Examination II

Once posterior fossa lesions have been ruled out by imaging, further examination for systemic signs associated with chronic ataxic disorders should be performed:

Hair	• Alopecia may be a sign of **thallium poisoning, hypothyroidism, or adrenoleukomyeloneuropathy.**
Skin	• Telangiectases, particularly in the conjunctivae, nose, and ears, or flexures, may be seen in **ataxia-telangiectasia.** Pigmentation may be seen in adrenoleukomyeloneuropathy.
HEENT	• Kayser-Fleischer rings appear as a brown border at the edge of the iris in **Wilson's disease.** Retinal angiomas seen on fundoscopic examination may be a part of **von Hippel–Lindau disease** that also includes cerebellar hemangioblastomas. Deafness in combination with short stature is often a sign of **mitochondrial encephalopathy.**
Heart	• Cardiomegaly, murmurs, arrhythmias, and heart failure may accompany **Friedreich's ataxia.** Conduction defects on electrocardiogram (ECG) may be present in mitochondrial encephalopathy.
Musculoskeletal	• Short stature is characteristic of mitochondrial encephalopathy and ataxia-telangiectasia. Other skeletal deformities may be a part of hereditary

ataxias and **hereditary motor and sensory neuropathy.**

■ MANAGEMENT II

Diagnostic Testing

Laboratory Investigation

Laboratory investigation should begin with an attempt to diagnose treatable or reversible causes of ataxia or gait failure. Laboratory tests to be performed include the following blood tests:
1. Chemistry panel, including electrolytes, glucose, and liver function tests
2. Urine and serum toxicology screen
3. Vitamin B_{12} and folate levels
4. Venereal Disease Research Laboratory (VDRL) test
5. Thyroid function tests
6. Anticonvulsant levels if the patient is taking anticonvulsants
7. Lithium level if the patient is taking lithium
8. Anti-Yo serum antibodies to investigate paraneoplastic cerebellar degeneration from ovarian, lung, or breast carcinoma, or Hodgkin's lymphoma (see Chapter 23)
9. Ceruloplasmin levels (Wilson's disease)

Other Diagnostic Tests

1. **Chest radiograph.** A chest radiograph may disclose occult neoplasm, raising the possibility of metastatic disease or a paraneoplastic cerebellar degeneration.
2. **Transcranial Doppler ultrasonogram or MR angiogram.** Vertebrobasilar transient ischemic attacks (TIAs) or vertebrobasilar insufficiency may be suggested if there is stenosis of the basilar or vertebral arteries.
3. **Visual evoked responses.** Delayed P100 suggests multiple sclerosis.
4. **Lumbar puncture.** Oligoclonal bands are present in multiple sclerosis. Abnormal cerebrospinal fluid (CSF) cell count, protein, or glucose may point to an infectious or neoplastic process. Elevated CSF protein without pleocytosis is found in the Miller-Fisher variant of Guillain-Barré syndrome. Cytology may be performed if a CNS- or meninges-based tumor is suspected.
5. **Electromyography (EMG)/nerve conduction studies (NCS).** The Miller-Fisher variant of the Guillain-Barré syndrome includes ataxia, oculoparesis, and areflexia. A typical demyelination pattern of slowed conduction velocities and prolonged F waves supports this diagnosis. Gait failure on the basis of neuropathy can also be diagnosed with EMG/NCS.

Treatment of Some of the Reversible Causes of Ataxia

1. **Acute sedative intoxication:** Administer **naloxone (Narcan) 0.4 to 2 mg IV** for opiate overdose; **flumazenil (Romazicon) 0.5 mg IV** for benzodiazepine overdose; admit for observation and supportive therapy.
2. **Anticonvulsant overdose:** Stop administering the anticonvulsant, admit for observation and cardiovascular monitoring, and follow anticonvulsant levels.
3. **Hypothyroidism:** Administer **Synthroid 0.05 to 0.15 mg every day.**
4. **Lithium toxicity:** Admit patient for cardiac monitoring, adjust dose, and follow lithium and electrolyte levels.
5. **Paraneoplastic disorder:** Treating the underlying malignancy may reverse the symptoms in some patients. Immunosuppressive therapy and plasmapheresis have not been proved to be effective.
6. **Vertebrobasilar TIAs:** Admit patient for workup for etiology of TIAs. Anticoagulation may be required (see Chapter 24).
7. **Multiple sclerosis:** Treat with IV methylprednisolone and interferon beta (see Chapter 21).
8. **CNS infections:** Treat with appropriate antimicrobial agents (see Chapter 22).
9. **Miller-Fisher variant of Guillain-Barré syndrome:** A several-day course of plasmapheresis or intravenous immune globulin (IVIG) early in the disease may be effective in halting progression and speeding recovery (see Chapter 15).

chapter 11 | Acute Visual Disturbances

No symptom may be as disturbing or dramatic to a patient as acute visual loss. Although acute ocular diseases such as glaucoma, uveitis, and retinal detachment may require urgent evaluation by an ophthalmologist, a high percentage of visual disturbances fall within the province of the neurologist. Neurologic visual symptoms may be reported as blurriness, focal obscurations, or positive visual phenomena. Because the visual pathway from the retina to the calcarine cortex is constant from individual to individual, anatomic localization can be made with a high degree of accuracy on physical examination. The progression, associated symptoms and signs, and clinical setting will help you make the correct diagnosis and suggest the proper acute management.

■ **PHONE CALL**

Questions

The following questions will need to be repeated during the selective history and physical examination of the patient. Nonetheless, these questions, asked prior to your arrival at the bedside, will form the starting point for your diagnostic and management algorithm.

1. Is the visual loss in one or both eyes?
This is the first point for anatomic localization. Visual disturbances affecting one eye indicate pathology between the retina and the optic chiasm. Binocular disturbances suggest lesions in the visual pathway between the chiasm and the calcarine cortex.

2. What is the nature of the visual disturbance?
This is an elaboration of question one. Vision can be altered in one of the following ways: monocular visual loss (temporary or permanent), bilateral blindness, a hemifield cut, diplopia, scotomata, or positive phenomena (e.g., flashes or lines). The first description of the disturbance will allow the visual problem to be categorized into specific disease entities.

3. How old is the patient?
Certain disorders, such as ischemic optic neuropathy or transient monocular blindness (TMB), are rare in patients under 45

years of age, whereas a first presentation of multiple sclerosis, pseudotumor cerebri, or migraine is much more common in a younger patient.

4. Is the patient still experiencing the visual symptom?
Although persistent acute visual loss may require immediate, specific therapy, transient visual loss may be no less ominous as a warning sign for further visual, cerebrovascular, or inflammatory events.

5. When did the visual disturbance begin?
Acute monocular blindness is a neuro-ophthalmologic emergency. Ischemia in the retina resulting from a central retinal artery occlusion may be irreversible after 105 minutes. Furthermore, even if the patient presents many hours after the onset of visual loss, efficient and accurate diagnosis may prevent contralateral visual loss due to temporal arteritis or stroke from carotid artery disease.

6. Was there any trauma or injury to the eyes?
Eye injury will nearly always require ophthalmologic evaluation. Because a dilated fundoscopic examination by an ophthalmologist will interfere with your ability to get an accurate assessment of pupillary reactivity, you should try to perform your assessment first.

Orders

If there has been eye trauma or if there is a pre-existing ophthalmologic condition such as glaucoma, call the ophthalmology service for consultation.

Inform RN

"Will arrive at the bedside in . . . minutes."

■ ELEVATOR THOUGHTS

What is the differential diagnosis of acute visual disturbance?
The differential diagnosis of acute visual disturbance can be divided into processes affecting one eye or both eyes.
1. Monocular visual loss
    - Retinal ischemia (central [or branch] retinal artery occlusion [CRAO])
      This occlusion is usually caused by an embolus from the ipsilateral internal carotid artery or from the heart or aortic arch. If the symptoms are transient (TMB or amaurosis fugax), the mechanism may be hemodynamic rather than

embolic. Hemodynamic TMB may be caused by perfusion failure in the retinal artery from high-grade carotid stenosis. Patients with vascular causes for retinal ischemia usually have risk factors for cerebrovascular disease, such as hypertension, diabetes, or a history of smoking.
- **Optic nerve head ischemia (anterior ischemic optic neuropathy [AION])**
  Although its pathophysiology is uncertain, this entity is often associated with arteritis. Patients in their 50s or 60s may have systemic lupus erythematosus, polyarteritis nodosa, sickle cell trait, or polycythemia. In patients over 60 years of age, the most common associated arteritis is giant cell (temporal) arteritis, which must be treated emergently.
- **Inflammatory/demyelinating optic neuritis**
  The most common cause for optic neuritis in a patient under 40 years of age is multiple sclerosis, but idiopathic forms and sarcoidosis can be present in older individuals.
- **Retrobulbar mass lesion**
  The lesion may be a **tumor, such as optic glioma, neurofibroma, meningioma, or metastasis, or a giant aneurysm in the cavernous segment of the carotid. Pseudotumor cerebri** (benign intracranial hypertension) can mimic a mass lesion, causing papilledema and visual loss in young women who are often obese and dysmenorrheic. Visual loss may begin unilaterally.

2. Binocular visual loss

   Binocular involvement with visual field defects implies pathology at or behind the optic chiasm. Acute binocular visual loss affecting the chiasm, the optic tracts, the thalamus (lateral geniculate body), the optic radiations, or the calcarine cortex is nearly always due to an anatomic lesion such as a **tumor, abscess, or stroke. Migraine** is a notable exception, in which "spreading depression" (a wave of depolarization) is thought to produce neuronal deactivation that moves slowly across the cortex and produces scotomata in one or both visual fields. **Pituitary adenomas** often produce bitemporal visual field defects as pressure from the mass disrupts midline-crossing fibers from both nasal retinae (Fig. 11–1). The farther back along the visual pathway the lesion is located, the more congruous is the visual field defect. Table 11–1 lists unusual visual syndromes associated with occipital cortex lesions.

3. Diplopia

   Double vision implies some form of oculoparesis. If diplopia persists when one eye is covered, the etiology is either factitious or an ophthalmologic condition such as retinal detachment, dislocated lens, or keratoconus. For true binocular diplopia, the lesion is almost always in the brain stem or

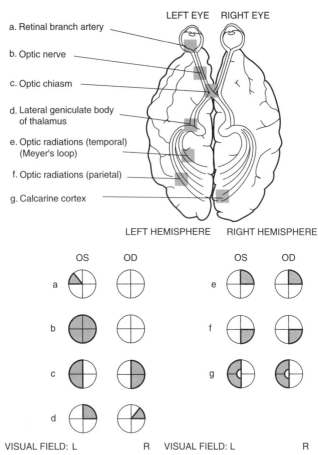

Figure 11–1 □ Visual field cuts produced by lesions at different points along the visual pathway. a. Monocular segmentanopia produced by a retinal artery branch occlusion in the left eye. b. Monocular blindness produced by a lesion in the left optic nerve. c. Bitemporal hemianopia produced by a mass lesion at the optic chiasm. d. Right segmentanopia produced by a lesion in the lateral geniculate body of the left thalamus. e. Right upper quadrantanopia produced by a lesion in the left temporal optic radiation (Meyer's loop). f. Right lower quadrantanopia produced by a lesion in the left parietal optic radiation. g. Left homonymous hemianopia produced by a lesion in the calcarine cortex of the right occipital lobe. Note that macular vision is sometimes spared because of middle cerebral artery collateral blood flow to the occipital pole. OS, Oculus sinister; OD, oculus dexter.

Table 11-1 □ UNUSUAL VISUAL SYNDROMES ASSOCIATED WITH OCCIPITAL CORTEX LESIONS

Syndrome	Localization	Description
Anton's syndrome	Bilateral calcarine	Bilateral loss of vision in which the patient denies blindness
Balint's syndrome	Bilateral occipito-parietal	Simultanagnosia, optic ataxia, and ocular apraxia
Bonnet's syndrome	Unilateral or bilateral calcarine	Lilliputian visual hallucinations in the absence of delirium
Dyschromatopsia	Lingual gyrus	Abnormal color perception contralateral to lesion
Pallinopsia	Incomplete injury or recovery in calcarine cortex	Visual persistence of afterimages
Prosopagnosia	Right or bilateral inferior calcarine (lingual gyrus)	Inability to recognize faces

involves CN 3, CN 4, or CN 6. The most common conditions affecting the brain stem are **stroke** and **multiple sclerosis,** although **brain stem tumors** and **progressive multifocal leukoencephalopathy (PML)** may rarely present with diplopia. The most common systemic condition that affects the ocular cranial nerves is **diabetes mellitus.** A **berry aneurysm** of the posterior communicating artery may also produce diplopia by stretching CN 3 as it passes over the artery on its way forward toward the cavernous sinus. Invasive or metastatic **tumor in the cavernous sinus region** or late **chronic meningitis** may cause oculomotor disturbances. Unilateral or bilateral CN 6 palsies can be a "false localizing" sign of **increased intracranial pressure** (see Chapter 12). **Hyperthyroidism** may cause diplopia by mechanical limitation of infiltrated, fibrotic ocular muscles. Finally, weakness of the extraocular muscles because of **myasthenia gravis** must be considered in the differential diagnosis of diplopia, particularly if the symptoms fluctuate or appear with fatigue.

Diagnoses for which immediate, specific therapy may arrest loss or restore vision are the following:
- CRAO
- Ischemic optic neuropathy from temporal arteritis

- Pseudotumor cerebri
- Acute glaucoma

Diagnoses for which urgent management may prevent further vision loss or stroke are the following:
- TMB with carotid stenosis
- Retrobulbar mass lesion (aneurysm or tumor)

■ MAJOR THREAT TO LIFE

Acute visual loss in the absence of other neurologic signs is rarely life threatening.

■ BEDSIDE

Quick Look Test

Are there any signs of trauma?

Is the patient in any pain or discomfort?

Is one eye affected or are both?

Selective History and Chart Review

Some of the questions asked in the initial telephone interview should be discussed with the patient.

1. **Was one eye affected or were both?**
   It may be difficult for a patient to distinguish between a visual field loss and monocular blindness. A patient will often refer to "the left eye" as being defective when in fact the left hemifield was affected. Ask if the symptoms improve if "the bad eye" is covered.

2. **When and how did the visual disturbance begin?**
   Ask the patient to describe the onset of the symptoms, with particular reference to the location and pattern of the visual disturbance. An obscuration that moves across the visual field "like a shade coming down" is a common description of an arterial occlusion. An altitudinal defect is common with ischemic optic neuropathy. An expanding blind spot may suggest worsening papilledema. Slowly marching lights, particularly the jagged-edged "fortification scotomata," is a common description of migraine, whether or not it is followed by headache. Sudden loss of vision over seconds to minutes suggests a vascular cause. Progression over hours to days may suggest ischemic optic neuropathy, demyelination, mass lesion, or pseudotumor cerebri.

3. **Was there pain?**
   Headache is common in temporal arteritis, pseudotumor cerebri, and migraine. Masticatory claudication and other myalgias may be a tip-off for arteritis. Pain with eye movement is the rule for the inflammatory optic neuritis of multiple sclerosis, but pain is usually absent with retinal embolism and ischemic optic neuropathy. The exception is in carotid artery dissection, which may cause pain in the side of the head or jaw, with radiation into the orbit.
4. **Were there any associated neurologic symptoms?**
   Dysarthria, vertigo, nausea, vomiting, and ataxia suggest stroke or mass lesion in the posterior fossa. Urinary incontinence, ataxia, diplopia, and patchy weakness or sensory loss are other presenting symptoms of multiple sclerosis.

Selective Physical Examination

General Physical Examination

Vital signs	• Fever may be a feature of temporal arteritis. Cardiac arrhythmia and hypertension are risk factors for cerebrovascular disease.
HEENT	• **Palpate the temporal arteries** just anterior and superior to the ear and along the side of the head. Exquisite tenderness strongly suggests temporal arteritis.
	• Listen for **carotid bruits.**
	• **Eye examination.** Check for **proptosis** by viewing the orbits from above. A retrobulbar mass lesion may cause the eye to protrude. Gentle palpation of the globe may disclose more resistance to posterior motion. The high pressure of glaucoma may also be detected, if present.

Neurologic Examination

- **Mental status**
  Aphasia or hemineglect may rarely accompany a disruption of optic radiations through the parietal lobe.
- **Cranial nerves**
  Check the following:
  1. **Pupillary reactivity.** Examine each pupil's direct and consensual response to light. Use low ambient light and a bright flashlight for the stimulus. A relative or absolute **afferent pupillary defect (APD)** may be detected by swinging the flashlight from one eye to the other. If the pupil enlarges when the flashlight swings to that eye **(Marcus Gunn pupil),** there is pathology in the retina or optic nerve.

2. **Visual fields.** Test for visual fields by having the patient visually fix on your nose and by holding your hands in two of the four visual quadrants, an arm's length from the patient. Move a finger or briefly display a number of fingers on one or both hands. Test all four quadrants. More subtle visual field loss may be tested by comparing the brightness of a red button or hatpin. Red desaturation may occur without frank blindness. Be sure to check macular vision in the central 6 degrees of vision. Figure 11-1 illustrates the visual field defects expected with lesions at various points along the visual pathway.
3. **Fundoscopic examination.** This can reveal a specific pathology, although an examination adequate to make a definitive diagnosis may require pharmacologic dilation of the pupil. Table 11-2 lists the fundoscopic features of the most important diagnoses of monocular blindness. **Hollenhorst (cholesterol) plaques** in retinal arteries are a sign of cholesterol emboli from atherosclerotic plaque in the aortic arch or carotid arteries.

Table 11-2 □ FUNDOSCOPIC FEATURES OF SOME NEURO-OPHTHALMOLOGIC ENTITIES

Diagnosis	Fundoscopic Appearance
Central retinal artery occlusion	White, ground-glass retina "Boxcar segmentation" (clumped red blood cells) in retinal veins (<1 hour) Macular cherry-red spot (hours to days)
Branch retinal artery occlusion	Embolic material (bright calcium flecks or lipid yellow Hollenhorst plaques) at arterial branch points Arcuate band of retinal infarction
Ischemic optic neuropathy	Disk head pallor, often in the superior or inferior half only Papilledema Superficial flame hemorrhages Optic disk cupping (late)
Optic neuritis	Disk pallor
Pseudotumor cerebri	Papilledema
Foster Kennedy syndrome	Optic atrophy ipsilateral to a retrobulbar mass Papilledema in contralateral eye due to increased retrobulbar pressure

4. Check **ocular motility** with the following steps:
   A. **Have the patient follow your finger through horizontal and vertical range of motion.** Note oculoparesis if it occurs. Simple observation of the eye movements may be sufficient to diagnose a CN 3 or CN 6 lesion.
   B. **Latent or subtle nonconjugate gaze may be revealed by the cover-uncover test.** Ask the patient to fix on one point such as your finger. Cover one eye, then uncover it. Repeat with the other eye. If the eyes shift when the eyes are uncovered, there is a nonconjugate gaze. Although a positive cover-uncover test may suggest brain stem or cranial nerve pathology, benign, latent phorias in patients with normal vision may cause a positive test.
   C. **Evaluate subtle oculoparesis using a Maddox rod.** If there is pre-existing amblyopia or if the patient is suppressing one eye's image, it may be difficult to identify diplopia without isolating the images from the two eyes. To check for horizontal diplopia, have the patient cover one eye with the Maddox rod, with the slats oriented horizontally, and then have the patient fix on a point light source. Two images should be seen: the point of light will be seen by the uncovered eye and a vertical red line will be seen by the covered eye. If gaze is conjugate, light should bisect the red line. As you move the light laterally, the light and line will move farther apart if there is a paresis of lateral gaze in one eye. This occurs as the image is projected onto the retina, away from the macula in the affected eye. The rules are as follows: (1) the "false" image is always the one on the outside, and (2) the false image always comes from the affected eye. Figure 11–2 diagrams the use of the Maddox rod. The same procedure can be used to check for a vertical nonconjugate gaze by orienting the slats of the Maddox rod vertically (making the red line horizontal), and moving the light up or down. Again, the image that is on the outside (farther up on upgaze or farther down on downgaze) comes from the affected eye. Impairment of abduction indicates CN 6 or lateral rectus palsy. Impairment of adduction indicates CN 3 or medial rectus palsy. If adduction palsy is accompanied by abduction nystagmus in the opposite eye, this is likely an **internuclear ophthalmoplegia,** suggesting multiple sclerosis in a younger patient or a paramedian midbrain infarct in an older person. *Nystagmus* is discussed in Chapter 13.

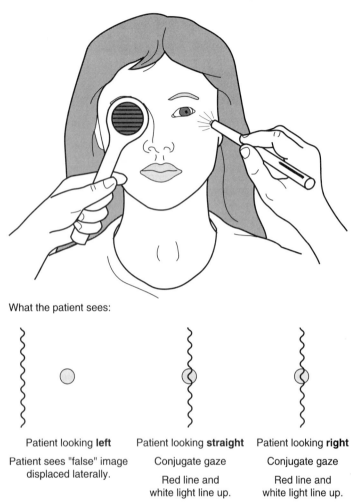

What the patient sees:

Patient looking **left**
Patient sees "false" image displaced laterally.

Patient looking **straight**
Conjugate gaze
Red line and white light line up.

Patient looking **right**
Conjugate gaze
Red line and white light line up.

Figure 11-2 □ Use of the Maddox rod in a patient with a right CN 3 palsy. Patient sees the red line to the left of the white light on left gaze. This occurs because the red line projects farther laterally onto the retina of the abnormal eye, giving a "false" image that appears displaced laterally. The gaze is conjugate on primary gaze and on rightward gaze. Right CN 3 palsy would be confirmed by holding the Maddox rod so that the red line is oriented horizontally and asking the patient to look upward. The red line would then appear above the white light.

- **Coordination and gait**
  Ataxia or dysdiadochokinesis may be a sign of multiple sclerosis or may suggest posterior circulation infarction affecting the cerebellum and the occipital cortex.
- **Sensation**
  Unilateral sensory loss may accompany visual field cuts produced by lesions in the thalamus or parietal lobe.
- **Reflexes**
  Asymmetry may be a subtle sign of brain injury.

■ MANAGEMENT

Order the following blood tests:
1. Erythrocyte sedimentation rate (ESR)
2. Complete blood cell count (CBC) with platelet count
3. Prothrombin time (PT) or International Normalized Ratio (INR)/partial thromboplastin time (PTT)
4. Chemistry panel including glucose and cholesterol levels

If there is monocular blindness or any suspicion of injury to the eye, have someone call for an ophthalmologic consultation to follow your assessment.

1. CRAO

Restoration of vision is usually possible only within the first 90 to 120 minutes after the occlusive event, although reversal of blindness has been reported up to 12 hours after embolus. Local intra-arterial thrombolysis with tissue-type plasminogen activator (t-PA) may be possible. Treatment between 12 and 24 hours would be considered heroic. Standard treatment in the hyperacute phase is aimed at dislodging the embolic particle and lowering the intraocular pressure. This is accomplished by laying the patient flat and applying **ocular massage** (intermittently, pressing firmly on the globe every 4 seconds). If segmentation can still be seen in the retinal veins, you should consult an ophthalmologist to perform an anterior oculocentesis. The presence of a cherry-red spot suggests that the retina has been infarcted.

Apart from treating the eye itself, CRAO requires a search for an embolic source. **Duplex Doppler ultrasonography** of the carotid arteries and echocardiography seeking a cardioembolic source should be performed urgently. **Intravenous (IV) heparin at 800 U/hour (no bolus), aiming for a PTT of 1.5 to 2.0 times the control value,** is recommended while the search for an embolic source is under way, provided there are no contraindications to anticoagulation therapy. **Patients with ipsilateral carotid stenosis greater than 70% should be referred for carotid endarterectomy** or **carotid angioplasty** to reduce the risk of stroke. Long-term anticoag-

ulation with warfarin (Coumadin) is probably indicated if a cardioembolic source is identified.
2. **Arteritic ischemic optic neuropathy**
Identifying temporal arteritis is of utmost importance. Because the prognosis for recovery of vision is less than 15% for the first eye, and because contralateral blindness may occur in up to 40% of patients, early recognition is important. Realistically, if visual loss is the presenting symptom, therapy is aimed at preventing involvement of the contralateral eye. Anorexia, fever, myalgias, and jaw claudication accompanying visual loss and headache in a patient over 65 years of age firmly establishes the diagnosis clinically. Less typical presentations are possible. Sedimentation rate and fibrinogen levels are usually markedly elevated. **Prednisone 100 mg by mouth (PO)** once a day should be started immediately, then tapered slowly after several weeks. **IV methylprednisolone 1 g per day** may also be used. Temporal artery biopsy should be arranged within a week. Corticosteroids generally have to be continued for 1 to 2 years. The ESR can be used as a marker of disease activity.
3. **Transient monocular blindness**
Patients with painless transient monocular visual loss, particularly those with risk factors for cerebrovascular disease, should be evaluated for risk of stroke. TMB is a classic warning sign for high-grade carotid stenosis. As in CRAO, the patient should be referred for duplex Doppler ultrasonography, echocardiography, and usually magnetic resonance (MR) angiography. Maintaining the patient on an antithrombotic agent, either **acetylsalicylic acid (aspirin) 325 mg once a day** or **IV heparin at 800 U/hour** if he or she is awaiting imminent endarterectomy, will reduce the risk of stroke or recurrent transient ischemic attack (TIA) (see Chapter 24).
4. **Retrobulbar mass lesion**
In a patient with a suspected retro-orbital mass, high-quality imaging is the key to accurate diagnosis. **MRI with gadolinium contrast enhancement** will help define soft-tissue masses. **Computed tomography (CT) scan with thin cuts through the orbits** can help define any bony erosion. Appropriate **surgical referral** to an ophthalmologist or neurosurgeon should be made.
5. **Inflammatory optic neuritis**
Optic neuritis is the presenting symptom for multiple sclerosis in about 15% of patients. Optic neuritis occurs at some point in the course of the disease in about 50% of patients with multiple sclerosis. As with treatment of other flares of multiple sclerosis (see Chapter 21), treatment of optic neuritis is **IV methylprednisolone 1 g for 7 to 10 days,** followed by a tapering dose of oral prednisone. Oral

prednisone as a first line of treatment for acute optic neuritis has been shown to be ineffective. Patients older than 45 years of age may have idiopathic optic neuritis that is steroid responsive.

6. **Pseudotumor cerebri**

   Visual loss is the most significant and dreaded complication of pseudotumor cerebri. Papilledema may occur with or without decreased acuity, but once visual loss begins, urgent therapy is imperative to prevent progression to blindness. Visual disturbance usually begins with an expanding blind spot or with constriction of the peripheral fields. Formal visual field testing may help evaluate the extent of loss. For mild visual loss, give **acetazolamide 500 mg PO two times a day.** This treatment is aimed at relieving increased intracranial pressure. For severe visual loss, the addition of **methylprednisolone 250 mg IV four times a day** (with an appropriate gastrointestinal protective medication such as ranitidine) may be vision saving. For patients whose visual loss is unresponsive to medical therapy, consult an ophthalmologist for **optic nerve sheath fenestration.** Periodic lumbar punctures or lumboperitoneal shunting has been advocated by some physicians, but the results of these treatments are inconsistent (see also Chapter 14).

chapter 12 | Increased Intracranial Pressure

Increased intracranial pressure (ICP) is not a symptom. Rather, intracranial hypertension is a pathologic state common to a variety of serious neurologic illnesses (Table 12–1). All conditions that result in increased ICP are characterized by an increase in intracranial volume. Accordingly, all therapies for ICP (hyperventilation, mannitol, etc.) are directed toward reducing intracranial volume.

Normal ICP is less than 200 mm H_2O, or 15 mm Hg. Because elevations beyond these levels can rapidly lead to brain damage and death, prompt recognition and treatment are essential. This chapter will be most useful in cases in which the pathology is known, and increased ICP is the suspected cause of clinical deterioration.

Table 12–1 □ CONDITIONS ASSOCIATED WITH INCREASED ICP

Intracranial mass lesions
  Subdural hematoma
  Epidural hematoma
  Intracerebral hemorrhage
  Brain tumor
  Cerebral abscess
Increased CSF volume (or resistance to outflow)
  Hydrocephalus
  Benign intracranial hypertension (pseudotumor cerebri)
Increased brain volume (cytotoxic cerebral edema)
  Cerebral infarction
  Global hypoxia-ischemia
  Reye's syndrome
  Acute hyponatremia
Increased brain and blood volume (vasogenic cerebral edema)
  Head trauma
  Meningitis
  Encephalitis
  Lead encephalopathy
  Eclampsia
  Hypertensive encephalopathy
  Dural sinus thrombosis

CSF, cerebrospinal fluid; ICP, intracranial pressure.

■ PHONE CALL

Questions

1. What is the patient's underlying neurologic problem?
2. Why is increased ICP suspected?
3. What is the patient's current level of consciousness?

■ BEDSIDE

Quick Look Test

Does the patient have clinical signs of increased ICP?

Increased ICP should be suspected in patients with known or suspected intracranial pathology (e.g., stroke, trauma, or neoplasm) who exhibit the following symptoms and signs:

Signs that are almost always present:
- Depressed level of consciousness (lethargy, stupor, coma)
- Hypertension, with or without bradycardia

Symptoms and signs that are sometimes present:
- Headache
- Vomiting
- Papilledema
- CN 6 palsies

Remember, however, that these signs may be nonspecific. For this reason, *the only way to confirm the diagnosis and properly treat increased ICP is to measure it.*

Does the patient have clinical signs of herniation?

Clinical signs of herniation, listed here, result from *brain stem compression:*
- Loss of pupillary reactivity
- Impairment of eye movements
- Hyperventilation
- Motor posturing (flexion or extension)

When ICP is differentially increased across the tentorium (as is usually the case with hemispheric mass lesions), pressure gradients lead to downward displacement of brain tissue into the posterior fossa. Herniation is often rapidly fatal but can be reversed in some cases by treatments that reduce intracranial volume and ICP.

■ MANAGEMENT I

Emergency Measures for Reduction of ICP

If the clinical signs described under **Bedside** are identified in a comatose patient, the emergency measures listed in Box 12–1 can

> **Box 12–1. EMERGENCY TREATMENT FOR ELEVATED ICP IN AN UNMONITORED PATIENT**
>
> 1. Elevate head of bed 30 to 45 degrees.
> 2. Intubate and hyperventilate (target partial pressure of carbon dioxide (P_{CO_2}) is 25 to 30 mm Hg).
> 3. Insert a Foley catheter.
> 4. Administer **mannitol 20% 1 to 1.5 g/kg intravenous (IV) rapid infusion.**
> 5. Administer **normal saline (0.9%) at 100 ml/hour (avoid hypotonic fluids).**
> 6. Consult the neurosurgery service.

"buy time" prior to computed tomography (CT) scan and a definitive neurosurgical procedure (craniotomy, ventriculostomy, or placement of an ICP monitor):

Placement of an ICP Monitor

Most clinicians would not treat a patient with suspected high blood pressure without measuring it. However, empirical therapy for increased ICP (i.e., repeated doses of mannitol) without monitoring is used all the time, to the great disadvantage of the patient. This approach is unsatisfactory because most ICP treatments are effective for a short time only, lose their efficacy with prolonged use, and have side effects. Optimally, therapy should be given when ICP is high and should be withheld when it is normal. Only use of an ICP monitor can make this possible.

Indications for ICP monitoring (all three conditions should be met):
1. The patient is in a coma (Glasgow Coma Scale score of ≤8).
2. Increased ICP is suspected.
3. The prognosis is such that aggressive treatment in the intensive care unit (ICU) is indicated.

ICP Monitors

If the decison has been made to treat the patient for suspected ICP, and surgical reduction of intracranial volume (i.e., ventriculostomy or craniotomy) is not feasible, an ICP monitor should be placed. There are three main types of monitors (Fig. 12–1):
  1. **Ventricular catheter**
     Once inserted, a ventricular catheter is connected to both a pressure transducer and an external drainage system via a three-way stopcock. The major advantage to ventricular catheters is that they allow treatment of increased ICP via drainage of cerebrospinal fluid (CSF). The main disadvan-

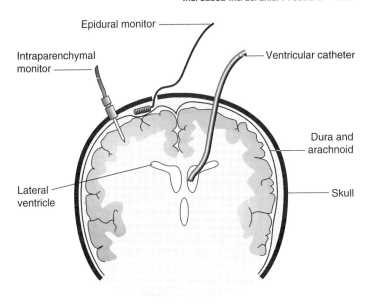

Figure 12-1 ▫ ICP monitoring devices.

tage is the high infection rate (10 to 20%), which increases dramatically after 5 days.

2. **Intraparenchymal probe (Camino, Codman)**
   These devices are easy to insert and very accurate and the infection rate is exceedingly low (approximately 1%).

3. **Epidural transducer (Gaeltec)**
   These devices are inserted deep to the inner table of the skull and superficial to the dura. They are associated with a minimal infection rate but have a tendency to malfunction and to have a baseline drift (>5 to 10 mm Hg) after more than a few days of use.

■ ELEVATOR THOUGHTS

What are the physiologic principles of ICP?

If you are caring for a patient with increased ICP, a firm understanding of intracranial physiology is essential.

Intracranial Anatomy

There are three principal components of volume within the cranium of the normal adult: brain (1400 ml), blood (150 ml), and

CSF (150 ml). CSF is produced by the choroid plexus within the ventricles at a rate of approximately 20 ml/hour, resulting in the formation of almost 500 ml/day. Normal ICP ranges from 50 to 200 mm H_2O (4 to 15 mm Hg). CSF is reabsorbed across the convexity of the meninges into the venous circulation via arachnoid granulations. These pathways normally offer little resistance to CSF outflow. For this reason, jugular venous pressure is normally the principal determinant of ICP.

Intracranial Compliance

Because the cranial vault is a rigid, fixed container, any increase in intracranial volume can lead to increased ICP. In clinical practice, the most common mechanisms of increased intracranial volume are **extrinsic mass lesions, hydrocephalus, and cerebral edema (brain swelling).** Initially, as volume is added to the intracranial space, increases in pressure are minimal because of the highly compliant nature of the intracranial contents; as intracranial volume increases, CSF is displaced through the foramen magnum into the paraspinal space, and blood is displaced from compressed brain tissue. When these mechanisms are exhausted, however, intracranial compliance decreases, and further increases in intracranial volume lead to dramatic elevations of ICP (Fig. 12–2).

Cerebral Perfusion Pressure

Cerebral perfusion pressure (CPP) is routinely monitored in conjunction with the ICP because it is an important determinant of cerebral blood flow (CBF). CPP is defined by the equation

$$CPP = MABP \text{ (mean arterial blood pressure)} - ICP$$

When autoregulation is intact, CBF is maintained at a constant level across a wide range of CPPs (50 to 150 mm Hg). However, in injured brain with impaired autoregulation, CBF approximates a straight-line relationship with CPP; that is, reductions of CBF are more severe at any given level of reduced CPP (Fig. 12–3). **CPP must be closely regulated within a relatively narrow range (70 to 120 mm Hg) in patients with increased ICP,** because reductions below this level can lead to secondary hypoxic-ischemic damage, whereas excessive increases can lead to "breakthrough" hyperperfusion and aggravation of cerebral edema.

ICP Waveforms

The normal ICP waveform (see Fig. 12–2) reflects a transient surge in cerebral blood volume that occurs with each heartbeat. As ICP rises and intracranial compliance decreases, the amplitude

Increased Intracranial Pressure 155

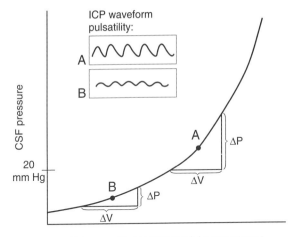

Figure 12–2 □ Intracranial pressure (ICP)-volume curve. At low pressures (point B) the intracranial compartment is compliant, meaning that large increases in volume (ΔV) lead to small increments in pressure (ΔP). At higher pressures (point A) the intracranial space becomes less compliant. As a result, the amplitude and pulsatility of the arterial reflection in the ICP waveform increases *(inset)*. CSF, cerebrospinal fluid.

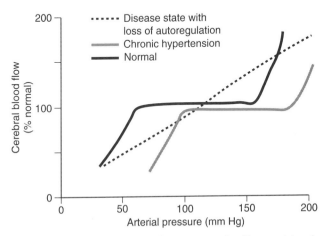

Figure 12–3 □ Cerebral autoregulation curve. In disease states (e.g., vasospasm or ischemia), cerebral blood flow becomes pressure passive *(dotted line)*. With chronic hypertension, the autoregulatory curve shifts to the right.

of the ICP waveform increases, and superimposed pathologic ICP elevations can occur. Two types of pathologic ICP waves have been described (Fig. 12–4):
1. **Lundberg A waves (plateau waves).** Plateau waves are dangerous elevations of ICP; they can reach levels of 20 to 80 mm Hg and are generally from 5 minutes to 1 hour in duration. When severe, they are associated with reduced CPP (less than 60 mm Hg) and CBF and with global hypoxic-ischemic injury.
2. **Lundberg B waves.** These waves are of lesser amplitude (10 to 20 mm Hg) and duration (1 to 5 minutes) than plateau waves and thus are less dangerous. Clinically, they are a useful marker of abnormal autoregulation and reduced intracranial compliance.

■ MANAGEMENT II

General Measures for Treating Patients with Increased ICP

1. **Elevate head of bed by 30 to 45 degrees and maintain a straight head position**
   Head elevation reduces ICP by reducing jugular venous pressure and by enhancing venous outflow. Sharp head an-

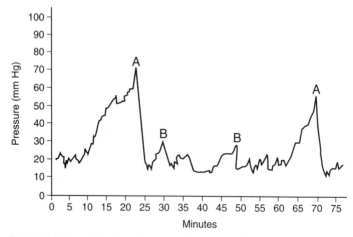

Figure 12–4 □ Pathologic intracranial pressure elevations. A = Lundberg A (plateau) waves; B = Lundberg B waves. (Redrawn from Chestnut RM, Marshall LF: Treatment of abnormal intracranial pressure. Neurosurg Clin North Am 1991;2:267–284.)

gulation should be avoided, because it may cause jugular venous compression, increased venous backpressure, and increased ICP.
2. **Prevent seizures**
   Seizures can lead to profound elevations of CBF, intracranial blood volume, and ICP, even in patients who are paralyzed. **Fosphenytoin (10 to 20 mg/kg loading dose; then 3 to 5 mg/kg per day)** is the preferred agent for seizure prophylaxis.
3. **Treat fever aggressively**
   Fever can exacerbate ICP, and it lowers the threshold for neuronal death. Treatment with **acetaminophen (650 mg every 4 hours), indomethacin (25 mg every 6 hours)**, or a **cooling blanket** can be effective.

Steps for Treating an "ICP Crisis" in an Intubated, Monitored Patient

Proper treatment of increased ICP requires an organized, stepwise approach (Box 12–2). Brief elevations of ICP (lasting only 1 to 5 minutes) occur frequently with suctioning, coughing, and repositioning and do not require aggressive treatment. **In general, the following measures should be instituted only when the ICP is elevated above 20 mm Hg for a period of 10 or more minutes.**
1. **Removal of intracranial mass or drainage of CSF**
   Remember that reduction of intracranial volume is the only definitive treatment for increased ICP. Consider a repeat CT scan in a patient with increasing ICP. If a ventricular catheter

---

Box 12–2. STEPWISE TREATMENT PROTOCOL FOR ELEVATED ICP IN A MONITORED PATIENT (ICP >20 mm Hg FOR >10 MINUTES)

1. Consider repeat CT scanning or definitive neurosurgical intervention (e.g., craniotomy or ventriculostomy)
2. Sedate patient to attain a quiet, motionless state
3. Optimize CPP with vasopressors to maintain >70 mm Hg, or with blood pressure lowering agents maintain <120 mm Hg
4. Mannitol 0.25 to 1.5 g/kg IV every 1–6 hours
5. Hyperventilate to maintain P_{CO_2} between 28 and 32 mm Hg
6. Pentobarbital infusion

is in place, the system should be opened for drainage, and 5 to 10 ml of CSF should be removed.
2. **Sedation and paralysis**
   In patients with reduced intracranial compliance, physical agitation or fighting the ventilator can lead to elevated ICP because of increased intrathoracic, jugular venous, and arterial pressures. *Before further measures are instituted, agitated patients with increased ICP should be sedated to the point at which they are motionless and quiet.*

   Note: Intravenous sedatives cause apnea and hypotension and thus require intubation and intravascular blood pressure monitoring. The following agents can be used:
   - **Morphine IV** is an opioid with sedative-hypnotic and analgesic effects. The dose is **2 to 5 mg IVP every hour.**
   - **Fentanyl IV** (supplied as 50 μg/ml) is also an opioid and is 100 times more potent than morphine. For rapid control of agitation, give **25 to 100 μg IVP.** For sustained sedation, give **fentanyl IV infusion 4 mg/250 ml normal saline (NS).** Start at 5 ml/hour (1.33 μg/min); the range is 8 to 23 ml/hour (2 to 6 μg/min).
   - **Propofol IV (10 mg/ml)** is a powerful sedative-hypnotic drug whose effect is more rapidly reversible than that of fentanyl. The typical maintenance dose is **5 to 50 μg/kg/min (0.3 to 3 mg/kg/hour);** this translates into 2 to 20 ml/hour for a 70-kg person.

3. **CPP optimization**
   If ICP remains elevated in a sedated patient, optimization of CPP should be attempted using vasoactive agents *before* mannitol and hyperventilation are administered.
   - If CPP is > 120 mm Hg and ICP is > 20 mm Hg, BP should be lowered. *However, CPP should not be allowed to fall to < 70 mm Hg.* Agents for controlling hypertension include the following:
     1. **Labetalol IV (5 mg/ml)** is a combined alpha-1 and beta-1 blocker. For immediate control of BP, **push 20 to 80 mg every 10 to 20 minutes.** Once the desired BP is attained, start **200 mg/200 ml NS (1 mg/ml) at 2 mg/min (120 ml/hour) and titrate.**
     2. **Nicardipine IV** is a rapidly titratable calcium channel blocker. Start with **25 mg/250 ml NS at 5 ml/hour (8 μg/min)** and titrate.
   - If CPP is < 70 mm Hg and ICP is > 20 mm Hg, BP should be elevated and CPP raised to > 70 mm Hg; this can lead to a reflex reduction of ICP by reducing the cerebral vasodilatation that occurs in response to inadequate perfusion. Pressor agents for raising CPP include
     1. **Dopamine (800 mg/500 ml NS)** at high doses is an alpha-, beta-, and dopamine receptor agonist. Start at

16 ml/hour (6 μg/kg/min in a 70-kg patient) and titrate upward.
2. Phenylephrine (10 mg/250 ml) is a pure alpha agonist. Start at 15 ml/hour (10 μg/min) and titrate upward.
4. Mannitol

Mannitol, an osmotic diuretic, lowers ICP via its cerebral dehydrating effects. The effects of mannitol are biphasic. Rapid infusion immediately creates an osmotic gradient across the blood-brain barrier, resulting in movement of water from brain to the intravascular compartment. The result is decreased brain tissue volume and, hence, reduced ICP. The secondary effect of mannitol results from its action as an osmotic diuretic. As mannitol is cleared by the kidneys, it leads to free water clearance and increased serum osmolality. As a result, even after the mannitol is gone, an intracellular dehydrating effect is maintained as water flows down the osmotic gradient, from the intracellular to the extracellular space.

- **The initial dose of mannitol 20% solution is 1 to 1.5 g/kg, followed every 1 to 6 hours with doses of 0.25–1.5 g/kg as needed.** The effect on ICP is maximal when mannitol is given rapidly (over 10 minutes).
- The effect of mannitol on ICP begins in 10 to 20 minutes, reaches its peak between 20 and 60 minutes, and lasts for 3 to 6 hours.
- Adverse effects of mannitol therapy include exacerbation of congestive heart failure (because of the initial intravascular volume load); volume contraction, hypokalemia, and profound hyperosmolality (after prolonged use); acute tubular necrosis (because of excessive hyperosmolality); and "rebound" increases in ICP.
- Patients treated repeatedly with mannitol require measurements of serum electrolytes and osmolality every 6 hours, and careful measurement of intake and output. Volume lost through urine should be replaced with NS (0.9%) to avoid volume depletion.

5. Hyperventilation

By acutely lowering the P_{CO_2} level to 26 to 30 mm Hg, *hyperventilation can lower ICP within minutes.* The alkylosis caused by hypocarbia leads to cerebral vasoconstriction, reduced cerebral blood volume, and decreased ICP.

- Hyperventilation is best accomplished by increasing the ventilatory rate (16 to 20 cycles/min) in mechanically ventilated patients, or by using a face mask with an Ambu bag in nonintubated patients.
- *The peak effect of hyperventilation on ICP is generally reached within 30 minutes.* Over the next 1 to 3 hours, the effect may

gradually diminish as compensatory acid-base buffering mechanisms correct the alkylosis, but exceptions can occur.
- Once ICP is stabilized, hyperventilation should be tapered slowly over 6 to 12 hours, because abrupt cessation can lead to vasodilatation and rebound increases in ICP.

Note: Beware that prolonged severe hyperventilation (P_{CO_2} less than 25 mm Hg) may actually exacerbate cerebral ischemia by causing excessive vasoconstriction.

6. Pentobarbital

High-dose barbiturate therapy, given in doses equivalent to those inducing general anesthesia, can effectively lower ICP in most patients refractory to the steps outlined above. The effect of pentobarbital is multifactorial but most likely stems from coupled decreases in cerebral metabolism, blood flow, and blood volume. In addition, pentobarbital causes profound hypotension and usually requires the use of vasopressors to maintain CPP at or higher than 70 mm Hg.

- **Pentobarbital typically requires a loading dose of 10 to 20 mg/kg, given in repeated 5 mg/kg boluses,** until a state of flaccid coma with preserved pupillary reactivity is attained. IV pressors (dopamine, phenylephrine) should be ready at the bedside to maintain BP and CPP.
- **Maintenance doses are usually 1 to 4 mg/kg/hour (order as 500 mg/250 ml NS, starting at 35 ml/hour).** Continuous or intermittent electroencephalogram (EEG) monitoring should be used, with the infusion rate titrated to a burst-suppression pattern.
- If ICP is adequately controlled with pentobarbital, it is generally maintained for 24 to 48 hours. It can then be discontinued abruptly, with a wash-out period lasting from 24 to 96 hours.
- Failure of ICP to respond to pentobarbital is an ominous sign. If ICP remains markedly elevated (higher than 30 mm Hg), discontinuation of all aggressive measures should be considered.

chapter 13 | Dizziness and Vertigo

Dizziness and vertigo are among the most common neurologic complaints. The etiology of these conditions may range from benign labyrinthitis to serious cardiac syncope to life-threatening cerebellar hemorrhage. Vertigo may be defined specifically as a sensation of movement—either of the environment or of the patient. A spinning sensation is most commonly described, but feelings of acceleration or other movement may also be reported. Dizziness, on the other hand, may be used to mean vertigo, but it may also mean lightheadedness, fatigue, or a general sense of illness.

■ PHONE CALL

Questions

1. **Does the patient have a normal level of consciousness?**
   Vertigo followed by a decreased level of consciousness may be a sign of impending herniation, a neurologic emergency.
2. **When did the dizziness or vertigo begin?**
   In general, a more acute onset requires a greater urgency in making a diagnosis.
3. **What are the vital signs?**
   Rapid, slowed, or irregular heart rhythm may suggest cardiac syncope or cardioembolic stroke. Fever may suggest infection. Tachypnea may be a sign of heart failure or an anxiety attack.

Orders

1. Obtain a finger stick glucose.
2. Obtain orthostatic blood pressure.
3. Obtain an electrocardiogram (ECG).

Inform RN

"Will arrive at the bedside in . . . minutes."

■ ELEVATOR THOUGHTS

What is the Differential Diagnosis of Dizziness and Vertigo?
The most common causes of dizziness and vertigo are or-

thostatic hypotension, medication side effect, **benign positional vertigo,** and **labyrinthitis.** A more complete differential diagnosis follows.

V (vascular): brain stem stroke (most often pontine, brachium pontis, or cerebellar), cerebellar hemorrhage, arteriovenous malformation (AVM) (rare), brain stem transient ischemic attacks (TIAs) resulting from vertebrobasilar stenosis ("insufficiency") or embolism, vasodepressor syncope, postural hypotension, cardiac arrhythmia

I (infectious): syphilis, viral or bacterial meningitis, otitis media with labyrinthitis, Lyme disease involving the vestibular cranial nerve, viral cerebellitis (mostly in children)

T (traumatic): head trauma or postconcussional syndrome

A (autoimmune): multiple sclerosis

M (metabolic/toxic): diabetes with hypoglycemia, dehydration, drug toxicity (Table 13–1)

I (idiopathic/iatrogenic): benign positional vertigo, Meniere's disease

N (neoplastic): neurofibroma, schwannoma, or meningioma of the acoustic nerve; brain stem glioma; posterior fossa metastasis

S (seizure/psychiatric)

■ MAJOR THREAT TO LIFE

- Cerebellar infarction or hemorrhage

■ BEDSIDE

Quick Look Test

Is the patient awake and alert?

Lethargy may indicate a brain stem or cerebellar stroke with potential for herniation or progression to coma.

Selective History and Chart Review

1. Is the dizziness lightheadedness or true vertigo?

Lightheadedness, a swimming sensation, faintness, or other similar symptoms point to a systemic disorder such as cardiac syncope, postural hypotension, or systemic infection. True **vertigo,** on the other hand, suggests neurologic dysfunction. The physical examination will help clarify the differential diagnosis, which will focus on distinguishing a peripheral cause from a central nervous system cause for vertigo.

Table 13-1 ▫ COMMON MEDICATIONS THAT CAUSE VERTIGO AND DIZZINESS*

Anticonvulsants: carbamazepine, phenytoin, primidone, ethosuximide, methsuximide
Antidepressants: nortriptyline and other tricyclic antidepressants
Antihypertensives: enalapril
Antihistamines: ranitidine, cimetidine
Antiarrhythmics: flecainide
Antibiotics: streptomycin, tobramycin, gentamicin
Analgesics: propoxyphene (Darvocet), naproxen, indomethacin
Neuroleptics: phenothiazines
Tranquilizers: diazepam, chlordiazepoxide, meprobamate
Aspirin
Digoxin

*Many medications have dizziness as a side effect. This is a partial list.

2. **What is the time course of the symptoms?**
   As already noted, an acute onset of vertigo may indicate posterior fossa stroke or hemorrhage. Rapid onset of lightheadedness can occur with cardiac disease. A more gradual onset may suggest medication toxicity, infection, tumor, or demyelinating disease. If this is an episode in a series of recurrences, Meniere's disease or benign positional vertigo may be the cause.
3. **Do the symptoms change with changes in head position?**
   Dizziness on standing may indicate orthostatic hypotension; dizziness or vertigo with head turning may be a sign of benign positional vertigo or labyrinthitis.
4. **Has the patient begun any new medications recently?**
   Table 13–1 shows common medications that cause vertigo. Dizziness without true vertigo is one of the most common side effects of medication. Refer to the *Physician's Desk Reference* for medications not listed in the table.
5. **Are there any accompanying symptoms?**
   Ask about symptoms specific to the brain stem, including diplopia, dysarthria, and ataxia. Tinnitus may localize the problem to the inner ear. If there is posterior neck or head pain, consider vertebral artery dissection and stroke.

Selective Physical Examination

General Physical Examination

HEENT   Be sure to look into the external auditory canal for vesicles of herpes zoster. Unilateral hearing loss and tinnitus are reliable signs of injury outside the brain stem.

Abdomen   Hepatomegaly, ascites, and caput medusae are signs of chronic alcohol abuse.

Neurologic Examination

1. **Mental status**

   Ensure that the patient is awake, alert, and attentive. Decreased attentiveness may suggest drug toxicity or metabolic disarray. If there is vertigo with decreased alertness, see Chapter 5 for further management.

2. **Cranial nerves**

   Any cranial nerve abnormality in combination with dizziness or vertigo should be considered a sign of brain injury until it is proved otherwise.

   a. Nystagmus

   When vestibular input to the brain stem is disrupted (e.g., damage to the vestibular nerve or inner ear apparatus), the eyes will drift toward the affected side. Repeated corrective saccades result in nystagmus, with the fast phase away from the lesion. The sensation of movement experienced with vertigo is the illusion of environmental drift as the eyes move through the slow phase of nystagmus in the other direction. Corrective saccades are suppressed by visual tracking systems so that there is a sensation of continued field shift in one direction. Oscillopsia—the illusion of the environment's jumping or oscillating—is actually quite rare. Nystagmus subtypes are listed in Table 13–2. A common and crucial differential diagnosis that arises in almost every case of vertigo is whether the process is peripheral, and often benign, or whether it represents a lesion in the brain stem or cerebellum. Certain characteristics of nystagmus can help identify the site of pathology (Table 13–3).

   (1) Look for nystagmus in the primary gaze by having the patient fix on your finger. More subtle nystagmus can be seen by looking for oscillations of the fundus on indirect ophthalmoscopy.

   (2) Have the patient follow your finger through the full range of horizontal and vertical gaze. The hand should be kept at a distance of 2 to 3 feet to minimize convergence, which should be tested separately.

   (3) Provocative tests may be helpful in distinguishing peripheral from central injury.

   (a) Nystagmus should be looked for with the patient in different positions, particularly if the patient notes a positional component to the vertigo. The Bárány maneuver is useful in helping to distinguish the positional vertigo of a benign vestibular disorder from a brain stem lesion (Fig. 13–1). A

Table 13-2 □ SUBTYPES OF NYSTAGMUS

Physiologic nystagmus
  Fine nystagmus at ends of gaze, extinguishes after a few beats
  Significance: none, if symmetric
Asymmetric horizontal nystagmus
  Horizontal or rotational
  Fast phase always in one direction
  Worse with gaze in one direction than in the other
  Often made worse with change in head position
  Significance: most often labyrinthine or vestibular disease (benign positional vertigo, labyrinthitis, Meniere's disease), but may be due to cerebellar or brain stem lesions
Vertical nystagmus
  Upbeat or downbeat nystagmus
  May be present with sedative or anticonvulsant medication
  Significance: if no drug toxicity is present, vertical nystagmus almost always means brain stem disease at the midbrain or craniocervical junction
Dissociated or abduction nystagmus
  Unilateral horizontal fast component in direction of gaze in the abducted eye
  Significance: internuclear ophthalmoplegia (e.g., in multiple sclerosis)
Convergence-retraction nystagmus
  Part of Parinaud's syndrome of impaired upgaze, impaired pupillary reaction, convergence insufficiency
  Fast component is convergence and retraction of both globes
  Significance: mass lesion compression of the tectum of the midbrain, for example, by pineal tumor, or a midbrain stroke in the region of the aqueduct of Sylvius
Pendular nystagmus
  Usually horizontal
  Sinusoidal waveform (oscillation, equal velocity in either direction)
  Significance: congenital; if acquired, most commonly multiple sclerosis; also cerebrovascular disease of the cerebellum or brain stem
Periodic alternating nystagmus
  Horizontal, with fast phase alternating directions in cycles of 1 to 3 minutes
  May coexist with downbeat nystagmus
  Significance: congenital or acquired lesions at the craniocervical junction
Ocular dysmetria
  Overshooting on attempt to refix on an eccentric target (e.g., moving from the examiner's nose to a finger held to the side)
  Overshooting may be followed by ever-shortening saccadic corrections
  Significance: cerebellar disease
Ocular bobbing
  Repetitive rapid conjugate downward movement followed by slow drift back to primary position
  Found in comatose patients
  Significance: severe central pontine destruction

Table 13-3 □ **CHARACTERISTICS OF NYSTAGMUS ARISING FROM PERIPHERAL OR CENTRAL CAUSES**

Nystagmus from peripheral causes
  Extinguishes with repetitive provocative maneuvers
  Exhibits latency of several seconds with provocative maneuvers
  Rotational nystagmus
  Hearing loss or tinnitus
  No accompanying brain stem signs
Nystagmus from central causes
  Any vertical nystagmus
  Accompanying brain stem signs
  Does not extinguish with provocative maneuvers
  No latency with provocative maneuvers

rotational component, a latency of a few seconds in onset of the nystagmus, and a lessening of the magnitude of the response with subsequent trials all suggest peripheral lesions.

(b) Injecting cold water into the ear on the side of an intact vestibular pathway (see Fig. 5–2) will result in nystagmus, with the fast component beating away from the stimulus. If the patient is comatose, cold water will induce the ipsiversive gaze with no contralateral corrective saccades. Be sure you view an intact tympanic membrane before attempting this test. Also be warned that the stimulus may produce nausea in an awake patient.

b. Diplopia, dysarthria, facial motor or sensory asymmetry, decreased gag response, or asymmetry of tongue protrusion

Any of these should alert you to the possibility of a CNS lesion.

3. **Cerebellar**
Evaluate for limb ataxia and gait ataxia.

■ MANAGEMENT

1. **Rule out a posterior fossa mass lesion.**
Because the consequences of missing a cerebellar hematoma or posterior fossa tumor can be serious, a **noncontrast computed tomography (CT) scan** should be obtained in all cases of first-time vertigo, particularly in the elderly, and certainly if there is any hint of brain stem involvement. CT is poor at identifying smaller lesions and infarcts in the posterior fossa because of the substantial bony artifact. If a

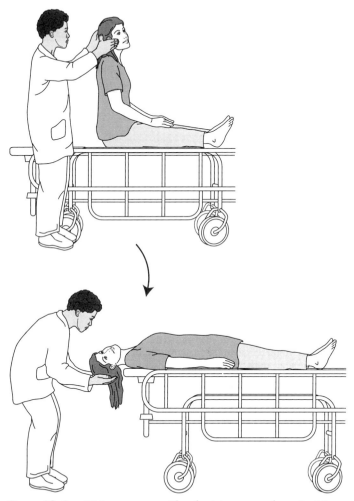

Figure 13–1 □ Bárány maneuver. The physician moves the patient from a sitting to a supine position, with the head rotated to one side and hyperextended 30 degrees. The test is positive if vertigo is re-created. Nystagmus should be seen with the onset of symptomatic vertigo.

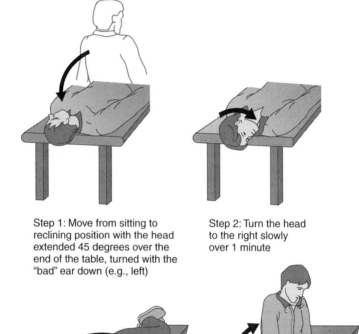

Step 1: Move from sitting to reclining position with the head extended 45 degrees over the end of the table, turned with the "bad" ear down (e.g., left)

Step 2: Turn the head to the right slowly over 1 minute

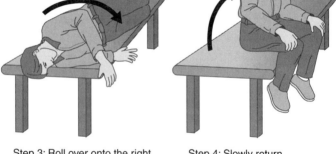

Step 3: Roll over onto the right side, with the head looking down at the floor

Step 4: Slowly return to sitting position with the chin tilted down

Figure 13–2 ◻ Four-step canalith repositioning procedure for benign positional vertigo (modified Epley maneuver). The clinician should support and rotate the patient's head in steps 1 and 2.

brain stem lesion is suspected but not identified on CT, a **magnetic resonance imaging (MRI) scan** should be obtained.
2. **Correct any obvious metabolic disorder,** or discontinue, taper, or substitute any toxic medication. Treat cardiac syncope if present.
3. **Identify a possible peripheral cause.**

    If no posterior fossa lesion and no metabolic abnormality is identified, a peripheral cause for vertigo may be present. Such causes include labyrinthitis (postinfectious congestion or inflammation of the labyrinths), Meniere's disease (recurrent attacks of severe vertigo, nausea and vomiting, tinnitus, and hearing loss) and benign positional vertigo (see below). An **electronystagmogram** may be useful in making a diagnosis of peripheral vestibulopathy. An audiogram may be useful in diagnosing Meniere's disease.
4. **Treat benign positional vertigo empirically.**

    Benign positional vertigo is a type of vertigo that occurs in adults over 50 years of age. This type of vertigo is thought to arise when particulate debris accumulates in the posterior semicircular canal. Particular head positions or head movement may cause the particles to stimulate hair cells and produce the sensation of movement. Benign positional vertigo may respond to **meclizine 25 mg by mouth (PO) three times a day.** Central causes of dizziness generally do not respond to meclizine. Nonmedicational treatment of benign positional vertigo has been successful in many cases. The two approaches are desensitization exercises, in which the patient moves through a series of repetitive head and body positions twice daily, and canalith repositioning procedures, such as the modified Epley maneuver, in which the head is rotated slowly from the bad side to the good side in an effort to move the particles out of the posterior semicircular canal (Fig. 13–2). Following the Epley maneuver, the patient is asked to sleep sitting up for two nights.

chapter 14 | Headache

Headache is one of the most common complaints presented to neurologists. In general, headaches can be grouped into two broad diagnostic categories. One group comprises the **primary headache disorders,** for example, migraine, tension, and cluster headaches. The second category comprises **symptomatic headache** resulting from intracranial lesions, systemic diseases, or local diseases of the eye or nasopharynx. The goal in evaluating headache is to establish the diagnosis and initiate effective treatment.

■ PHONE CALL

Questions

1. **How severe is the headache?**
2. **Was the onset sudden or gradual?**
    Sudden onset of extremely severe headache is suggestive of subarachnoid hemorrhage or meningitis.
3. **When did the headaches begin?**
    Recent-onset headaches or headaches that have become progressively worse over time suggest a symptomatic etiology such as subdural hematoma or brain tumor.
4. **What are the vital signs?**
5. **Has there been a change in level of consciousness?**
6. **Is the patient experiencing nausea or vomiting?**
    Nausea and vomiting can occur with severe migraine or with conditions associated with increased intracranial pressure (ICP).

Orders

1. Place the patient in a quiet, darkened room.
2. Start **D5NS IV at 80 ml/hour if** nausea and vomiting are severe.
3. Obtain a temperature if this has not already been obtained.
4. Order an erythrocyte sedimentation rate (ESR) if the patient is older than 50 years of age.
5. If you are confident that the headache represents a chronic, previously diagnosed problem, the patient can be treated with an agent that has previously relieved the headache or with **acetaminophen 650 mg.**

ELEVATOR THOUGHTS

What causes headache?

Primary Headache Disorders

1. Tension headache
2. Migraine headache
3. Cluster headache
4. Paroxysmal hemicrania
5. Trigeminal neuralgia
6. Occipital neuralgia (cervical osteoarthritis)

Symptomatic Headache Disorders

1. Vascular
    - Subarachnoid hemorrhage
    - Intracerebral hemorrhage
    - Cerebral infarction
2. Infectious
    - Meningitis
    - Sinusitis
3. Posttraumatic (postconcussion) headache
4. Increased intracranial pressure
    - Intracranial mass lesions (brain tumor, hemorrhage, etc.)
    - Malignant hypertension
    - Idiopathic intracranial hypertension (pseudotumor cerebri)
5. Decreased intracranial pressure
    - Spontaneous intracranial hypotension
    - Post–lumbar puncture headache
6. Temporal arteritis
7. Drug exposure or withdrawal
    - Nitrate exposure
    - Caffeine withdrawal

MAJOR THREAT TO LIFE

- **Subarachnoid hemorrhage**
  Aneurysmal subarachnoid hemorrhage, if not properly diagnosed, can lead to fatal rebleeding.
- **Bacterial meningitis**
  Bacterial meningitis must be recognized early if antibiotic treatment is to be successful.
- **Herniation from intracranial mass lesions**
  Herniation may occur as a result of a tumor, subdural or epidural hematoma, abscess, or any other mass lesion.

■ BEDSIDE

Quick Look Test

Does the patient look well (comfortable), sick (uncomfortable), or critical (about to die)?

Most patients with chronic headache look well, whereas those with severe migraines, subarachnoid hemorrhage, or meningitis look sick.

Airway and Vital Signs

What is the temperature?

Fever associated with headache suggests meningitis. However, headache can also represent a nonspecific reaction to a systemic febrile illness.

What is the blood pressure (BP)?

Contrary to popular belief, headache is rarely caused by hypertension, unless the hypertension is acute and severe (diastolic pressure greater than 120 mm Hg). Hypertension may also reflect subarachnoid hemorrhage, acute stroke, or increased ICP from an intracranial mass lesion.

Selective History and Chart Review

A detailed, well-focused history is the most important tool in diagnosing the cause of headache. The following questions are important:

1. **What is the quality of the pain?**
   Tension headache is frequently described as tight, aching, and band-like. Migraine often has a throbbing quality.
2. **Where is the pain located?**
   Tension headache is usually generalized and most prominent in the occiput and forehead. Alternating unilateral headaches suggest migraine. Cluster headaches are periorbital.
3. **What time of day do the headaches occur?**
   Tension headaches typically develop in the late morning or the early afternoon and go away with sleep. Cluster headaches frequently strike *after* the patient has gone to sleep and tend to occur at the same time every day.
4. **Do warning symptoms occur before the headaches begin?**
   Migraine is often preceded by prodromal symptoms of hunger, restlessness, or moodiness. Classic migraine is preceded by an aura that is usually visual. Neurologic symptoms that persist once the headache has started are unusual in migraine and suggest a structural lesion (i.e., neoplasm or arteriovenous malformation).

5. **Do any factors precipitate the headaches?**
   Migraine is frequently precipitated by emotional stress, fatigue, foods containing tyramine (e.g., red wine or cheese), or menstruation.
6. **Are any symptoms associated with the headache?**
   Nausea, vomiting, photophobia, and phonophobia are highly characteristic of migraine. Ipsilateral tearing or nasal congestion occur with cluster headache.
7. **Is there a history of chronic or recurring headaches?**
   The longer a headache has lasted in its present form, the more likely it is to be benign. Headaches that are qualitatively different from previous headaches should raise suspicion for a symptomatic etiology.
8. **Do headaches run in the family?**
   Migraine is familial in approximately 50% of cases.

Selective Physical Examination

In most patients with headache, the neurologic and physical examinations are normal. The primary purpose of the initial screening examination is to check for signs of *meningismus, increased intracranial pressure, or neurologic focality.*

General Physical Examination

HEENT	• Sinus tenderness (sinusitis)
	• Temporal artery tenderness (temporal arteritis)
	• Conjunctival injection (cluster headache)
	• Cranial bruit (arteriovenous malformation)
Neck	• Neck rigidity (subarachnoid hemorrhage, meningitis)
	• Neck muscle spasm (tension headache)
	• Kernig's and Brudzinski's signs (Fig. 14–1)

Neurologic Examination

- Level of consciousness
- Confusion or disorientation
- Pupil symmetry
- Papilledema and spontaneous venous pulsations
- Retinal hemorrhages (flame or subhyaloid)
- Pronator drift
- Deep tendon and plantar reflexes
- Gait

■ DIAGNOSTIC TESTING

Diagnostic testing is not necessary if the patient has a long history of characteristic primary headaches (migraine, tension,

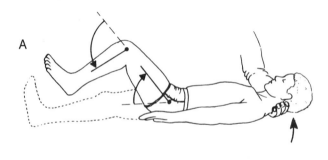

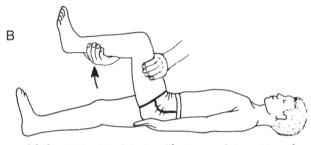

Figure 14–1 □ *A*, Brudzinski's sign. The test result is positive when the patient actively flexes the hips and knees in response to passive neck flexion by the examiner. *B*, Kernig's sign. The test result is positive when pain or resistance prevents full extension of the knee from the 90-degree hip/knee flexion position. (From Marshall SA, Ruedy J: On Call: Principles and Protocols, 2nd ed. Philadelphia, WB Saunders Co, 1993.)

or cluster), a normal neurologic examination, and no fever or meningismus.

1. **Obtain a CT scan in patients with the following:**
   - Acute, extremely severe headache ("thunderclap headache")
   - Headache with progressive onset over days to weeks that is not similar to previous headaches
   - Altered mental status (even if intoxicated)
   - Focal neurologic signs
   - Papilledema
2. **If subarachnoid hemorrhage or meningitis is suspected and the CT scan is negative, a follow-up lumbar puncture (LP) is mandatory.**

   Fifteen percent of patients with aneurysmal subarachnoid hemorrhage have a negative CT scan. In these instances, the diagnosis can be made only by cerebrospinal fluid (CSF) examination (increased numbers of red blood cells and xanthochromia are present).

When bacterial meningitis is suspected, it is generally a good idea to obtain a CT scan before performing an LP, as long as administration of antibiotics is not delayed. *CT scanning prior to LP is mandatory in patients with depressed level of consciousness, neurologic focality, papilledema, or acquired immune deficiency syndrome (AIDS), because of the high likelihood of detecting a mass lesion in these patients.* As long as the patient does not look terribly ill, antibiotics should be held until after the LP, as long as both the CT and LP can be performed **within 1 hour.** Otherwise, treat first, keeping in mind that the CSF culture results may be negative. **Empirical treatment of suspected meningitis consists of ceftriaxone 1 g intravenously (IV) every 12 hours and ampicillin IV 2 g every 6 hours.**

■ MANAGEMENT: SPECIFIC DISORDERS AND THEIR TREATMENT

Migraine Headache

The term "migraine" is often used to describe any severe headache. However, migraine is a specific clinical syndrome with a distinct pathophysiology. *The diagnosis of migraine is based not on the quality of the pain (i.e., throbbing) but on the characteristic symptoms associated with the headache.*

Common Migraine (Migraine Without Aura). This is defined by the following criteria.
1. Recurrent headaches of 4 to 72 hours' duration with *at least two* of the following characteristics:
   - Unilateral location
   - Pulsating quality
   - Severe enough in intensity to limit daily activity
   - Aggravated by light physical activity (e.g., walking)
2. In addition, *at least one* of the following characteristics must be present:
   - Nausea or vomiting
   - Photophobia and phonophobia

Classic Migraine (Migraine with Aura). This resembles common migraine except that it is preceded by an aura—a fully reversible symptom indicative of focal cerebral dysfunction. Common types of aura include the following:
- Homonymous visual disturbance
- Unilateral paresthesias or numbness

- Unilateral weakness
- Aphasia or other speech disorder

In the typical patient with classic migraine, a visual aura precedes the headache by 10 to 20 minutes. The aura is usually characterized by scintillations (shimmering, geometric patterns known as fortification spectra), migrating scotomata, or waving and blurring of vision. In some patients, aura may occur without the subsequent headache.

Complicated Migraine. This refers to a migraine headache with particularly severe or persistent sensorimotor deficits, suggestive of cerebral infarction. In these patients, vasoconstrictors such as ergotamine should be avoided because of the risk of precipitating cerebral infarction.

Treatment

Start with **identifying and eliminating inciting factors.** Many women experience fewer migraines after discontinuing oral contraceptives. Mild migraine headaches may respond to symptomatic treatment with **nonsteroidal anti-inflammatory drugs (NSAIDs)** such as ibuprofen or naproxen. Adjunctive therapy with **antiemetics (metoclopramide 10 to 15 mg PO four times a day; prochlorperazine 5 to 10 mg PO four times a day or 25 mg PO twice a day)** may also be used to reduce nausea and vomiting. Therapy with simple analgesics should be tried prior to using combination medications (Fioricet, Midrin). Moderate-to-severe migraine headaches may require **abortive therapy** with an *ergot-containing agent* or a *triptan*, which should be taken as soon as possible after the start of the headache in an attempt to cut it short. Sumatriptan and zolmitriptan are generally most effective, with 60 to 70% of patients responding within 2 hours, but zolmitriptan lasts longer and has a lower frequency of "rebound" headache. Agents used for abortive therapy in migraine are listed in Table 14–1.

Patients with frequent disabling attacks of migraine (more than one per week) who fail to respond to abortive therapy alone should be considered for **preventive therapy.** Agents used for migraine prevention are listed in Table 14–2. *Beta blockers or tricyclic antidepressants* are the usual first-line agents; valproic acid may be particularly effective for patients who fail first-line therapy.

A protocol for the **emergency room treatment of severe migraine** is shown in Table 14–3. Intravenous hydration is important for patients with intractable vomiting. If sumatriptan is unsuccessful, "cocktail" treatment with *prochlorperazine, dihydroergotamine,* and *dexamethasone* can break the cycle of intractable migraine in most patients. In severe cases, the migraine headache can last for days (**status migrainosus**).

Tension Headache

Tension headaches are also known as "muscle contraction headaches," although muscle contraction has little to do with the pathogenesis. Because most people experience tension headaches to some degree, those who present for medical evaluation (less than 5% of the population) either have unusually frequent or severe symptoms or are depressed. Headache that never goes away or that grows worse as the day progresses is suggestive of tension headache. The pain is usually bilateral, most prominent in the occiput and frontal regions, and is described as tight, pressing, or band-like. Associated eye strain or neck and scalp muscle tightness is common. **Chronic daily headache** refers to tension headaches associated with overuse of NSAIDs or other analgesic agents, in which medication withdrawal contributes significantly to the pathogenesis.

Treatment

Most patients respond to **relaxation techniques** and **NSAIDs** such as ibuprofen or naproxen (see Table 14–1). If the patient is depressed, an antidepressant may be helpful. If the patient has chronic daily headache, it may be necessary to taper the analgesics.

Cluster Headache

Cluster headache is characterized by excruciating unilateral head pain, often localized to the orbit, associated with ipsilateral tearing, conjunctival injection, and nasal congestion. The pain is described as sharp, boring, and piercing and occurs in brief episodes (15 minutes to 2 hours) without prodrome. The headaches are distributed into "clusters," occurring daily for 3 weeks to 3 months, then remitting for months or years. Cluster headaches are most common early in the morning or late at night, and they frequently occur with regularity at a particular time of day. Men are affected five times more often than are women. Ipsilateral facial flushing, Horner's syndrome, and exacerbation of symptoms by alcohol are seen in some patients.

Treatment

Any abortive treatment for migraine can be used to abort a cluster headache, but the following agents are particularly effective:

1. **Ergotamine 1 to 2 mg PO**
2. **Sumatriptan 6 mg SC**
3. **Oxygen 100% at 7 to 10 L/min**
4. **Dihydroergotamine (D.H.E.) 1 mg IV**
5. **Lidocaine 4% 1 ml intranasally**

Table 14-1 □ SELECTED MEDICATIONS USED FOR ABORTIVE THERAPY OF MIGRAINE HEADACHE*

Drug	Dosage
Nonsteroidal anti-inflammatory agents (NSAIDs)	
Acetaminophen (Tylenol)	325–650 mg PO q4h prn (325-mg tabs)
Aspirin	325–650 mg PO q4h prn (325-mg tabs)
Celecoxib (Celebrex)†	100 mg PO bid (100-, 200-mg tabs)
Diclofenac (Voltaren)	50 mg PO q8h prn (50-mg tabs)
Indomethacin (Indocin)	25–50 mg PO/PR q8h prn (25-, 50-mg caps, 50-mg supp)
Ibuprofen (Motrin, Advil)	400–800 mg q6h prn (200-, 400-, 600-, 800-mg tabs)
Ketorolac (Toradol)	10 mg q4h prn, up to 5 days total duration (10-mg tabs)
Naproxen (Naprosyn, Anaprox)	500–750 mg at onset, 250–375 mg q4h prn (250-, 375-, 500-mg tabs)
Piroxicam (Feldene)	20 mg PO qd (10-, 20-mg tabs)
Rofecoxib (Vioxx)†	12.5–50 mg PO qd (1.5-, 25-mg tabs)
Sulindac (Clinoril)	150–200 mg PO qd (150-, 200-mg tabs)
Non-narcotic analgesic combinations	
Acetaminophen/butalbital/caffeine 325/50/40 mg (Fioricet)	1–2 tabs q4h prn, maximum 6 per day
Aspirin/butalbital/caffeine 325/50/40 mg (Fiorinal)	1–2 tabs q4h prn, maximum 6 per day
Isometheptene/acetaminophen/dichloralphenazone 65/325/100 mg (Midrin)	2 capsules at onset, repeat 1 q1h prn, maximum of 5 per day, 10 per week

Ergot medications

Ergotamine tartrate (Ergomar) — 2 mg SL at onset, repeat q 30 min prn, max 6 mg per attack or 10 mg per week (2-mg tabs)

Ergotamine/caffeine 1/100 mg (Cafergot, Ercaf, Wigraine) — 1-2 tabs PO at onset, repeat q 30 min prn, max 6 tabs/attack; suppositories 2/100 mg PR, up to 2 per attack

Dihydroergotamine (DHE-45, Migranal nasal spray) — 1 mg IV/IM/SC, repeat q1h prn, max 2 mg IV or 3 mg SC/IM qd; nasal spray 1 in each nostril, repeat q15 min prn, max 6 sprays/day (0.5 mg per spray)

Serotonin (5-HT1) receptor agonists

Naratriptan (Amerge) — 1-2.5 mg PO, may repeat after 4h, max 5 mg qd (tabs 1, 2.5 mg)
Rizatriptan (Maxalt) — 5-10 mg PO, may repeat after 2h, max 30 mg qd (tabs 5, 10 mg)
Sumatriptan (Imitrex) — 6 mg SQ, may repeat after 1h, max 12 mg qd; 25-100 mg PO, repeat q2h prn, max 300 mg qd (tabs 25, 50 mg); 5-20 mg nasal spray, repeat q2h prn, max 40 mg qd (spray 5, 20 mg)

Zolmitriptan (Zomig) — 1.25-2.5 mg PO q2h, max 10 mg qd (tabs 2.5, 5 mg)

---

*Medication classes are listed in general order of preference.
†Cox-2 inhibitor with minimal gastrointestinal side effects.

Table 14-2 □ DRUGS USED FOR PREVENTIVE THERAPY OF MIGRAINE*

Beta blockers
Propranolol (Inderal, Inderal LA): 40–320 mg daily (10-, 20-, 40-, 60-, 80-mg tabs qid; 60-, 80-, 120-, 160-mg long-acting tabs bid)
Nadolol (Corgard): 20–120 mg qd (20-, 40-, 80-, 120-mg tabs)
Atenolol (Tenormin): 25–100 mg qd (25-, 50-, 100-mg tabs)

Tricyclic antidepressants
Amitriptyline (Elavil): 50–200 mg qhs (10-, 25-, 50-, 75-mg tabs)
Nortriptyline (Pamelor): 25–150 mg qhs (10-, 25-, 50-, 75-mg tabs)

Anticonvulsant
Valproic acid (Depakote, Depakene): 125–750 mg PO tid (125, 250, 500 mg tid)

Calcium-channel blocker
Verapamil (Calan, Calan SR): 80–160 mg daily (40-, 80-, 120-mg tabs q8h; sustained release 120-, 180-, 240-mg qd)

Anti-serotonin drugs
Methysergide (Sansert): 2 mg qd-tid (2-mg tabs)
Cyproheptadine (Periactin): 4–8 mg tid (4-mg tabs)

MAO inhibitor
Phenelzine (Nardil): 15–30 mg PO tid (15-mg tabs)

*Medications are listed in general order of preference.

Table 14–3 ◻ PROTOCOL FOR THE EMERGENCY ROOM TREATMENT OF MIGRAINE

Mild to moderate migraine
Administer sumatriptan 6 mg SC
Severe or refractory migraine
1. Insert IV line or Hep-Lock.
2. Premedicate with **promethazine (Phenergan) 50 mg** or **prochlorperazine (Compazine) 10 mg IV.**
3. Administer **dihydroergotamine (D.H.E. 45 1 mg IV push over 2 minutes).**
4. Follow with **dexamethasone (Decadron) 4 to 12 mg IV.**
5. Repeat 1 mg D.H.E. 45 every 1 to 2 hours as needed (maximum 3 mg/day).

In some patients, the cluster headache can be managed with purely abortive treatment. In many cases, however, daily prophylactic medication must be given. Commonly used preventive agents include the following:
1. Prednisone 20 to 40 mg per day
2. Methysergide 2 mg four times a day (limit to 6 months)
3. Cyproheptadine 2 to 4 mg four times a day
4. Verapamil 80 mg three times a day
5. Lithium 300 mg three to four times a day
6. Ergotamine 1 mg two times a day
7. Valproate 200 to 500 mg every 6 hours

Postconcussion Headache

After concussion, patients may complain of headache, dizziness, poor concentration, and irritability (postconcussional syndrome). Brain imaging is normal, as is the neurologic examination, except for the occasional finding of nystagmus. In many cases, there is coexisting depression, anxiety, or potential for secondary gain, such as a disability claim or litigation.

Treatment

Begin with **NSAIDs** (see Table 14–1) and provide reassurance; in most cases, the symptoms remit over a period of weeks to months. In protracted cases with depressive symptoms, a tricyclic agent may be helpful.

Idiopathic Intracranial Hypertension (Pseudotumor Cerebri)

Also known as benign intracranial hypertension, this illness is characterized by the triad of *headache, papilledema, and increased ICP* in the absence of an intracranial mass lesion or hydrocephalus. The disease occurs almost exclusively in obese young women. The key to establishing the diagnosis is excluding other causes of increased ICP. These include dural sinus thrombosis, chronic meningitis, hypervitaminosis A, and tetracycline or steroid exposure. Depressed level of consciousness and focal neurologic deficits do not occur, except for occasional CN6 palsies.

The main hazard in idiopathic intracranial hypertension is **visual loss** that results from optic nerve damage, which can be permanent. If this diagnosis is suspected, MRI with magnetic resonance venography should be performed to rule out a mass lesion, hydrocephalus, or dural sinus thrombosis. If the MRI is normal, LP establishes the diagnosis by the finding of normal CSF under increased pressure (greater than 20 cm H_2O).

Treatment

About one third of patients have spontaneous remission of headache after the first LP. Many patients will respond to repeated lumbar taps and removal of CSF, performed every few days to every few weeks. In the extremely obese, weight reduction is recommended. If the patient does not respond to serial LPs, start **acetazolamide 250 to 500 mg three times a day. Prednisone 40 to 60 mg PO per day** or **dexamethasone 6 to 12 mg per day** may be added with additional benefit in patients who do not respond to acetazolamide alone. All patients should have baseline **visual field and acuity testing.** If visual loss progresses despite medical therapy, a lumboperitoneal shunt or optic nerve sheath decompression may be necessary.

Temporal (Giant Cell) Arteritis

Temporal arteritis, a sytemic illness of elderly patients, is characterized by inflammatory infiltrates of lymphocytes and giant cells in cranial arteries. It occurs almost exclusively in patients older than 50. Most patients have systemic symptoms of low-grade fever, diffuse myalgias, weight loss, weakness, and malaise (*polymyalgia rheumatica*). The ESR is elevated in all patients, usually to high levels (60 to 120 mm/hour). Jaw claudication is an uncommon, but useful, diagnostic clue.

Treatment

The main hazard in temporal arteritis is *visual loss* (ischemic optic neuropathy; see Chapter 11), which occurs in 10 to 30% of untreated patients because of involvement of the ophthalmic artery. If the diagnosis is suspected, start **prednisone 100 mg every day** immediately and schedule the patient for a **temporal artery biopsy.** Because false-negative biopsy results are common, biopsy should be repeated on the opposite side if the initial biopsy result is negative. In most patients, prednisone will abolish all symptoms and normalize the ESR in 2 to 4 weeks. Because the illness is self-limited, steroids (10 to 20 mg per day) can usually be discontinued within 6 months to 2 years.

Trigeminal Neuralgia

Also known as tic douloureux, this illness is characterized by brief, sharp, lancinating paroxysms of pain in the distribution of the trigeminal nerve. The maxillary (V2) and mandibular (V3) divisions are most frequently affected, and specific trigger points can often be found on the face. For this reason, the pain is often related to activities such as toothbrushing, shaving, or eating. More than 90% of patients present after age 40, and women are more often affected than men. If trigeminal neuralgia is associated with trigeminal sensory loss, other cranial nerve deficits, or onset before age 40, MRI should be performed to rule out neoplasm, multiple sclerosis, or vascular compression of the trigeminal nerve. **Glossopharyngeal neuralgia,** a rare disorder similar to trigeminal neuralgia, is characterized by lancinating pains in the oropharynx that radiate to the ear. The pain is triggered by swallowing, yawning, sneezing, or coughing. Treatment is the same as for trigeminal neuralgia.

Treatment

The most effective treatment is **carbamazepine, 400 to 1200 mg per day given four times a day.** The initial dose of **200 mg two times a day** is gradually increased to the minimal effective dosage. **Baclofen (10 to 20 mg three times a day)** or **gabapentin (100 to 600 mg three times a day)** may also be effective in some patients. **Phenytoin (300 to 400 mg a day)** may be used as adjunctive treatment to either carbamazepine, baclofen, or gabapentin. In refractory cases, radiofrequency surgical ablation or microsurgical vascular decompression of the trigeminal ganglion may be required.

Spontaneous Intracranial Hypotension

This unusual disorder, which resembles **post-LP headache,** is characterized by headache that worsens after standing. Associated symptoms include nausea, vomiting, tinnitus, and vertigo. The pathogenesis is related to spontaneous leakage of CSF along the craniospinal axis, most often in the thoracic spine. By definition, CSF pressure is low (less than 6 cm H_2O), and the diagnosis is confirmed by meningeal enhancement on MRI (because of traction) and demonstration of CSF leakage by CT myelography.

Treatment

If prolonged bed rest fails to relieve the symptoms, most patients will respond to autologous epidural blood patch at the level of CSF leakage.

Chapter 15 | Neuromuscular Respiratory Failure

Generalized weakness is the primary problem in patients with severe neuromuscular disease. Weakness of the bulbar or respiratory muscles leads to life-threatening respiratory compromise by two mechanisms: (1) lack of upper airway protection and (2) hypoventilation because of respiratory muscle weakness. The most common diseases presenting as acute paralysis and ventilatory failure are **myasthenia gravis** and **Guillain-Barré syndrome** (acute inflammatory polyneuropathy). Your management should be directed toward stabilizing the patient, assessing the need to intubate and ventilate, and establishing a diagnosis. Because patients with neuromuscular disease can deteriorate rapidly, close observation and meticulous airway and ventilatory management in the early stages are critical.

■ PHONE CALL

Questions

1. **What are the vital signs?**
2. **Is the patient in respiratory distress?**
   Rapid, shallow breathing is a danger sign of impending ventilatory failure. Patients with acute weakness who are in obvious respiratory distress should be intubated immediately.
3. **Over what time period has the weakness developed?**
   Fluctuating weakness that has been present for weeks or months is characteristic of myasthenia gravis. Progressive ascending paralysis over hours to days is suggestive of Guillain-Barré syndrome.
4. **Has the patient had difficulty swallowing?**
   Dysphagia (coughing or choking after swallowing) is a symptom of bulbar muscle weakness. Affected patients are at risk for aspiration and should be given nothing by mouth (NPO).

Orders

1. **Administer oxygen.**
   For mild to moderate respiratory distress, order 40% oxy-

gen via face mask and reassess oxygen requirements on arrival at the bedside.
2. **Perform bedside pulmonary function tests.**
   - *Vital capacity* is the maximal exhaled volume after full inspiration and is normally 60 ml/kg (approximately 4 L in a 70-kg person). Patients generally require intubation when vital capacity falls below 15 ml/kg (approximately 1 L).
   - *Peak inspiratory pressure* (normally greater than 50 cm H_2O) measures the force of inhalation generated by contraction of the diaphragm and is an index of the ability to maintain lung expansion and avoid atelectasis.
   - *Peak expiratory pressure* (normally greater than 60 cm H_2O) correlates with the strength of cough and the ability to clear secretions from the airway.
3. **Measure arterial blood gas levels on room air.**
   Hypercarbia (partial pressure of carbon dioxide [P_{CO_2}] greater than 45 mm Hg) results from alveolar hypoventilation.
   Hypoxia (partial pressure of oxygen [P_{O_2}] less than 75 mm Hg) is indicative of impaired ventilation-perfusion matching and is usually related to atelectasis or pneumonia.
4. **Obtain a chest radiograph.**
5. **Keep the patient NPO.**
6. **Insert an intravenous line.**
   IV access should be established in the event of an acute deterioration.

■ ELEVATOR THOUGHTS

What can cause generalized weakness leading to respiratory failure?
An anatomic approach is the most useful way to classify causes of generalized weakness. Further discussion of many of the entities listed here can be found later in this chapter.
1. **Spinal cord lesion**
   - Cervical cord compression
   - Tranverse myelitis
2. **Motor neuron lesion**
   - Amyotrophic lateral sclerosis
   - Polio
3. **Peripheral nerve lesion**
   - Guillain-Barré syndrome (acute inflammatory polyneuropathy)
   - Chronic inflammatory demyelinating polyneuropathy
   - Diphtheritic polyneuropathy

- Acquired immunodeficiency syndrome (AIDS)–related demyelinating polyneuropathy
- Toxic neuropathy (lead, arsenic, hexacarbons, dapsone, nitrofurantoin)
- Lyme disease
- Tick paralysis
- Critical illness polyneuropathy
- Acute intermittent porphyria

4. **Neuromuscular junction lesion**
   - Myasthenia gravis
   - Lambert-Eaton syndrome
   - Botulism
   - Organophosphate poisoning

5. **Muscle lesion**
   - Polymyositis or dermatomyositis
   - Critical illness myopathy
   - Hyperthyroid myopathy
   - Mitochondrial myopathy
   - Acid maltase deficiency (Pompe's disease)
   - Periodic paralysis (hyperkalemic or hypokalemic)
   - Congenital myopathy (muscular dystrophy)

■ MAJOR THREAT TO LIFE

- **Hypoxia**
  Inadequate oxygenation is the most worrisome end result of any process leading to shortness of breath. Hence, your initial assessment should be directed toward ascertaining whether significant hypoxia is present.

■ BEDSIDE

Quick Look Test
Does the patient look well (comfortable), sick (uncomfortable), or critical (about to die)?

Agitation, diaphoresis, difficulty finishing sentences, accessory respiratory muscle contraction, and rapid or labored breathing may signal impending respiratory failure.

Airway and Vital Signs
Is the upper airway clear?
- Weakness of the tongue and oropharyngeal muscles can lead to upper airway obstruction, which increases resistance to

airflow and the work of breathing. *Stridor* is indicative of potentially life-threatening upper airway obstruction.

- Weakness of the laryngeal and glottic muscles can lead to impaired swallowing and aspiration of secretions. A *wet, gurgled voice* and *pooled oropharyngeal secretions* are the best clinical signs of significant dysphagia.

What is the respiratory rate?

Check for *paradoxical respirations* (Fig. 15–1), inward movement of the abdomen on inspiration, which is indicative of diaphragmatic paralysis.

What is the heart rate and blood pressure?

Sinus tachycardia, hypertension, or BP lability can result from dysautonomia in Guillain-Barré syndrome.

What is the temperature?

Fever should raise suspicion for aspiration pneumonia.

Selective History

To make the diagnosis, it is important to establish the time course and distribution of weakness. Key questions to keep in

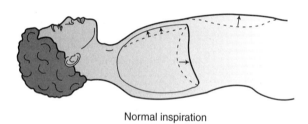

Normal inspiration

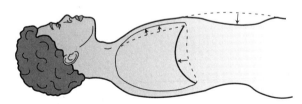

Paradoxical respiration

Figure 15–1 □ Paradoxical respirations. With normal inspiration *(top)*, contraction and downward movement of the diaphragm cause the abdomen to move outward. With paradoxical respiration *(bottom)*, outward expansion of the chest leads to passive upward movement of the diaphragm and inward movement of the abdomen.

mind when obtaining a history in patients with generalized weakness include the following: (1) Is a spinal cord lesion a possibility? (2) Is the process purely motor or is sensation involved? (3) Is the patient at risk for sudden respiratory failure?

1. **When did the weakness develop?**
   Early symptoms of weakness can be subtle. Ask about difficulty arising from a chair, climbing stairs, lifting packages, combing or brushing hair, or turning keys or doorknobs.
2. **Was there an antecedent illness?**
   Approximately 70% of cases of Guillain-Barré syndrome are triggered by an antecedent viral illness or *Campylobacter jejuni* gastroenteritis. Respiratory crisis in myasthenia gravis is triggered by infection in approximately 40% of patients.
3. **Does the weakness fluctuate?**
   Fluctuating weakness (on an hourly basis) is almost pathognomonic for myasthenia gravis.
4. **Has there been any blurred or double vision?**
   Blurred vision occurs with botulism.
5. **Has there been any neck or back pain?**
   Neck pain should raise suspicion for a cervical cord lesion. Low backache occurs frequently with Guillain-Barré syndrome.
6. **Has there been any numbness or tingling?**
   Distal paresthesias are common in Guillain-Barré syndrome.
7. **Have there been any muscle aches, cramps, or tenderness?**
   Aching and tenderness generally occur with myopathy. Cramps can occur with motor neuron disease or with severe electrolyte derangements.
8. **Has there been any exposure to toxins or insecticides?**
   Organophosphate is the most common toxin that can lead to respiratory failure.

Selective Physical Examination

Once the patient has been stabilized, the goal is to identify signs of airway or respiratory compromise and to search for clues to the diagnosis.

General Physical Examination

HEENT
- **Oropharynx:** Check for *pooled secretions,* which are diagnostic of impaired swallowing and ability to handle secretions. *Exudative pharyngitis* occurs with diphtheria.

	• **Swallow test:** Give the patient a small amount (3 oz) of water to drink. Coughing after swallowing is diagnostic of aspiration.
	• **Speech:** Check for *dysphonia*. A nasal voice results from palatal paralysis. A soft, strangulated voice results from vocal cord paralysis. Evaluate *dysarthria* by checking the buccal (ma, ma), lingual (la, la), and pharyngeal (ga, ga) components of articulation.
Respiratory	• **Lungs:** Auscultate for wheezes, rales, rhonchi, or consolidation.
	• **Diaphragm:** Palpate for normal, outward abdominal movement during inspiration.
	• **Cough:** Check the strength of the patient's cough.
	• **Ventilatory reserve:** Ask the patient to inhale fully and count from 1 to 25. A patient with adequate ventilatory reserve should be able to do this in a single breath.
Skin	• **Rashes:** Check for a rash (Lyme disease, dermatomyositis).

Neurologic Examination

- **Pupils:** Pupillary reactivity may be lost with botulism or in the Miller-Fisher variant of Guillain-Barré syndrome (triad of ophthalmoplegia, ataxia, and areflexia).
- **Extraocular muscles:** *Ptosis and ocular muscle weakness* is characteristic of myasthenia gravis but can occur with the Miller-Fisher variant of Guillain-Barré syndrome, botulism, diphtheria, polymyositis, Graves' disease, mitochondrial myopathy, or critical illness myopathy.
- **Face, palate, tongue, and neck strength**
- **Limb strength**
- **Fasciculations:** Fasciculations are seen with motor neuron disease or organophosphate poisoning.
- **Reflexes:** *Areflexia* is **always** seen with Guillain-Barré syndrome.
- **Coordination:** Ataxia occurs with the Miller-Fisher variant of Guillain-Barré syndrome.
- **Sensation:** A cervical or upper thoracic *sensory level* associated with quadraparesis suggests a cervical cord lesion. Mild sensory loss in the distal extremities is common in Guillain-Barré syndrome.

■ MANAGEMENT

Airway Management and Mechanical Ventilation

Criteria for Intubation

A number of factors must be considered when deciding when to intubate and ventilate. The most important factor, perhaps, is the overall comfort level of the patient. Decisions must be individualized, but the following criteria may be helpful:

- *Reduction of vital capacity to 15 ml/kg (approximately 1 L in a 70-kg person)*
- *Po_2 less than 70 mm Hg on room air*
- *Pco_2 greater than 50 mm Hg associated with acidosis (pH less than 7.35)*
- *Severe oropharyngeal paresis with inability to protect the airway*

Remember that conservative, early intubation and institution of positive-pressure ventilation can minimize the development of atelectasis and pneumonia and may lead to earlier extubation.

Initial Ventilator Management

The initial goals of ventilator management immediately after intubation are (1) to provide rest and (2) to promote lung expansion. These goals are best accomplished using *synchronized intermittent mandatory ventilation (SIMV)* at a rate of 6 to 8 breaths per minute, using tidal volumes of 10 to 15 ml/kg. *Positive end-expiratory pressure (PEEP)* aids in the expansion of collapsed alveoli and should be used in all patients at levels of 5 to 15 cm H_2O.

Patients with long-standing weakness and CO_2 retention should be intentionally hypoventilated (Pco_2 at or higher than 45 mm Hg). Overventilating to normal or reduced Pco_2 levels will result in alkalosis and renal serum bicarbonate wasting, which in turn will make it more difficult to successfully wean the patient.

Bronchoscopy

Fiberoptic bronchoscopy for pulmonary toilet should be performed aggressively in patients with hypoxia, severe atelectasis, or lobar collapse because of mucus plugging.

Tracheostomy

After the patient has been on mechanical ventilation for approximately 2 weeks, tracheostomy should be performed. Compared to prolonged (more than 2 weeks) endotracheal intubation, tracheostomy (1) is more comfortable, (2) poses less risk of permanent laryngeal or tracheal injury, (3) facilitates weaning from mechanical ventilation by reducing dead space and airway resistance, and (4) makes it easier to clear airway secretions by cough or suctioning.

> Box 15–1. CRITERIA FOR WEANING TO EXTUBATION
>
> 1. Vital capacity greater than 15 ml/kg
> 2. Peak inspiratory pressure greater than 25 cm H_2O
> 3. Po_2 greater than 80 mm Hg on 40% oxygen
> 4. No adverse medical conditions: infection, fever, hypotension, anemia, gastric distention, volume overload, or cardiac arrhythmias

Weaning to Extubation

Criteria to be met before weaning is initiated are listed in Box 15–1.

Continuous positive airway pressure (CPAP) with pressure support is the preferred initial mode for weaning patients with respiratory muscle weakness. Each time the patient inhales, "pressure support" delivers additional inspiratory volume until a preset level of pressure is reached. The amount of inspiratory pressure support given (range, 5 to 15 cm H_2O) should be initially adjusted to attain tidal volumes of approximately 300 to 500 ml in an adult. We advocate daytime weaning trials and "resting" the patient on SIMV overnight (Box 15–2).

Extubation can be performed once the patient has demon-

> Box 15–2. WEANING TRIAL PROTOCOL
>
> 1. Begin the weaning trial by switching the ventilator mode from SIMV to CPAP with pressure support.
> 2. After 15 to 30 minutes, record the respiratory rate and mean tidal volume.
> 3. Every 2 to 4 hours, the level of pressure support may be decreased by 1 to 2 cm H_2O if the patient remains comfortable.
> 4. In general, the weaning trial should be continued up to 12 hours or until signs of respiratory fatigue occur. *An increasing respiratory rate combined with falling tidal volumes is the most reliable indicator of respiratory fatigue.* At this point, an arterial blood gas measurement may be desirable.
> 5. When the weaning trial is over, return to SIMV mode overnight.

strated the ability to tolerate long periods (e.g., overnight) on CPAP with pressure support equal to 5 cm H_2O without fatigue. Fluctuating pulmonary function tests, excessive secretions, or concurrent medical problems (i.e., infection or cardiovascular instability) are relative contraindications to extubation. Extubation should always be performed early in the day.

General Care of the Patient with Neuromuscular Respiratory Failure

1. **Elevate the head of the bed**
   With diaphragmatic weakness, lung volumes become diminished and work of breathing increases in the supine position.
2. **Chest physical therapy**
   Chest percussion and airway suctioning are essential for preventing mucus plugs and aiding in the clearing of secretions. Prescribe *incentive spirometry* every 6 hours if the patient is not intubated.
3. **Serial measurements of vital capacity**
   Vital capacity should be checked every 4 to 6 hours in nonintubated patients and every 12 to 24 hours in intubated patients.
4. **Prophylaxis for deep vein thrombosis (DVT)**
   Order **heparin 5000 U SQ every 12 hours.**
5. **Nutrition**
   Patients with bulbar weakness should be made NPO and fed via a *small-bore nasoduodenal tube.* When attempting to wean a CO_2 retainer, use a nutritional supplement with a high ratio of carbohydrate to lipid (e.g., Pulmocare) to minimize CO_2 production.
6. **Fluids and electrolytes**
   Hypokalemia and *hypophosphatemia* can exacerbate muscle weakness and should be periodically checked for and treated.
7. **Bowel and bladder care**
   Paralysis predisposes to constipation and can be prevented with **docusate sodium (Colace) 100 mg three times a day and milk of magnesia 30 ml every night.** Intermittent straight catheterization carries a lower risk of infection than an indwelling Foley catheter.

■ SPECIFIC DISORDERS

Guillain-Barré Syndrome

Guillain-Barré syndrome is a monophasic, acute inflammatory demyelinating polyneuropathy. The etiology is related to an autoimmune attack directed against surface antigens on peripheral nerves, resulting in focal segmental demyelination.

Onset

In approximately 70% of cases, the syndrome follows a respiratory or gastrointestinal infection by 5 days to 3 weeks. Viral upper respiratory infection and *Campylobacter jejuni* gastroenteritis are the most common precipitating infections. Other causes include human immunodeficiency virus (HIV) infection, immunization, pregnancy, Hodgkin's disease, and surgery.

Clinical Features

The syndrome usually begins with rapidly progressive ascending paralysis, associated with cranial nerve and respiratory muscle weakness, loss of deep tendon reflexes, and distal paresthesias and sensory loss. Unlike other neuropathies, proximal muscles are often affected more than distal muscles. The weakness progresses over 7 to 21 days; the median duration from onset to maximal weakness is 12 days. Respiratory failure requiring intubation occurs in 20% of patients. Papilledema, autonomic disturbances (e.g., hypertension, hypotension, urinary retention, sinus tachycardia, cardiac arrhythmias), and syndrome of inappropriate antidiuretic hormone (SIADH) are seen in some patients.

Laboratory Data

The cerebrospinal fluid (CSF) classically shows dissociation between albumin levels and cytologic findings, with elevated protein levels and normal white blood cell counts (5 cells/μl or fewer). The elevation in the protein level can sometimes take up to 2 weeks to develop. A mild lymphocytic or monocytic pleocytosis is sometimes seen (10 to 100 cells/mm^3) and should raise suspicion for an infectious polyradiculopathy (e.g., HIV, cytomegalovirus [CMV], West Nile virus, or Lyme disease) or poliomyelitis. Nerve conduction studies show loss of F waves and reduced conduction velocities. Reduced motor fiber amplitudes reflect secondary axonal damage and imply a worse prognosis for recovery.

Treatment (Box 15–3)

Patients with signs of respiratory muscle weakness should be admitted to an ICU for observation until it is clear that the illness has stabilized. **Plasmapheresis,** when initiated within 10 days of the onset of symptoms, can speed the onset of recovery. A total of five treatments is performed every 1 to 2 days, with a total of 2 to 4 L of plasma exchanged for 5% albumin during each treatment. High-dose **intravenous immune globulin (IVIG), 0.4 g/kg per day for 5 consecutive days,** has been shown to be as effective

Box 15–3. CHECKLIST FOR THE MANAGEMENT OF GUILLAIN-BARRÉ SYNDROME

1. *Diagnostic work-up:* Lumbar puncture, electromyography/nerve conduction studies, hepatitis and Lyme disease serologies, CMV, Epstein-Barr virus (EBV), herpes simplex virus (HSV), and HIV titers, urine porphyrin levels, urine heavy metal screen, stool analysis for *Campylobacter.*
2. *Pain management:* Pain can be severe and may result from meningeal inflammation or neuropathic mechanisms. Nonsteroidal anti-inflammatory drugs **(NSAIDs) (ketorolac 30 mg IM every 6 hours)** and **narcotics (morphine 10 mg every 2 to 4 hours as needed)** are most effective.
3. *Dysautonomia:* The most frequent cardiovascular manifestation of dysautonomia is sustained hypertension and tachycardia. Treatment with beta blockers (propranolol **PO 10 to 40 mg every 6 hours** or **labetolol infusion)** may be desirable in older patients with coronary artery disease.

as plasmapheresis and may be slightly superior. "Rebound" deterioration after completing a course of IVIG can sometimes occur.

Prognosis

Features shown to have a poor prognosis in Guillain-Barré syndrome include (1) advanced age, (2) very low distal motor amplitudes, (3) rapidly progressive weakness occurring over the first week, and (4) respiratory failure requiring intubation.

Myasthenia Gravis

Myasthenia gravis is caused by an antibody-mediated attack on nicotinic acetylcholine receptors, resulting in a defect in neuromuscular transmission. This phenomenon manifests clinically as *fluctuating weakness* and *muscle fatigability*, the hallmarks of myasthenia gravis.

Clinical Features

Fluctuating weakness is typical of myasthenia gravis; it tends to involve the eyes (in 90% of patients), face, neck, and oropharynx (in 80% of patients), and limbs (in 60% of patients). The age distribution at onset is bimodal, with an early peak between ages 20 and 40 (primarily in women) and a later peak between ages

50 and 80 (in both sexes). The limbs are almost never affected in isolation. Sensation is always normal, and reflexes are preserved unless the muscle is plegic. Most patients reach the maximum severity of their disease within the first 1 to 2 years; thereafter, spontaneous remission is common (in approximately 30% of patients), and the disease process tends to become less severe. *Malignant thymoma* is present in approximately 15% of patients with myasthenia and is associated with more severe disease.

Myasthenic crisis is defined by respiratory failure requiring intubation and mechanical ventilation. Crisis is most often provoked by infection (in 40% of patients) but can also occur spontaneously (in 30% of patients) or result from aspiration, surgery, pregnancy, medications (Table 15–1) or emotional upset. Approximately 25% of patients can be extubated within 1 week, 50% within 2 weeks, and 75% within 1 month. One third of patients intubated for crisis will proceed to experience a second crisis. Although a crisis is by definition life-threatening, with modern ICU management, death (approximately 5% mortality rate) results only from overwhelming medical complications (e.g., myocardial infarction, sepsis).

Laboratory Data

The diagnosis of myasthenia gravis can be established with the following tests:

1. *Edrophonium (Tensilon) testing* reveals transient improvement in patients with ocular and facial weakness. **Edrophonium 10 mg** is used in adults; infuse 2 mg initially and observe for severe cholinergic muscarinic effects such as nausea, bradycardia, and hypotension. **Atropine 0.4 mg** should be kept at the bedside and can be used to reverse these symptoms. If there are no severe effects, inject the remaining 8 mg and observe for improvement, which generally occurs within 2 to 10 minutes.
2. *Repetitive nerve stimulation* at 2 to 3 Hz characteristically produces a greater than 10% decrement in amplitude between the first and fifth compound muscle action potential. Sensitivity and specificity are 90% when weak, proximal muscles are tested; however, sensitivity falls to less than 50% in myasthenic patients without limb weakness.
3. *Single-fiber EMG* reveals "jitter," variation in the time interval between firing of muscle fibers in the same motor unit. Single-fiber EMG is highly sensitive (sensitivity greater than 95%) for myasthenia gravis but is not specific.
4. *Acetylcholine receptor antibodies* are present in 80 to 90% of patients with generalized myasthenia but in only 50% of patients with ocular myasthenia. Titers do not correlate with the severity of illness.

> **Box 15–4. CHECKLIST FOR THE MANAGEMENT OF MYASTHENIC CRISIS**
>
> 1. Eliminate and avoid all contraindicated medications (see Table 15–1).
> 2. *Diagnostic work-up:* Edrophonium test, acetylcholine receptor antibody level, repetitive nerve stimulation, single-fiber EMG, thyroid function tests, chest computed tomography (CT) scan.
> 3. *Treatment:* Anticholinesterase medications should be *discontinued* while patients are mechanically ventilated because they lead to excessive stimulation of secretions (see Table 15–2). A course of plasmapheresis or IVIG is indicated in all patients.

Treatment (Box 15–4)

Therapeutic options for treating myasthenia gravis can be divided into three categories: *symptomatic therapy* (with acetylcholinesterase inhibitors), *short-term disease suppression* (with plasmapheresis and IVIG), and *long-term immunosuppression* (with thymectomy, steroids, or chemotherapy).

Symptomatic Therapy. Acetylcholinesterase inhibitors (Table 15–2) improve myasthenic weakness by allowing acetylcholine to accumulate at the neuromuscular junction. **Pyridostigmine (Mestinon) is started at 30 mg PO three times a day, increased to 60 to 120 mg every 4 to 6 hours as a maintenance dose, and increased to 120 mg every 3 hours as a maximal dose.** A long-acting 180-mg tablet (Mestinon Timespan) can be given at bedtime for patients with nocturnal or morning weakness. Excessive muscarinic side effects (e.g., pulmonary secretions, diarrhea) can be controlled by concurrently giving an antimuscarinic agent such as **glycopyrrolate (Robinul) 1 to 2 mg PO three times a day** or **propantheline bromide (Pro-Banthīne) 15 mg PO four times a day.**

Short-term Disease Suppression. This is indicated to hasten clinical improvement in hospitalized patients. **Plasmapheresis (five exchanges of 2 to 4 L every 1 to 2 days)** can lead to improvement within days, but the effect is short-lived, lasting only 2 to 4 weeks. Similar benefits have been reported in 70% of patients treated with **IVIG (0.4 g/kg daily for 5 days),** but experience with this therapy remains limited.

Long-term Immunosuppression. This treatment is indicated when weakness is inadequately controlled with anticholinesterase

Table 15-1 □ DRUGS THAT CAN EXACERBATE WEAKNESS IN MYASTHENIA GRAVIS

Antibiotics
  Aminoglycosides (gentamicin, streptomycin, others)
  Peptide antibodies (polymyxin B, colistin)
  Tetracyclines (tetracycline, doxycycline, others)
  Erythromycin
  Clindamycin
  Ciprofloxacin
  Ampicillin
Antiarrhythmics
  Quinidine
  Procainamide
  Lidocaine
Neuromuscular junction blockers (vecuronium, pancuronium, others)
Quinine
Steroids
Thyroid hormones (thyroxine, levothyroxine, others)
Beta blockers (propranolol, timolol, others)
Phenytoin

---

medications. **Prednisone** is most commonly prescribed; to use the lowest dose possible, start with **15 to 20 mg per day** and gradually increase to **40 to 100 mg per day over 4 to 8 weeks** until an adequate response is achieved. Temporary worsening of symptoms within the first 2 weeks of starting steroids can be expected in up to 40% of patients. **Azathioprine 1 to 2 mg/kg PO per day** can also be used for long-term immunosuppression in patients who cannot tolerate the side effects of steroids. **Thymectomy** leads to disease remission in 40% of patients and clinical improvement in another 40%, but these benefits can take months or years to occur. Thymectomy is indicated in any patient between the ages of 15 and 60 with thymoma or with generalized myasthenia.

Uncommon Causes of Paralysis and Respiratory Failure

Botulism

Botulism is caused by an exotoxin produced by *Clostridium botulinum,* an anaerobic, gram-positive, spore-forming rod that contaminates food. Weakness occurs because the toxin is a potent inhibitor of presynaptic acetylcholine release. Clinical symptoms begin within 12 to 24 hours of ingestion and are characterized by gastrointestinal complaints, dilated and nonreactive pupils, blurred vision, and weakness that begins with the extraocular and oropharyngeal muscles before becoming generalized. Urinary retention, dry mouth, and anhidrosis may also occur. **Botulism**

Table 15-2 □ ANTICHOLINESTERASE DRUGS USED FOR MYASTHENIA GRAVIS

	Route	Equivalent Dosage	Onset	Maximal Response	Dosage Range
Pyridostigmine bromide (Mestinon)	PO*	60 mg	30 to 60 minutes	1 to 2 hours	30 to 120 mg every 3 to 8 hours
	IM, IV†	2 mg	5 to 10 minutes	20 to 30 minutes	—
Pyridostigmine long-acting (Mestinon Timespan)	PO	—	1 to 2 hours	3 to 5 hours	180 mg per day at night
Neostigmine bromide (Prostigmin)	PO	15 mg	30 minutes	1 hour	15 to 30 mg every 2 to 3 hours
Neostigmine methylsulfate (Prostigmin injectable)	IV†	0.5 mg	1 to 2 minutes	20 minutes	0.5 to 1 mg every 2 hours
	IM	1.5 mg	30 minutes	1 hour	1.5 to 3 mg every 2 to 3 hours

*Can be given as a tablet or as a liquid.
†Equivalent IV dose of pyridostigmine or neostigmine is one thirtieth of the oral dose.

trivalent antitoxin (one vial IV and one vial IM every 2 to 4 hours) should be given as soon as possible. **Guanidine hydrochloride (40 mg PO every 4 hours)** is an acetylcholine agonist that can counteract the presynaptic blockade caused by the toxin.

Poliomyelitis

Poliovirus is an enterovirus that can cause selective destruction of motor neurons in the spinal cord and brain stem, resulting in flaccid, areflexic paralysis. Modern vaccination has made the disease a clinical rarity. Acute paralysis from poliomyelitis is differentiated from that caused by Guillain-Barré syndrome by the presence of headache, high fever, mental status changes, asymmetric weakness, and neutrophils in the CSF.

Tetanus

Tetanus results from an exotoxin produced by *Clostridium tetani,* an anaerobic gram-positive coccus that can infect soft-tissue wounds. The toxin results in neuronal hyperexcitability; the result is seizures, autonomic instability, and sustained "tetanic" muscle contractions involving the jaw ("lockjaw"), neck, back, and respiratory muscles. Treatment is directed toward (1) assisting ventilation, which may require intubation and administration of neuromuscular blocking agents; (2) neutralizing the toxin with intramuscular or intrathecal **tetanus immune globulin 250 units (single dose);** and (3) eradicating the soft-tissue infection with **procaine penicillin 1.2 million units every 6 hours for 10 days.**

chapter 16 | Syncope

Syncope is brief loss of consciousness caused by a sudden reduction of cerebral blood flow. *Presyncope* refers to the situation in which there is reduction of cerebral blood flow and a sensation of impending loss of consciousness, although the patient does not actually pass out. Presyncope and syncope represent degrees of the same disorder and should be addressed as manifestations of the same underlying problem. Your task is to discover the cause of the syncopal attack.

■ PHONE CALL

Questions

1. Did the patient actually lose consciousness?
2. Is the patient still unconscious?
3. What are the vital signs?
4. Was the patient standing, sitting, or lying down when the attack occurred?
    Syncope in the recumbent position is almost always cardiac in origin. Syncope that occurs immediately after standing up suggests orthostatic hypotension.
5. Was any seizure-like activity witnessed?
6. Did the patient sustain any injury from the fall?

Orders

- If the patient is still unconscious, give the following orders:
   1. Administer IV D5W to keep the vein open (KVO) if IV is not already in place.
   2. Turn the patient onto the left side (this maneuver minimizes the risk of upper airway obstruction and aspiration).
   3. Order a stat 12-lead electrocardiogram (ECG) and rhythm strip.
   4. Obtain a finger stick glucose level.
- If the patient has regained consciousness, if there is no evidence of head or neck injury, and if the vital signs are stable, do the following:
   1. Instruct the RN to keep the patient supine for at least 10 to 15 minutes, until the patient feels comfortable. To return

the patient to bed, slowly raise the patient to the sitting position, and then to a standing position.
2. Have the RN check orthostatic vital signs (blood pressure [BP] and heart rate with the patient lying down and standing).
3. Order an ECG and rhythm strip.
4. Have vital signs taken every 15 minutes until you arrive at the bedside. Instruct the RN to call you back immediately if the patient becomes unstable before you are able to perform your assessment.

■ ELEVATOR THOUGHTS

What causes syncope?
A comprehensive list of the differential diagnoses for syncope and the approximate relative frequency of each of the main categories in an emergency room (ER) population are given here. **Note that neurologic and psychiatric causes are at the bottom of the list and in combination account for only 5% of all patients presenting with syncope.** In the majority of patients (90%), syncope results from a transient drop in systemic BP and can be explained on the basis of reflex vasodilation, cardiac disease, orthostatic hypotension, or medications. *Accordingly, your initial evaluation should focus on excluding these conditions before a neurologic diagnosis is seriously considered.*

1. **Reflex vasodilation (60% of ER patients)**
   a. Vasodepressor (vasovagal, neurocardiogenic) syncope
   b. Carotid sinus syncope
   c. Situational syncope
      (1) Micturition syncope
      (2) Defecation syncope
      (3) Cough syncope
2. **Cardiac causes (25% of ER patients)**
   a. Arrhythmias
      (1) Tachycardias
         (a) Ventricular tachycardia/fibrillation
         (b) Supraventricular tachycardia
      (2) Bradycardias
         (a) Sick sinus syndrome
         (b) Second- and third-degree heart block
         (c) Pacemaker malfunction
   b. Flow failure
      (1) Obstruction to left ventricular outflow
         (a) Aortic or mitral stenosis
         (b) Hypertrophic obstructive cardiomyopathy
         (c) Aortic dissection

(2) Obstruction to pulmonary outflow
      (a) Pulmonary stenosis
      (b) Pulmonary embolism
   (3) Pump failure
      (a) Myocardial infarction
      (b) Cardiac tamponade
3. **Orthostatic (postural) hypotension (10% of ER patients)**
   a. Volume depletion (anemia, dehydration)
   b. Drug induced (Table 16–1)
   c. Autonomic dysfunction
      (1) Central: Shy-Drager syndrome
      (2) Peripheral: autonomic neuropathy
4. **Neurologic causes (5% of ER patients)**
   a. Seizure (technically not syncope but mimics syncope)
      (1) Unwitnessed tonic-clonic seizure
      (2) Atonic seizure (drop attack)
   b. Transient ischemic attack (TIA)
      (1) Brain stem ischemia
         (a) Vertebrobasilar stenosis/occlusion
         (b) Subclavian steal syndrome

Table 16–1 □ **DRUGS AND MEDICATIONS THAT CAN CAUSE SYNCOPE**

Antihypertensive agents
  Nitrates
  Calcium channel blockers
  Diuretics
  Angiotensin-converting enzyme inhibitors
  Beta blockers
  Others (hydralazine, prazosin)
Antiarrhythmic agents (prolonged QT interval syndrome, torsades de pointes)
  Quinidine
  Procainamide
  Disopyramide
  Sotalol
  Amiodarone
Tricyclic antidepressants
Monoamine oxidase inhibitors
Phenothiazines
Levodopa
Digoxin
Ethanol
Marijuana

(2) Bilateral hemispheric ischemia from carotid artery stenosis or occlusion
c. Increased intracranial pressure (ICP)
(1) Subarachnoid hemorrhage (SAH)
(2) Space-occupying lesion (e.g., brain tumor)
5. **Psychiatric causes (less than 1% of ER patients)**
a. Hyperventilation
b. Conversion disorder (technically not syncope but mimics syncope)

■ MAJOR THREAT TO LIFE

- *Aspiration* **is the main threat if the patient is still unconscious.**
  Remember that syncope generally lasts only a few minutes. If the patient remains persistently unconscious (longer than 15 minutes), the diagnosis is coma, and your evaluation should proceed as outlined in Chapter 5.
- *Fatal cardiac arrhythmia* **is the main hazard once the patient has regained consciousness.**
  If a cardiac rhythm disturbance is suspected, the patient should be attached to an ECG monitor, and consideration should be given to observing the patient in an intensive care unit (ICU). Other potentially life-threatening illnesses that can present with syncope include subarachnoid hemorrhage, gastrointestinal bleeding, pulmonary embolism, aortic dissection, and myocardial infarction.

■ BEDSIDE

Quick Look Test

Does the patient look well (comfortable), sick (uncomfortable), or critical (about to die)?

Most cases of syncope are brief (loss of consciousness less than 5 minutes), and many patients look well shortly after regaining consciousness. Others may appear nauseated, pallid, and diaphoretic—these signs represent the systemic autonomic response to hypotension and should resolve rapidly.

Are there any external signs of head or neck trauma?

Significant head injury is unusual after syncope but should be checked for. In most cases, a period of presyncope warns the patient that something is amiss and allows him or her to avoid a hard fall. **Cardiac syncope often occurs without warning and is more likely to lead to traumatic injury.**

Airway and Vital Signs

Abnormal vital signs can help make your diagnosis of the specific cause of syncope much easier.

Is the airway clear?
If the patient is still unconscious, ensure that he or she is lying on the left side and that respirations are adequate.

What is the heart rate?
Supraventricular or ventricular tachycardia should be documented on ECG tracings. If the patient is hypotensive, call for a cardiac arrest team and treat immediately with electrical cardioversion.
Sinus bradycardia implicates vagally mediated vasodepressor syncope. In this case, both the heart rate and the BP should normalize quickly as the patient remains supine.

What is the BP?
Persistently low BP or significant orthostatic hypotension combined with normal sinus rhythm or sinus tachycardia implicates volume depletion. Begin IV volume resuscitation with D5NS and order a stat hematocrit. Rule out gastrointestinal (GI) bleeding and ruptured aortic aneurysm, which rarely present with syncope.
Hypertension, if found in association with headache, stiff neck, or altered level of consciousness, may indicate subarachnoid hemorrhage.

What is the temperature?
Patients with syncope are rarely febrile. If *fever* is present, it is usually due to a concomitant illness not related to the syncopal attack. If the syncopal attack was unwitnessed, be careful to exclude meningitis or encephalitis associated with a seizure.

Selective History

History should be obtained from the patient as well as from witnesses, if available. Focus on events immediately preceding and following the attack.
1. **Has this ever happened before?**
   If it has, ask the patient if a diagnosis was made after the previous attack.
2. **What do the patient or witnesses recall from the period immediately before the syncope?**
   - Syncope occurring while changing from the supine or the

sitting position to the standing position suggests *orthostatic hypotension*.
- Palpitations or the complete absence of prodromal symptoms suggest *cardiac arrhythmia*.
- A prodrome of dizziness, lightheadedness, pallor, diaphoresis, and dimming of vision (i.e., presyncope) is highly characteristic of *reflex vasodepressor syncope*.
- Syncope after turning the head to one side, especially if the patient is wearing a tight collar, may represent *carotid sinus syncope*.
- Syncope during or immediately following Valsalva's maneuver (coughing, micturition, defecation) can result from mechanical disruption of venous return and is termed *situational syncope*.
- One or more episodes of vertigo, diplopia, dysarthria, numbness, weakness, or ataxia preceding the attack, alone or in combination, are suggestive of *vertebrobasilar insufficiency*.
- An aura (unusual smell or taste, abdominal sensations, visual or sensory hallucinations) may point to a *seizure* as the cause of an unwitnessed attack.

3. **How does the patient feel upon waking from the syncopal attack?**
   - Headache suggests *subarachnoid hemorrhage*.
   - Persistent lethargy and confusion are atypical for true syncope and suggest an unwitnessed *seizure* or *subarachnoid hemorrhage*.

4. **Were any shaking movements observed?**
   Loss of consciousness associated with simultaneous generalized tonic-clonic activity is diagnostic of seizure. *Caution:* Be aware that minor twitching, myoclonic activity, or a single convulsion that **follows** loss of consciousness is common and reflects *secondary* consequences of cerebral hypoxia-ischemia.

5. **Was the patient incontinent of stool or urine?**
   If the attack was unwitnessed, incontinence is highly suggestive of seizure. Be aware that incontinence can also occur with true syncope.

6. **Is there any history of cardiac disease, seizure, stroke, or TIA?**
   These may point to an obvious cause of syncope.

7. **Has the patient been feeling ill recently?**
   Ask about symptoms of infection, diarrhea, peptic ulcer, chest pain, palpitations, or neurologic dysfunction, which may point to a predisposing illness.

8. **What are the medications?**
   Refer to Table 16–1 for a list of medications that can cause syncope.

Selective Physical Examination

Your physical examination is directed toward finding a cause for the syncope. However, a search for evidence of injuries sustained by a fall is equally important at this time.

General Physical Examination

Vital signs	• Repeat now, including *orthostatic* tests if not performed yet
HEENT	• Fundoscopy: look for subhyaloid hemorrhages (SAH)
	• Tongue lacerations, especially at lateral borders (seizure)
	• Ecchymoses, abrasions, lacerations
Neck	• Neck stiffness (SAH)
Cardiac	• Heart murmur (mitral, pulmonic, or aortic stenosis)
	• Pericardial rub (cardiac tamponade)
GU	• Urinary incontinence (seizure)
Rectal	• Heme-positive stool (GI bleeding)
Extremities	• Palpate for evidence of fracture

Neurologic Examination

- Lethargy, confusion, or disorientation (seizure, SAH)
- Hemianopia or aphasia (stroke, CNS mass lesion)
- Diplopia, nystagmus, facial weakness or numbness, dysarthria or dysphonia (vertebrobasilar ischemia)
- Hemiparesis/pronator drift (Todd's paralysis, stroke, CNS mass lesion)
- Cogwheel rigidity (Shy-Drager syndrome)
- Stocking-glove sensory loss and areflexia (peripheral and autonomic neuropathy)
- Appendicular or gait ataxia (vertebrobasilar ischemia)

■ DIAGNOSTIC TESTING

Apart from an ECG, there are no laboratory tests that are routinely indicated for the evaluation of syncope. In approximately 50% of cases, a careful history, examination (including orthostatic BP), and ECG are all that are needed to establish a diagnosis (for instance, a clear-cut case of vasovagal syncope in a patient having blood drawn).

If the cause of syncope is unexplained and the history and examination are not suggestive of a neurologic cause, further workup should be directed toward ruling out a cardiac cause of syncope. The reason for this is that cardiac causes of syncope carry a substantially higher risk of subsequent sudden death than

do noncardiac causes (approximately 30% compared to 10% over 12 months) and thus are important to rule out. Tests to rule out a cardiac cause of syncope may include the following:
- Echocardiography
- Cardiac telemetry
- Holter monitoring
- Head-up tilt table testing
- Signal-averaged electrocardiography (SAECG)
- Electrophysiologic (EP) studies
- Cardiac stress testing
- Coronary angiography
- Ventilation-perfusion scan

If a neurologic cause of syncope is suggested by history or examination, specific testing may include the following (refer to the next section on specific neurologic causes of syncope to guide your selection):
- 3-minute trial of hyperventilation
- Electroencephalogram (EEG) (with and without sleep)
- Head CT or MRI
- Transcranial Doppler ultrasonography (intracranial vertebral and basilar arteries)
- Duplex Doppler ultrasonography (extracranial carotid and vertebral arteries)
- Magnetic resonance angiography
- Cerebral angiography
- Electromyography (EMG)/nerve conduction studies (NCS)

■ MANAGEMENT

Approach to Syncope: A Neurologist's Perspective

Step 1: Rule out medical causes of syncope

As stated previously, neurologic causes of syncope are unusual. When called in consultation to evaluate for a possible neurologic etiology, the first step is to verify that the more common and easy-to-identify medical causes have been excluded. Important tests to rule out a medical cause of syncope in the ER include the following:
- Orthostatic BP
- ECG
- Cardiac auscultation
- Hematocrit
- Arterial blood gas measurement (rule out pulmonary embolism)
- Review of medications (Table 16–1 lists medications that can cause syncope)
- Toxicology screen and serum ethanol level

Step 2: Know what you are looking for
Syncope results from temporary reduction of cerebral blood flow, and in the majority of cases, the cause is a drop in systemic BP. True neurologic causes of syncope follow the same principle and result from only two basic mechanisms:
1. **Transient focal reduction of cerebral blood flow related to stenosis or embolism of a cerebral artery (i.e., TIA).** With rare exceptions, the only brain region in which transient focal ischemia can lead to loss of consciousness is the brain stem. Hence, *vertebrobasilar TIA* is the main consideration.
2. **Reduction of cerebral blood flow caused by a transient elevation of ICP.** *Subarachnoid hemorrhage* and an ICP wave associated with a *pre-existing mass lesion* are the main considerations.

Seizures are not a cause of syncope. However, generalized seizures lead to sudden, temporary loss of consciousness and thus can be confused with syncope. As the consulting neurologist, you may be asked to corroborate or rule out the diagnosis.

■ SELECTED DISORDERS THAT CAN CAUSE OR MIMIC SYNCOPE

Nonneurologic Causes

Vasovagal (Vasodepressor, Neurocardiogenic) Syncope

Also known as "the common faint," vasodepressor syncope is apt to occur in the setting of a strong emotional or painful stimulus. A prodrome of presyncope (dizziness, pallor) is the rule. Bradycardia may be identified shortly after the episode, and recovery is usually rapid. If the clinical picture is unclear, *head-up tilt table testing* can be used to provoke vasovagal syncope and establish the diagnosis, with a sensitivity and specificity of approximately 80%. Sudden head-up tilting in patients with vasovagal syncope produces an increase in myocardial contractility, which in turn leads to excessive stimulation of left ventricular mechanoreceptors (C fibers) and an exaggerated reflex vagal response. Isolated episodes require no specific intervention, and the prognosis is excellent. Eighty percent of patients with recurrent vasovagal syncope respond to treatment with a **beta blocker (propranolol 10 to 60 mg four times a day** or **pindolol 5 to 20 mg three times a day)** that blunts the cardiac inotropic response to a fall in BP and thus prevents the overly sensitive reflex vagal response.

Carotid Sinus Syncope

This unusual disorder is seen almost exclusively in older individuals and results from hypersensitivity of baroreceptors in the carotid sinus. External pressure of the neck (e.g., turning the head while wearing a tight collar) results in an exaggerated vagal response and fall in BP. *Carotid massage* with ECG monitoring can be used to establish the diagnosis, but this should be performed with caution.

Neurologic Causes

Transient Ischemic Attack

As stated previously, **vertebrobasilar stenosis or occlusion** is a rare cause of syncope. The diagnosis is suggested by symptoms or signs of focal brain stem ischemia (diplopia, vertigo, ataxia, nystagmus, dysarthria, facial numbness, unilateral or bilateral weakness, or sensory loss) either before or after the event. Deficits referable to the posterior cerebral artery, particularly hemianopia, may also occur. Syncope following prolonged head extension ("beauty parlor syncope") in patients with atherosclerotic vertebrobasilar disease has been described. *Transcranial and duplex Doppler ultrasonography, magnetic resonance angiography,* or *conventional angiography* is required to establish the diagnosis. Management is discussed in Chapter 24.

Subclavian steal syndrome is an unusual cause of vertebrobasilar insufficiency. It results from occlusion of one of the subclavian arteries proximal to the origin of the vertebral artery. The distal subclavian artery is hence supplied by retrograde flow from the ipsilateral vertebral artery, which "steals" flow from the basilar and contralateral vertebral arteries, resulting in intermittent hemodynamic flow failure in the posterior circulation.

Unilateral **carotid stenosis or occlusion** does not cause syncope. However, in very rare instances, syncope may result from severe bilateral disease, particularly with superimposed reduction of blood pressure.

Seizures

Generalized tonic-clonic seizures always result in loss of consciousness and can easily be mistaken for syncope if the event is unwitnessed. **Atonic (akinetic) seizures** manifest as sudden loss of consciousness and muscle tone and thus are clinically indistinguishable from true syncope. They represent an unusual form of generalized-onset seizure and occur most often in children with severe epilepsy, in combination with other seizure types. Atonic seizures are exceedingly rare in adults. If seizures are suspected, identification of interictal epileptiform activity on *EEG* can establish the diagnosis. Refer to Chapter 4 for information regarding the management of seizures.

Subarachnoid Hemorrhage

This frequently presents with sudden loss of consciousness due to a brief surge in ICP. However, in most cases, severe headache and nuchal rigidity are the predominant symptoms once the patient awakens, and these complaints easily point to the diagnosis. *Head CT and LP* are required to establish the diagnosis. Management is discussed in Chapter 24.

Intracranial Mass Lesions

In rare instances, syncope can result from an ICP wave in a patient harboring an unsuspected intracranial mass lesion or in a patient with obstruction to cerebral venous outflow resulting from dural sinus thrombosis. The diagnosis should be evident by the presence of abnormalities on the neurologic examination and can be confirmed with *neuroimaging studies (CT or MRI).*

Autonomic Dysfunction

Syncope or near-syncope due to autonomic impairment is *always* associated with orthostatic hypotension. **Peripheral neuropathy** from diabetes, amyloidosis, paraneoplastic disease, and other causes can involve the sympathetic nerves, which normally mediate a compensatory pressor response when BP declines upon standing. **Shy-Drager syndrome** is a multiple-system atrophy (MSA) characterized by parkinsonism (tremor, rigidity, bradykinesia, postural instability) and central autonomic failure that manifests primarily as orthostatic hypotension. Idiopathic isolated central and peripheral autonomic failure have also been described but are rare. Autonomic failure leading to orthostatic hypotension can be treated with **support stockings** and **fludrocortisone (Florinef) 0.1 mg one to three times a day,** a pure mineralocorticoid that induces sodium retention and intravascular volume expansion. The alpha-agonist **midodrine 5 to 10 mg three times a day** can be used as an alternative to fludrocortisone.

Conversion Disorder

"Hysterical faints" generally occur as a dramatic loss of consciousness in the presence of other people, without changes in BP or pulse. Patients may betray their state by having complete or partial memory of the spell. The diagnosis should be suspected when pre-existing psychiatric disease (anxiety or personality disorder) is present and the workup is negative. *Caution:* Many psychiatric medications can cause true syncope.

Hyperventilation

Hypocapnia resulting from hyperventilation leads to syncope or presyncope by decreasing cerebral blood flow because of cerebral vasoconstriction. Acute lowering of P_{CO_2} to 25 mm Hg is sufficient to produce symptoms. Tetany or carpopedal spasm can result from the associated alkalosis and may or may not precede the event. The diagnosis is established by a *3-minute trial of hyperventilation,* which reproduces the symptoms of presyncope or syncope. Hyperventilation usually results from **anxiety or panic disorder;** further management should be directed toward treatment of these conditions. If the problem is recurrent, acute episodes can be managed by having the patient breathe into a paper bag (CO_2 rebreathing).

chapter 17 | Pain Syndromes

Pain is the chief complaint in many patients. Both nociceptor and spinothalamic sensitization may contribute to the development of chronic pain. Although pain may arise from a variety of nonneurologic causes, this chapter will cover the diagnosis and management of six pain syndromes that are uniquely neurologic. Headache is covered in Chapter 14. Treatment of pain, independent of the underlying cause, is usually possible with appropriate therapeutic agents, but rational management decisions can be made only after identification of the site of the pain-producing lesion and recognition of the pathophysiology of the particular pain syndrome. Figure 17–1 outlines the possible sites and mechanisms of pain. This chapter will address the following pain syndromes:

- Complex regional pain syndrome (reflex sympathetic dystrophy, causalgia, sympathetically maintained pain [SMP])
- Facial pain (tic douloureux)
- Postherpetic neuralgia
- Painful peripheral neuropathy
- Cervical or lumbar root compression
- Brachial neuritis

■ PHONE CALL

Questions

Questions to be asked at the time of initial contact depend on the pain syndrome. Localization will determine the subsequent path of questioning, but certain questions are pertinent to all pain syndromes. The first three questions can be asked over the phone to prepare for the history taking and examination.

1. **Where is the pain?**
   Is the pain localized, or does it radiate from one region to another, suggesting an anatomic territory?
2. **When did it begin?**
   Acute pain may respond well to specific analgesics, whereas chronic pain may require a combination of therapies, including strong psychologic support.
3. **Is there a history of injury or underlying neurologic disease?**
   Acute injury from lifting or from a mechanical task is common for radicular pain. Traumatic injury to a limb usually precedes complex regional pain syndrome. A vari-

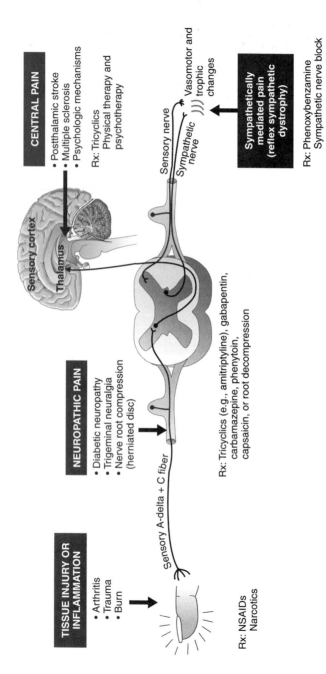

Figure 17-1 □ Sites of origin of pain within the nociceptive pathway.

ety of underlying medical conditions predisposes to painful peripheral neuropathies, including diabetes mellitus, alcoholism, acquired immunodeficiency syndrome (AIDS), and exposures to environmental toxins. Some medications can produce painful neuropathies as well.

Orders

No orders should be given over the phone. Although analgesia may be required in order to obtain an adequate history and perform an adequate physical examination, it is best to evaluate the patient yourself first.

Inform RN

"Will arrive at the bedside as soon as possible."

■ ELEVATOR THOUGHTS

What is the differential diagnosis based on the location of pain?
Face: trigeminal neuralgia (tic douloureux), herpes zoster ophthalmicus (or herpes zoster oticus), temporomandibular joint disease, atypical facial pain, carotid artery dissection
Neck: rheumatoid arthritis, osteoarthritis, meningitis, subarachnoid hemorrhage, vertebral artery dissection, carotid artery dissection, glomus jugulare tumor, tension headache
Low back: herniated nucleus pulposus, epidural abscess, vertebral metastasis, osteomyelitis, osteoarthritis, disk infection, herpes zoster, spinal stenosis, myofasciitis, musculoligamentous strain, ankylosing spondylitis, retroperitoneal disease (referred pain from neoplasm, pancreatitis, ulcer, aortic aneurysm, etc.)
Arms/shoulders: cervical radiculopathy, brachial plexitis, SMP, ischemic heart disease, entrapment syndromes (suprascapular syndrome, radial nerve entrapment, interosseous syndrome, lateral epicondylitis)
Hands/feet (painful peripheral neuropathies): diabetes mellitus, alcoholic neuropathy, AIDS-associated neuropathy, toxin exposure (arsenic, thallium, chloramphenicol, metronidazole), amyloidosis, carpal tunnel syndrome, de Quervain's disease, SMP, paraneoplastic sensory neuropathy, multiple myeloma, inherited neuropathies (Fabry's disease, Tangier disease, dominantly inherited sensory neuropathy)

■ MAJOR THREAT TO LIFE

Neck pain is the only category in which a missed early diagnosis could lead to significant disability or death. Etiology of pain syndromes in this category include carotid artery dissection, meningitis, and subarachnoid hemorrhage.

■ BEDSIDE

Quick Look Test

Does the patient appear acutely ill?
Tachypnea, jaundice, or a decreased level of alertness suggests that the medical illness should be attended to before the pain syndrome is addressed.

How severe does the pain appear to be?
Pain tolerance varies widely from individual to individual. Psychologic factors mediate the response to pain. You should try to get an impression of the relationship between the complaints and the true degree of disability. When you walk into the room, is the patient lying or sitting comfortably in bed or is he or she rolling about, grimacing, moaning, or holding the body in an unmoving posture?

Vital Signs

Fever suggests infection. Tachypnea may mean diabetic ketosis or hyperventilation in response to pain. Tachycardia and elevated blood pressure often accompany acute pain.

Selective History and Chart Review

1. **Define the character of the pain.**
   The questions posed during the phone call should be asked directly (Where is the pain? When did the pain begin?). It is then important to try to determine whether the pain is due to involvement of neural or nonneural tissue.

   Injury to nonneural structures (muscle, bone, or joint) is often abrupt in onset, is continuous or recurrent in specific focal regions, and is usually relieved by rest. Pain caused by injury to neural structures, by contrast, can be delayed or gradual in onset, is often paroxysmal, and is often present at rest. Numbness or tingling between episodes of pain is common. The pain is often described as burning or lancinating. Particularly when the pain is caused by injury to the peripheral nervous system, the pain may be induced by

normally innocuous stimuli such as the touch of a shirt or spray from a shower.
2. **What makes the pain better or worse?**
   Dysesthesias from light tactile stimuli suggest injury to peripheral nerves. "Shooting" (radiating) pains induced by movement of the arm or leg suggest cervical or lumbosacral radiculopathy.
3. **What is the patient's medical history?**
   Ask specifically about diabetes, renal disease, and risk for human immunodeficiency virus (HIV) infection when probing for causes of peripheral neuropathy. Any history of trauma may lead to a diagnosis of nerve or root compression or complex regional pain syndrome. Malignancy may produce neural pain either by compression from a mass or by neural infiltration. Chemotherapeutic agents such as vincristine can produce a painful neuropathy. A previous stroke, particularly in the thalamus, the lateral medulla, or the parietal lobe, may produce a late pain syndrome.
4. **What medications is the patient taking?**
   See Table 17–1 for a list of medications that have pain as a potential side effect.

Selective Physical Examination I

Specific points on examination are discussed under the individual pain syndromes. Certain general principles of examination hold for all pain syndromes, however.

General Physical Examination

Musculoskeletal   If there is pain in or around a joint, look for signs of inflammation, palpate for tenderness, and test the joint for active

Table 17–1 □ COMMON MEDICATIONS THAT CAN CAUSE PAIN OR PARESTHESIA

Antimicrobials	Psychoactive agents
Chloramphenicol	Amitriptyline
Metronidazole	Phenelzine
Streptomycin	Other medications
Nalidixic acid	Acetazolamide
Isoniazid	Pyridoxine
Antineoplastic agents	Ergotamine tartrate
Vincristine	Sulindac
Procarbazine	
Cisplatin	
Cytosine arabinoside	

Skin	and passive range of motion. Be sure to percuss the spine to check for spinal involvement from infection or neoplastic disease. Rash may accompany an infection or a drug reaction. Vesicles of herpes zoster may precede or follow the associated neuralgia.
Abdomen	Organomegaly may suggest chronic ethanol abuse. Abdominal or pelvic masses may produce pain that is referred to the back or the legs.

Neurologic Examination

Focus on the motor and sensory examinations in the location of the pain. A straight leg raise test should be done when there is low back or leg pain (Fig. 17–2). A straight leg raise test is positive when raising the leg reproduces the pain (by stretching the nerve root), particularly if the pain occurs with straight leg raise of the contralateral leg. Look for muscular atrophy in the distribution of the pain to suggest chronic sensorimotor neuropathy or local nerve entrapment or compression. Sensory loss will

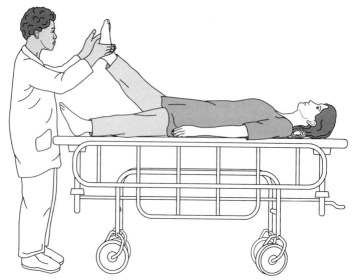

Figure 17–2 □ Straight leg raise. The physician raises each of the patient's legs, in turn, while the patient is supine. A positive test occurs when the pain is reproduced as a result of stretch on a nerve root. Pain of muscle stretch in the posterior thigh does not constitute a positive test.

often map to the same territory as the pain. Hyporeflexia usually accompanies peripheral neuropathy.

■ MANAGEMENT

Management of individual pain syndromes is discussed later. There are, however, some general principles of pain management that apply in any symptomatic treatment of pain.

1. **Treat acute pain aggressively and early.**

    A common error in managing pain is to wait to see whether the pain will go away or become less intense on its own. The problem with this approach is that peripherally induced central mechanisms may intensify and prolong the pain. Partial treatment of acute pain may also be counterproductive. **For severe, acute pain, opioids are the drug of first choice** (Table 17–2). They are quick acting, and their actions may be reversed pharmacologically if necessary. Doses should be increased for maximal pain control and should be limited only by undesirable side effects. **Nonsteroidal anti-inflammatory drugs (NSAIDs), tricyclic antidepressants (TCAs), amphetamine, or hydroxyzine** may be useful adjuncts to opioids if only partial pain control is achieved (see Table 17–2 for opioid dosing).

2. **Avoid "as-needed" dosing for chronic or frequently recurring pain.**

    Regular dosing schedules achieve better pain control in chronic pain and minimize the anxiety from uncertainty about the next attack.

3. **Tailor the therapy to the type, location, and duration of pain.**

    Specific pharmacologic therapy remains the cornerstone of treatment, but nonpharmacologic treatment such as transcutaneous electric nerve stimulation (TENS), local or regional anesthetic blocks, or physical therapy may be useful in specific instances. Psychologic support is especially important in management of chronic pain.

■ SELECTED PAIN SYNDROMES

Complex Regional Pain Syndrome (Reflex Sympathetic Dystrophy, Causalgia)

Clinical Presentation

This relatively rare entity usually occurs after trauma to a limb, either soft-tissue injury (type 1, formerly called reflex sympathetic dystrophy) or neural injury (type 2, formerly called causalgia).

Table 17-2 □ NARCOTIC EQUIVALENCE DOSES

Drug	IM/IV Dose (mg)	PO Dose (mg)	Duration of Action (hours)
Codeine	130	200	4-6
Fentanyl	0.1	—	1-2
Hydrocodone	—	5-10	4-5
Hydromorphone (Dilaudid)	1.3	7.5	4-5
Meperidine (Demerol)	75	300	3-5
Methadone	10	20	4-6
Morphine	10	60	4-5
Oxycodone (Percocet)	—	5-10	4-5
Oxymorphone	1	—	4-6
Pentazocine (Talwin)	30	—	4-6

The natural history is one of persistent pain, with the development of signs of sympathetic involvement occurring days to weeks later. Sympathetic signs may include vasoconstriction and sweating, with red, glossy skin and abnormalities of the hair and nails. Hyperpathia or allodynia to light touch or cold are present on examination. Long-term consequences may be fixed joints and osteoporosis.

Diagnosis

The symptoms and signs resolve following sympathetic blockade. Blockade may be achieved by sympathetic ganglion blocks with local anesthetic, regional alpha-adrenergic blockade with guanethidine, or systemic alpha-adrenergic blockade with IV phentolamine.

Treatment

1. Pharmacologic: begin with **phenoxybenzamine** (systemic alpha-adrenergic blocker) **10 mg two times a day, tapering up to 120 mg per day** maximum or until unacceptable side effects (impotence, postural hypotension) occur. Alternatives are **clonidine 0.1 mg up to three times a day** or **prazosin 2 mg two times a day.**
2. Repeated regional sympathetic blockade with guanethidine.
3. Surgical sympathectomy.
4. Treatment with **gabapentin 900 mg to 3600 mg divided into three doses** is often effective for neuropathic pain in general. Gabapentin or another antiepileptic drug such as phenytoin or carbamazepine may be helpful as an adjunct in any of the first three treatments.

Trigeminal Neuralgia (Tic Douloureux)

This disorder of the sensory division of the trigeminal nerve usually occurs in the middle and late stages of life. The cause is unknown. Degenerative or fibrotic changes in the gasserian ganglion have been reported. In some cases, the trigeminal nerve has been found to be compressed by a tumor or a blood vessel.

Clinical Presentation

Paroxysmal unilateral lightning-like jabs of pain occur in one or more divisions of the trigeminal nerve, most commonly in the second or third division. Paroxysms usually last 1 to 2 minutes but may last up to 15 minutes. The frequency of pain ranges from several times daily to once or twice a month. Typically, patients describe a trigger that induces the paroxysm, for example, chewing, facial movements, or light touch. Patients may avoid nourishment or conversation in a desperate attempt to avoid triggering an attack. There is generally no objective sensory loss or weakness in the distribution of the pain, although patients may refuse to be examined for fear of inducing a paroxysm.

Diagnosis

Because of an absence of signs, the diagnosis of trigeminal neuralgia is made on the basis of history and observation. The differential diagnosis includes dental and sinus pain, as well as herpes zoster. Herpes (and postherpetic neuralgia) most commonly involves the first division, however. The appearance of vesicles verifies the diagnosis of herpes infection.

Treatment

Carbamazepine 200 mg two to five times a day is the first-line treatment, and it induces remissions in a high percentage of patients. Phenytoin or lamotrigine may be a medical alternative. Radiosurgery of the trigeminal ganglion may be successful in refractory cases.

Herpetic Neuralgia (Shingles), Postherpetic Neuralgia

Clinical Presentation

Herpes zoster infection causes a painful neuropathy in a dermatomal distribution, thought to result from the reactivation of a latent infection of the virus in sensory ganglion cells (i.e., from childhood chickenpox). It occurs during the lifetime of 10 to 20% of the general population, but this incidence is mostly in the elderly and in those who are immunocompromised. A thoracic dermatome is the most common site of occurrence, followed by the cervical and then the lumbosacral dermatome. Herpes zoster ophthalmicus results from infection in the first division of the trigeminal ganglion, producing a painful vesicular eruption over the upper face and the eyes. The rash of herpes zoster appears 1 to 4 days after a prodrome of fever, malaise, and dysesthesias. The vesicular eruption becomes pustular in 3 to 4 days and then crusts over by 7 to 10 days. In the normal host, the lesions resolve without sequelae in 2 to 3 weeks. In immunocompromised hosts, however, the infection may linger.

Postherpetic neuralgia is the persistence of pain after the resolution of the rash. This occurs in 10 to 20% of patients with herpes zoster, with the bulk of occurrences in the elderly and the immunocompromised. Fifty percent of patients with postherpetic neuralgia will have a resolution of the pain in 2 months, and 70% of patients are better in 1 year. In some patients, however, the neuralgia may persist for many years.

Diagnosis

You can make the clinical diagnosis on the basis of the typical dermatomal rash. Pain and mild sensory loss should follow the same dermatomal distribution. For confirmatory diagnosis, consultation from the infectious disease or dermatology service may be helpful. Vesicles may contain polymorphonuclear leukocytes. A scrape biopsy may show giant cells and intranuclear inclusions. Varicella-zoster virus antibody titers may increase fourfold.

Treatment
1. **Acute herpes zoster infection**
   Acyclovir 5 mg/kg IV (infuse over 1 hour) three times a day for 7 days will shorten the period of acute dermatomal pain and accelerate healing of the rash but will not reduce the incidence or severity of postherpetic neuralgia. A newer antiviral agent, **famciclovir, given orally for 7 days** may reduce the duration and severity of the neuralgia. **Prednisone 60 mg PO per day for 7 days** may reduce acute pain and potentially reduce the incidence of postherpetic neuralgia. Beware of using prednisone in immunocompromised hosts.
2. **Postherpetic neuralgia**
   This condition is notoriously difficult to treat, and a variety of anticonvulsants and antidepressants have been tried. **Amitriptyline 50 to 150 mg PO per day in divided doses, gabapentin 300 to 900 mg PO three times a day,** and **oxycodone/acetaminophen (Percocet) 1 to 2 tablets every 6 hours** may reduce the burning pain. Lidoderm (5% lidocaine) patch has been shown to be an effective topical treatment. Intrathecal treatment with methylprednisolone (60 mg) plus 3% lidocaine (3 ml) has been shown to be effective in patients with refractory pain.

Painful Peripheral Neuropathy

Clinical Presentation
Systemic disease affecting the peripheral nervous system produces symptoms in the longest nerves first. Dysesthesias and sensory loss in a symmetric, stocking-glove distribution are typical for early peripheral neuropathy. The patient may describe "burning" on the soles of the feet or hypersensitivity to touch in the feet more than in the hands. There may be gait disturbance from the pain of walking or from early sensory loss.

During the examination, look for wasting of the muscles, sensory loss (vibratory sense may be the first to be lost), and hyporeflexia in the distal extremities.

Diagnosis
The clinical diagnosis may often be made from the history and physical examination. Be sure to ask about diabetes mellitus, ethanol use, renal disease, and HIV risks. Occupational history may reveal exposure to toxins.

If the patient has an obvious cause (e.g., post–vincristine chemotherapy), no further workup may be needed. *Electromyography (EMG) and nerve conduction studies* can confirm a diagnosis of peripheral neuropathy and distinguish between demyelinating and axonal pathology (most painful neuropathies are axonal). Initial laboratory tests to order should include fasting glucose level with full chemistry panel including liver and thyroid function tests, rheumatologic screen (erythrocyte sedimentation rate [ESR], antinuclear antibodies [ANA], and rheumatoid factor [RF]) serum protein electrophoresis (SPEP [screen for multiple myeloma]), complete blood count (CBC), and serum vitamin B_{12} level.

Treatment

1. Treat any underlying metabolic disorder or malignancy or remove any offending neurotoxins.
2. Symptomatic treatment of painful peripheral neuropathy consists of anticonvulsaants, tricyclic antidepressants, or topical agents. Begin with **gabapentin 100 mg three times a day** (lower dosage for elderly patients) and taper up to 1800 to 3600 mg per day divided in three doses. Tricyclic antidepressants, such as amitriptyline 25 to 100 mg daily, are an alternative.
3. For topical treatment, use **capsaicin (0.075% to 0.25%) three to four times per day or Lidoderm (5% lidocaine)-impregnated occlusive dressing.**
4. Anti-inflammatory agents such as **ibuprofen 400 to 800 mg PO every 6 hours** may be a useful adjunct to more specific therapies, particularly when the cause of the neuropathy may be inflammatory. A 10- to 14-day tapering course of oral steroids such as **dexamethasone 6 mg PO four times a day** can be a useful analgesic while chemotherapy is being initiated.
5. Nonpharmacologic therapies such as TENS can supplement the treatment regimen.

Cervical or Lumbosacral Root Compression

Clinical Presentation

Acute low back or neck pain from root compression is often precipitated by a specific physical event such as lifting a heavy weight or twisting in an unusual way during housework or gardening. The differential diagnosis includes neck or back strain without neural injury. Radicular pain usually presents as shooting pain into an arm or leg. There is almost always perispinal pain because of reactive muscle spasm. With lumbosacral disk herniation, the pain is often increased by coughing or sneezing. Lumbar disks tend to herniate posterolaterally and cervical disks tend to herniate centrally. Disk herniation is therefore more likely to produce radicular syndromes in the low back as opposed to signs of myelopathy in the neck. Root compression in the neck, therefore, is more often seen with cervical degenerative disease. Osteoarthritis can produce cervical spondylitic ridges and osteophytes, facet joint arthritis, and neural foraminal narrowing.

Diagnosis

The typical symptom for lumbar radiculopathy is **sciatica**, or radiation of pain into the back and side of the leg. The most commonly affected roots are L5 (produced by herniation of the L4–L5 disk) and S1 (produced by herniation of the L5–S1 disk). Upper lumbar root compressions are less common. In the cervical region, C5 and C6 are the roots most affected by cervical spondylosis; C7 is the root most affected by disk lesions. Higher cervical involvement or thoracic radiculopathies warrant further investigation for neoplastic disease or neurofibromatosis. Table 17–3 lists the pain, sensory, and reflex changes for common cervical and lumbosacral radicular syndromes. Also see the **dermatome and myotome charts** in Appendices A–1, A–2, and A–5. Clinical diagnosis can usually be made from the history and examination. Be sure to check motor, sensory, and reflex function in the distribution of the pain. For lumbosacral pain, putting stretch on the root with a straight leg raise test (the exact pain syndrome should be reproduced by ipsilateral or contralateral straight leg raise) supports the diagnosis of radiculopathy (see Fig. 17–2). *Cervical or lumbosacral spinal magnetic resonance imaging (MRI)* is the diagnostic test of choice to visualize the spinal cord, the vertebrae, the disks, and the nerve roots. If there is any suspicion of a neoplastic or infectious lesion, a gadolinium MRI should be obtained.

Treatment

1. **Conservative management** with rest and analgesia usually suffices to achieve good recovery. Even if there is evidence for disk herniation, long-term recovery will be better if the condition resolves without operation. For cervical radiculopathy, a soft collar in combination with **ibuprofen 600 mg PO every 4 to 6 hours** may be enough to promote recovery. For cervical or lumbosacral root disease, the addition of narcotics such as **acetaminophen with codeine 1 to 2 tabs PO every 4 to 6 hours** may be necessary, particularly in the first few days. The addition of **diazepam 2 to 5 mg every 6 hours** may also be helpful in the short term to relieve reactive muscle spasm.
2. **Surgical intervention** should be reserved for three indications: (1) bowel or bladder involvement with lumbosacral radiculopathy, (2) severe neurologic deficit, such as a com-

Table 17-3 □ CLINICAL FEATURES OF CERVICAL AND LUMBOSACRAL ROOT COMPRESSION SYNDROMES

Root	Area of Pain	Sensory Loss	Motor Loss	Reflex
C5	Lateral upper arm and medial scapula	Lateral upper arm	Shoulder abduction, internal and external rotation, and elbow flexion	Biceps jerk
C6	Lateral forearm, thumb, and index finger	Lateral forearm and thumb	Elbow supination	Supinator jerk
C7	Over the triceps, mid-forearm, and middle finger	Middle fingers	Elbow extension and wrist extension	Triceps jerk
C8	Medial forearm and little finger	Medial forearm and little finger	Finger flexion and finger extension	Finger jerk
L4	Knee to medial malleolus	Medial knee and leg	Foot inversion and knee extension	Knee jerk
L5	Back of thigh, lateral calf, and dorsum of foot	Dorsum of foot	Foot and toe dorsiflexion	None
S1	Back of thigh, back of calf, and lateral foot	Behind lateral malleolus, sole of foot	Foot plantar flexion and foot eversion	Ankle jerk

plete footdrop or more than mild weakness in the upper extremity, and (3) failure to control pain or reverse a neurologic deficit with medical management for at least 3 weeks. Referral should be made to a neurosurgeon experienced with spine disease.
3. Local injections of corticosteroids at the nerve roots may obviate the need for sugery.

Brachial Neuritis (Neuralgic Amyotrophy, Brachial Neuralgia, Parsonage-Turner Syndrome)

Clinical Presentation

This rare syndrome typically begins with pain localized to the C5 and C6 dermatomes. Pain in the shoulder may have an aching quality that radiates into the arm. Some patients have mild sensory loss in the distribution of the axillary nerve. Within a few days, the shoulder girdle musculature becomes weak and atrophic, affecting the C5 and C6 myotomes. The disease is idiopathic and sporadic, affecting men more than twice as frequently as women. Most cases occur after the third decade. The syndrome may be associated with trauma, infection, or vaccination and is usually unilateral, rarely bilateral. Guarding of the shoulder may lead to a frozen shoulder.

Diagnosis

The clinical pattern of relatively rapid onset of pain followed by weakness is typical for brachial neuritis. The differential diagnosis at the early stage in which pain is the only complaint includes inflammatory and orthopedic involvement, as well as cervical radiculopathy and root compression from a rudimentary cervical rib. **EMG/nerve conduction studies usually show evidence of denervation in the affected myotomes and decreased amplitude of sensory nerve action potentials.** Subtle signs may also be present on the "unaffected" side in up to 25% of patients.

Treatment

Because the cause of brachial neuritis is unknown, there is no specific therapy. **Immobilization of the shoulder girdle** can help minimize the pain caused by movement, but gentle physical therapy with **passive range-of-motion exercises** should be used to avoid a frozen shoulder. **Ibuprofen 600 mg every 4 to 6 hours** may be used as the first therapy for analgesia. If there is no relief in 24 hours, **acetaminophen with codeine 1 to 2 tabs PO every 4 to 6 hours,** or a 2-week, tapering course of steroids, beginning with **prednisone 60 mg PO per day**, may be used. The prognosis is good, with 90% of patients making a good recovery. The prognosis is poor if the EMG shows no voluntary motor units.

Chapter 18 | Amnesia and Dementia

Memory dysfunction may be variable in its presentation and ranges from the highly functioning senior citizen complaining of forgetfulness to the patient brought in by a relative for bizarre behavior and "confusion." **Amnesia** is defined as a pure loss of memory without other cognitive dysfunction. **Dementia** implies chronic, progressive cognitive loss including chronic loss of memory to a degree sufficient to interfere with occupational or social performance. Dementia should not be confused with **delirium,** which is an acute, global disorder of thinking and perception, characterized by impaired consciousness and inattention. **Retrograde amnesia** refers to loss of memory for events before a specific point in time. **Anterograde amnesia** is the inability to lay down new memory. Memory is often categorized into **immediate recall** (seconds), **short-term memory** (minutes to hours), and **long-term memory** (days to years), with short-term memory being the most vulnerable to pathologic processes, both in acute amnestic states and in dementia syndromes. The hippocampi and parahippocampal structures, and dorsomedial thalamus along with the dorsolateral prefrontal cortex, have been implicated in short-term memory function. Verbal memory is mediated predominantly by the left hemisphere, and visuospatial memory is mediated by the right hemisphere.

■ PHONE CALL

Questions

1. **What is the patient's predominant neurologic condition? In addition to memory loss, is there confusion, agitation, delirium, or stupor?**

    Although dementia or amnesia may be one element of a patient's presentation, memory loss may be part of an acute confusional state, decreased level of consciousness, or stroke.

2. **Is this new memory dysfunction, or does the patient have known dementia?**

    Much of your differential diagnosis will depend on the acuteness of onset. Acute-onset memory dysfunction suggests a vascular, epileptic, infectious, or toxic/metabolic etiology, whereas gradual onset suggests degenerative disease.

3. **How old is the patient?**
   The most common causes of dementia—Alzheimer's disease, vascular dementia, and Parkinson's disease with dementia—are diseases of the elderly. In patients younger than 60 years of age, Huntington's disease, acquired immunodeficiency syndrome (AIDS), and a variety of metabolic disorders must be considered.
4. **Does the patient have acute medical problems?**
   Although the evaluation of the dementia or amnesia may be your primary role in the patient's care and does not preclude your making an initial assessment, chronic dementia, in particular, is not a medical emergency. The acute medical illness may be a more pressing issue. Furthermore, treatment of an intervening illness may reverse a worsening of dementia.

Orders

1. Check the vital signs.
2. Obtain a finger stick glucose level.
3. If the patient is agitated, keep him or her under close observation. Avoid the use of sedative medications until an initial neurologic assessment can be made.
4. Make sure a family member or a health-care person is available to provide a history.

Inform RN

"Will arrive at the bedside in . . . minutes."

■ ELEVATOR THOUGHTS

What is the differential diagnosis of amnesia and dementia?
V (vascular): cerebral infarction, multiple strokes, diffuse white-matter ischemia, bilateral thalamic infarctions, amyloid angiopathy
I (infectious): syphilis, chronic meningitis (tubercular or fungal), AIDS, progressive multifocal leukoencephalopathy, herpes simplex encephalitis, subacute sclerosing panencephalitis, Whipple's disease
T (traumatic): subdural hematoma, dementia pugilistica, head injury
A (autoimmune): central nervous system (CNS) vasculitis, multiple sclerosis, systemic lupus erythematosus (SLE)
M (metabolic/toxic): renal failure, hepatic failure, hypothyroidism, hypercalcemia, benzodiazepine and other tranquilizer intoxication, chronic alcohol use (Wernicke-Korsakoff syn-

drome), vitamin B_{12} deficiency, nicotinic acid deficiency (pellagra), lead exposure, carbon monoxide exposure

I (idiopathic/inherited): transient global amnesia (TGA), Alzheimer's disease, Huntington's disease, Parkinson's disease, Lewy body disease, Pick's disease, progressive supranuclear palsy, amyotrophic lateral sclerosis–parkinsonism–dementia complex of Guam, Wilson's disease

N (neoplastic): brain tumor, paraneoplastic limbic encephalitis, meningeal carcinomatosis, postradiation effects

S (seizure, psychiatric, structural): complex partial seizure, postictal state, depression ("pseudodementia"), normal-pressure hydrocephalus

■ MAJOR THREAT TO LIFE

If the patient is awake, alert, and attentive, memory loss or other cognitive dysfunction is unlikely to indicate a life-threatening condition. For alterations in level of consciousness or delirium, see Chapter 5 or 8.

■ BEDSIDE

Quick Look Test

Is the patient agitated?

Patients with primary dementia can be agitated, particularly in the evening (evening disorientation and agitation is often referred to as "sundowning"), but you should be sure you are not dealing with delirium.

Does the patient look medically ill?

As mentioned earlier, medical illness can produce or exacerbate dementia. Attention may first need to be directed toward treating an acute medical condition such as hypoxia, hyperglycemia, or an infection.

Selective Physical Examination

General Physical Examination

HEENT	Look for external signs of head trauma.
Cardiopulmonary	Listen for rales to suggest congestive heart failure. Atrial fibrillation predisposes to cardioembolic stroke.
Abdomen	Hepatomegaly and ascites may be signs of liver failure or chronic alcohol abuse.

Extremities Clubbing may indicate chronic disease. Asterixis is a nonspecific sign of metabolic disarray.

Neurologic Examination
1. **Mental status**
   Is the patient lethargic, inattentive, or aphasic? If there is a decreased level of consciousness, inattention, or aphasia, then memory deficits and other cognitive function cannot be accurately assessed. Dementia can be screened for with the standardized "Mini Mental State Examination" (MMSE) (Appendix A–6). A score less than 28 out of 30 in a younger person or less than 24 out of 30 in an older person is abnormal. The MMSE yields a quantitative score, which can be used to monitor the patient over time.
   a. **Alertness and attentiveness**
      Have the patient count backward from 20 to 1 or recite the months of the year backward. Serial sevens (serially subtracting 7 from 100) can be used also, but the test may be influenced by education level.
   b. **Aphasia**
      Check for the following:
      (1) **Fluency**
         Listen for effortful, nonfluent speech with loss of grammar and syntax, not just word-finding difficulties.
      (2) **Naming**
         Anomia is a nonspecific finding common to all types of aphasia.
      (3) **Auditory comprehension of single and multistep commands**
         For example, commands such as "Show two fingers" or "With your eyes closed, tap your right knee with two fingers of your left hand."
      (4) **Repetition of unfamiliar phrases**
         When testing repetition, avoid stock phrases such as "no ifs, ands, or buts," which may be overlearned, practiced utterances. Using a sentence such as "The spy fled to Greece" for testing both repetition and reading aloud may yield a clinically important dissociation (e.g., conduction aphasia versus pure alexia).
      (5) **Reading aloud**
      (6) **Writing**
         Have the patient write his or her name, a dictated sentence, and a spontaneous sentence.
      (7) **Listen for phonemic paraphasias** (substitution of one phoneme for another within a word: e.g., "tadle" for

"table") **or semantic paraphasias** (substitution of one semantically related word for another: e.g., "door" for "window").

c. **Memory**

Check for **immediate recall** by asking the patient to repeat number strings ("digit span"). Reciting less than six numbers forward or four numbers backward is abnormal for younger patients; reciting less than six numbers forward or three numbers backward is abnormal for patients over 65 years of age. Check **short-term memory** by asking the patient to repeat three words and then to recall them after 5 minutes. **Long-term memory** can be tested by asking the current month and year or the patient's address and phone number and by asking the patient to name present and past presidents, mayors, or sports players. Be sure to take into account education level and interests (the patient may follow sports but not politics, or vice versa).

d. **Calculations**

Ask the patient to do two-digit addition or multiplication, based on his or her education level, or to tell you how many quarters are in $1.75.

e. **Hemineglect**

Have the patient bisect a horizontal line. Average deviation from the true midline greater than 10% on six lines is abnormal. Ask the patient to perform a target cancellation task (e.g., to circle all letter As in an array of letters); look for left-right asymmetry in targets missed.

f. **Apraxia**

Apraxia is impairment of the execution of a learned or imitated movement in the absence of weakness, sensory loss, or incoordination. Ask the patient to pantomime or imitate striking a match or opening a lock with a key. Abnormal performance on this task (ideomotor apraxia) may be seen in Alzheimer's disease and other dementias. In more severe dementia, inability to use real objects in a sequence of acts may be seen (ideational apraxia), for example, inability to put on and button a shirt.

g. **Drawing**

Have the patient copy a complex figure, for example, the Rey Complex Figure shown in Figure 18–1. Dyspraxia for drawing may be found in dementia. Evidence of hemineglect may also be picked up by this test (e.g., the left side of the drawing is incomplete or less organized than the right).

2. **Motor**

Look for signs of hemiparesis that may suggest a focal lesion such as subdural hematoma, stroke, or tumor. **Adventitial movements** such as myoclonus, chorea, and tremor often ac-

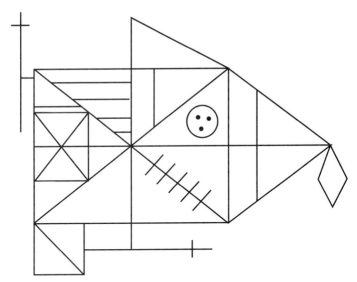

Figure 18–1 □ Rey Complex Figure.

company degenerative dementias, particularly in the later stages. Signs of parkinsonism may accompany Alzheimer's disease or be a part of the dementia of Lewy body disease, progressive supranuclear palsy, amyotrophic lateral sclerosis–parkinsonism–dementia complex of Guam, or idiopathic Parkinson's disease.

3. **Coordination and gait**

    Ataxia may be present with **Wernicke-Korsakoff syndrome**. A **"magnetic gait,"** characterized by hesitancy and shuffling in initiation of gait and difficulty in turning 180 degrees, is seen in **normal-pressure hydrocephalus** (triad of urinary incontinence, gait dysfunction, and dementia).

4. **Frontal "release" signs**

    Frontal lobe dysfunction may produce a disinhibition of motor and behavioral functions, signaled by the appearance of persistent blinking when the examiner taps the forehead just above the bridge of the nose (Myerson's or glabellar sign) or the snouting, rooting, and palmomental reflexes (Fig. 18–2).

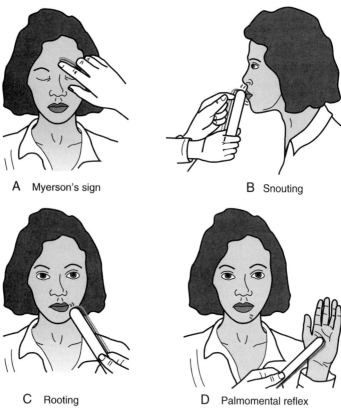

Figure 18–2 □ Frontal release signs. *A*, Myerson's sign. Patient displays persistent blinking (does not habituate) to repeated taps to the brow above the bridge of the nose. *B*, Snouting. Patient purses lips reflexively in response to tapping with a pen or tongue blade. *C*, Rooting. Patient's lips and mouth deviate toward a light scratch to the side of the mouth. *D*, Palmomental reflex. Patient's chin twitches when the palm is scratched.

■ MANAGEMENT I

1. **Check the vital signs.**
    If the patient is in respiratory distress, check an arterial blood gas measurement.
2. **Check the finger stick glucose level.**
3. **Order the following laboratory tests stat:**
    - Complete blood cell count (CBC)
    - Chemistry panel
    - Erythrocyte sedimentation rate (ESR)

- Electrocardiogram (ECG)
- Chest x-ray
- Urinalysis
- Toxicology screen and ethanol level (if indicated)
4. **If the patient is too agitated to examine, follow the algorithm for delirium in Chapter 8.**

    Haloperidol (Haldol) 2 to 10 mg IM may be used unless there is alcohol use, benzodiazepine withdrawal, or hepatic encephalopathy, in which case, **lorazepam 1 to 2 mg IM or IV** may be used initially.

Selective History and Chart Review

Because of the nature of the disease, a detailed and reliable history may need to come from a relative of the patient or a home health aide who knows the patient well rather than the patient.

1. **What was the time course of onset of the patient's memory dysfunction?**

    Has there been a gradual progression, for example, from minor forgetfulness to getting lost around town to being unable to fulfill basic needs? Or was the change relatively sudden, occurring over minutes, hours, or days? As discussed earlier, an insidious course suggests a chronic, degenerative process such as Alzheimer's disease. Be warned, however, that a patient may compensate in daily activities for some time before problems become manifest, particularly in the eyes of a loved one. If the onset was truly acute, consider a vascular, epileptic, infectious, or metabolic/toxic etiology.

2. **Has the patient started any new medications within the time frame of the memory loss?**

    Review the chart for any recent change in medications. Table 18–1 shows medications that may be associated with memory impairment.

3. **Is there any underlying medical illness?**

    Review the patient's medical history for underlying medical illness such as renal failure, hepatic failure, hypothyroidism, or other metabolic disorders.

Table 18–1 ◻ MEDICATIONS THAT MAY BE ASSOCIATED WITH MEMORY IMPAIRMENT

Corticosteroids	Chlorpromazine
Isoniazid	Anticonvulsants (overdose)
Benzodiazepines	Interleukins
Barbiturates	Methotrexate
Bromides	Clioquinol (antifungal)

4. **Have there been other cognitive or behavioral changes besides memory loss, such as difficulty making change in the grocery store, change in reading habits, or disorientation, particularly in the evening?**

    The differential diagnosis for an acute pure amnestic syndrome is limited. If the patient is awake, alert, and attentive and has no focal neurologic deficits, consider the diagnosis of TGA, particularly if there is no acute medical illness and no suspected drug toxicity.

5. **Is there any history of head trauma?**

    Boxers may develop chronic traumatic encephalopathy (dementia pugilistica). For the general population, head trauma may produce acute or chronic subdural hematoma, may predispose to the development of hydrocephalus, and may have an association with idiopathic Alzheimer's disease.

■ MANAGEMENT II

Diagnostic Testing

After acute medical illness has been eliminated as a cause of memory dysfunction, the evaluation of dementia should proceed with the following laboratory tests:

1. **Blood tests**
    - Thyroid function tests
    - Venereal Disease Research Laboratory (VDRL) test
    - Vitamin B_{12} level
    - HIV testing (if risk factors are present)
2. **Imaging**
    - Computed tomography (CT) or magnetic resonance imaging (MRI) scan to identify structural and potentially treatable causes such as subdural hematoma, tumor, or hydrocephalus
    - Single photon emission computed tomography (SPECT) or positron emission tomography (PET) scan: Alzheimer's disease produces posterior parietotemporal hypometabolism; Pick's disease may show frontal hypometabolism; and TGA may show transient unilateral or bilateral hypoperfusion in the parieto-occipital region.
3. **Electroencephalogram (EEG)**

    EEG may help identify seizure or metabolic encephalopathy.

4. **Lumbar puncture**

    Lumbar puncture may be useful for diagnosing infection (e.g., syphilis, chronic meningitis, or herpes simplex encephalitis), carcinomatous meningitis, or hydrocephalus.

Treatment

Treatment of dementia may be possible by treating the underlying disease (infection, stroke, head trauma, intoxication, metabolic disarray, tumor, or seizure). For treating primary dementias, the management is two-pronged:

Treatment of Behavioral Dysfunction

1. Agitation, delusions, or hallucinations/illusions
   Treat initially with **haloperidol 0.5 to 2.0 mg PO every night or two times a day up to 10 mg per day** or **thioridazine 50 to 100 mg PO three times a day up to 800 mg per day.**
2. Insomnia
   Diphenhydramine 25 to 50 mg PO at night or **zolpidem (Ambien) 5 to 10 mg PO at night** can be used. Behavioral side effects may occur.
3. Anxiety
   Treat with **lorazepam 0.5 to 1.0 mg PO up to three times a day** or **alprazolam 0.025 to 0.5 mg PO one or two times a day.**
4. Depression
   Nortriptyline 10 to 25 mg PO up to 75 mg every day, fluoxetine 20 mg per day, or **sertraline 50 to 100 mg per day** can be used.

Disease-Specific Treatment of the Pathophysiologic Process

1. Alzheimer's disease
   Now known to be associated with abnormal production of the amyloid precursor protein, particularly in individuals with the apolipoprotein ϵ-4 genotype, the presence of beta amyloid plaques and neurofibrillary tangles in the brains of Alzheimer's patients plays an unknown role in the pathophysiology of the disease. No agent has been proved effective in altering the brain pathology of Alzheimer's disease; however, the limited success in treatment has come with cholinergic-enhancing medications. **Donepezil hydrochloride 5 to 10 mg PO per day,** an acetylcholinesterase inhibitor, appears to slow the progression of mild to moderate Alzheimer's disease with minimal side effects. Other cholinesterase inhibitors show promise as well.
2. Parkinson's disease, Lewy body disease, and progressive supranuclear palsy
   A common feature of these diseases is extrapyramidal signs from dopamine depletion. Motor dysfunction responds better than cognitive deficits to dopamine agonists. See Chapter 25 for drugs used in the treatment of Parkinson's

disease. Anticholinergics should be avoided in all patients with dementia in this category. Administration of dopamine agonists may be limited by the development of psychosis.

3. Normal-pressure hydrocephalus

A ventriculoperitoneal shunt may produce a reversal of the urinary incontinence and gait disturbance. Reversal of the dementia is less common. Improvement of symptoms, particularly the gait, may be seen minutes to hours after a large-volume tap—removal of 25 to 40 ml of CSF—or placement of a lumbar drain for 48 to 72 hours. A positive response to the CSF drainage may indicate a better response to ventriculoperitoneal shunting.

4. Huntington's disease

No specific treatment is available for this disease. Antidepressants can be helpful. Propranolol may be helpful in reducing impulsive behavior.

5. AIDS dementia complex

Zidovudine (AZT) 200 mg every 4 hours has been shown to improve cognitive function better than placebo can. Newer combination antiretroviral drug regimens (reverse transcriptase inhibitors and protease inhibitors) have reduced the incidence of AIDS dementia complex. Treatment with tricyclic antidepressants and psychostimulants such as **methylphenidate 10 to 30 mg daily** in divided doses and **dextroamphetamine tapering up from a dose of 5 mg daily** in divided doses may help with symptoms of apathy and abulia.

6. Transient global amnesia

Patients with TGA are middle-aged or older, often with hypertension, prior ischemic episodes, or atherosclerotic heart disease, but are otherwise healthy. Typically, they are brought in by a relative or friend because they are "confused." On examination, there are no focal neurologic deficits. Cognitive function and language are intact, except for a profound anterograde amnesia and a retrograde amnesia for the preceding several hours or days. Patients typically appear agitated and will repeat the same question over and over, such as "What am I doing here?" The anterograde amnesia clears gradually after minutes to hours and usually resolves completely within 24 to 48 hours. A residual retrograde amnesia for the hours immediately surrounding the event is often permanent. TGA often appears in the setting of an emotional or physical stress. The pathophysiology is unknown; both epileptic mechanisms and vascular mechanisms have been proposed but have not been proved. The differential diagnosis includes unwitnessed head trauma or seizure, drug intoxication, stroke, dissociative states, and Wernicke-Korsakoff syndrome. The EEG is usually negative.

MRI should be obtained to evaluate for a seizure-producing lesion. The condition is self-limiting and there is no specific treatment, although some physicians have advocated using **aspirin 325 mg per day** for secondary prophylaxis. Recurrence occurs in less than one fourth of the patients.
7. **Wernicke-Korsakoff syndrome**
   Wernicke-Korsakoff syndrome is a nutritional thiamine deficiency occurring in chronic alcoholics. The acute component (Wernicke's encephalopathy) is characterized by inattentiveness, lethargy, truncal ataxia, and ocular dysmotility (nystagmus—horizontal with or without a vertical or rotary component; and gaze palsy—horizontal or lateral rectus palsy, progressing to complete external ophthalmoplegia). Other signs of nutritional deficiency may be present, such as skin changes or redness of the tongue. If left untreated, the condition is fatal in 10% of patients. Treatment is **thiamine 100 mg IV, IM, or PO daily for 3 days,** along with magnesium and multivitamins. Although the ataxia, inattentiveness, and ocular dysmotility may resolve, the more purely amnestic Korsakoff's syndrome persists in greater than 80% of patients. Korsakoff's syndrome is characterized by moderate to severe anterograde amnesia and patchy long-term memory loss. Unlike patients with TGA, patients with Korsakoff's syndrome are not distressed by their amnesia. Confabulation is often present. Even with good nutrition, the amnesia of Korsakoff's syndrome rarely resolves. Histopathologic examination shows cell loss and degenerative changes in the dorsomedial thalami, the mamillary bodies, the periaqueductal midbrain, and the Purkinje cell layer of the cerebellar vermis.

chapter 19 | **Brain Death**

Brain death describes a condition of complete and irreversible cessation of all cortical and brain stem activity. Although death has traditionally been defined by the irreversible cessation of cardiorespiratory function, technologic advances have led to formal recognition of death on the basis of complete and permanent brain destruction in individuals on life support. In turn, legislative and hospital policies recognizing cerebral death as the equivalent of cardiac death have enabled physicians to save thousands of lives through organ transplantation.

The most common causes of brain death are trauma, intracranial hemorrhage, and hypoxic-ischemic injury from cardiac arrest. Whatever the inciting cause, in the end, brain death ultimately results from widespread cerebral necrosis and edema, herniation, increased intracranial pressure (ICP), and the complete absence of cerebral blood flow.

■ CLINICAL SIGNIFICANCE OF BRAIN DEATH

It is important to identify and diagnose brain death **quickly** for the following reasons:
1. To prevent prolonged anguish and suffering on the part of the patient's loved ones.
2. To avoid the needless waste of valuable medical resources in an unequivocal no-win situation.
3. To create an opportunity for organ donation. Because circulatory collapse and homeostatic disarray begin as soon as brain death occurs, delays in declaration of brain death can lead to the loss of organ viability.

Although the clinical criteria for brain death outlined in the following section are widely agreed upon, policies vary by state and institution regarding (1) the need for examination by a concurring physician, (2) the timing of examinations or a required observation period, and (3) the requirements for confirmatory testing. If you are unsure of the policy at your institution, find out. The declaration of death is a serious issue and must be made with care and precision.

■ CRITERIA FOR THE CLINICAL DIAGNOSIS OF BRAIN DEATH

To make the clinicial diagnosis of brain death, the following conditions must be met:

1. **CEREBRAL FUNCTION MUST BE ABSENT.**
   This means that the patient must be in deep coma, with no behavioral or reflex responses to painful stimuli mediated above the level of the foramen magnum. Triple flexion responses, deep tendon reflexes, or other primitive movements (back arching, extensor plantar responses) resulting from spinal reflex activity are compatible with brain death. In most cases, the patient with brain death is in a state of flaccid and areflexic paralysis, with isolated lower-extremity triple flexion responses to deep pain. Decerebrate or decorticate posturing is incompatible with brain death, because these reflexes are mediated at the brain stem level.
2. **BRAIN STEM FUNCTIONS MUST BE ABSENT.**
   a. **Pupils**
      The pupils must be unreactive to bright light. Size is not critical, as pupils may be small, midposition, or large. Exposure to mydriatic agents must be excluded.
   b. **Ocular movements**
      Ocular responses must be absent to passive head turning (the oculocephalic or "doll's eye" reflex) and caloric irrigation of the ear canals with 50 ml of ice water (the oculovestibular reflex). Care must be taken that the stimulus reaches the tympanic membrane. Testing using passive head turning alone is not adequate.
   c. **Facial sensation and motor response**
      Corneal reflexes should be tested with a cotton-tipped applicator. Reflex or spontaneous facial or eyelid movements must be completely absent.
   d. **Pharyngeal and tracheal reflexes**
      Cough and gag responses must be absent in response to manipulation of the endotracheal tube or bronchial suctioning.
3. **THE PATIENT MUST BE APNEIC.**
   Spontaneous respirations must be absent in response to a hypercarbic stimulus, as documented by formal apnea testing (Box 19–1).
4. **A PROXIMATE AND UNTREATABLE CAUSE OF BRAIN DEATH MUST BE ESTABLISHED.**
   a. **The cause of coma should be clearly evident and sufficient to account for the loss of brain function.**
      Examples include documented structural disease (e.g., massive intracranial hemorrhage) or severe brain anoxia resulting from cardiopulmonary arrest.
   b. **Potentially reversible conditions must be excluded.**
      These conditions may include hypothermia (core temperature less than 32°C), drug intoxication or poisoning, hypo-

> **Box 19–1. PROTOCOL FOR APNEA TESTING**
>
> 1. Adjust minute ventilation to attain partial pressure of carbon dioxide (P_{CO_2}) levels of 35 to 45 mm Hg and document with a **baseline arterial blood gas measurement.**
> 2. **Preoxygenate** with 100% oxygen for 5 minutes.
> 3. Place the patient on a **T-piece with 100% oxygen flow-by** at 6 to 10 L/min for 4 to 6 minutes. Because P_{CO_2} increases 3 to 4 mm Hg per minute of apnea, a *4- to 6-minute period of observation* should allow the P_{CO_2} to rise to levels of hypercarbia (greater than 55 mm Hg) sufficient to provide an adequate respiratory stimulus.
> 4. **Observe for respiratory movements.** Abort the test and place the patient back on mechanical ventilation if cardiac arrhythmia, hypotension, or significant oxygen desaturation occurs.
> 5. At the end of the observation period, **perform a second ABG measurement** to document the level of hypercarbia attained and place the patient back on **mechanical ventilation.**
> 6. **Write a note** in the chart documenting that no respiratory movements were observed. Record the duration of the observation period and the postobservation arterial blood gas level.

tension (systolic blood pressure [BP] less than 90 mm Hg), and severe acid-base or electrolyte abnormalities. If these conditions are present, the patient may require rewarming, treatment with IV pressors, or correction of acid-base and electrolyte disorders in order to proceed with the declaration of brain death. A toxicology screen should be performed in all patients.

c. **Loss of all brain function should persist for an appropriate period of observation.**

If the cause of coma is established and is adequate to account for brain death, an extended period of observation is not required. A period of observation of 6 to 24 hours may be appropriate if the cause of brain death is not absolutely clear (for example, suspected but unwitnessed cardiac arrest). Some institutions require a period of observation of 6 to 24 hours in all patients.

■ CONFIRMATORY TESTING

Brain death is a clinical diagnosis. *Confirmatory tests such as EEG are not essential to the declaration of brain death but may be required according to state laws or institutional policy.* In circumstances in which the clinical diagnosis of brain death cannot be made with certainty, a confirmatory test may be needed. Examples may include severe facial or limb trauma, pre-existing pupillary abnormalities, or severe pulmonary disease resulting in chronic retention of carbon dioxide.

Tests Commonly Used for the Confirmation of Brain Death

1. **Electroencephalography (EEG)**
   Confirmation of neocortical death should be documented by at least 30 minutes of electrocerebral silence, using a 16-channel instrument with increased gain settings, according to guidelines developed by the American Electroencephalographic Society. If any brain wave is present, the diagnosis of brain death cannot be made.
2. **Angiography**
   Complete absence of intracranial blood flow in a four-vessel angiogram confirms the diagnosis of brain death.
3. **Radioisotope cerebral imaging**
   The complete absence of cerebral perfusion can also be established using radionuclide angiography or single photon emission computed tomography (SPECT).
4. **Transcranial Doppler ultrasonography**
   A velocity profile showing systolic spikes with absent or reversed diastolic flow is consistent with the cessation of cerebral blood flow and brain death.

■ PSYCHOSOCIAL ISSUES

The emotional and psychosocial impact of death is always stressful for those who survive the patient; this can be even more difficult in the setting of brain death. Communication of the concept and meaning of brain death to the patient's family is paramount. This communication, however painful, should be initiated as early as possible in order to give those involved time to adjust to the situation. Although family permission is generally *not* required to discontinue life support once a patient is declared legally brain dead, their consent and understanding is extremely important. Misunderstanding, bereavement, emotional upset, and religious or moral beliefs may lead family members to object to "pulling the plug" in some cases. In these instances, third-party mediation by a medical ethics consultant or member of the clergy may be desirable.

■ MANAGEMENT OF THE POTENTIAL ORGAN DONOR

Brain death eventually leads to severe homeostatic derangements and cardiac arrest, despite mechanical ventilation and aggressive life-support measures. This inexorable progression toward multisystem organ failure creates a challenge in managing the potential organ donor, in whom the goal is to maintain and optimize organ viability for transplantation.

Most patients become hypotensive and require IV pressors at the time brain death occurs, and soon thereafter they develop diabetes insipidus (because antidiuretic hormone secretion ceases). As the situation deteriorates, hypothermia, refractory hypoxia, disseminated intravascular coagulation, and metabolic acidosis can occur. The key to management is to be ready for these complications. Even with meticulous attention to cardiovascular, acid-base, and electrolyte homeostasis, organ viability in most adult patients with brain death can be maintained for only 72 to 96 hours.

Protocol for Management of the Potential Organ Donor in the Intensive Care Unit

1. Insert a central venous catheter or two large-bore peripheral IV lines.
2. Insert an arterial line for continuous BP monitoring.
   a. Maintain systolic BP at or higher than 100 mm Hg with stepwise intervention:
      (1) **500 ml 0.9% saline fluid bolus (two times at 10-minute intervals)**
      (2) **Dopamine 800 mg/500 ml NS (start at 13 ml/hour, 5 µg/kg/min), titrated to maintain systolic BP at or higher than 100 mm Hg**
      (3) If refractory hypotension (systolic BP less than 90 mm Hg) or tachyarrhythmia occurs with dopamine treatment, start vasopressin (Pitressin) drip (see item 6)
3. Start baseline IV flow: **0.9% saline at 150 to 200 ml/hour.**
   a. Check serum sodium levels every 6 hours:
      (1) If sodium level is 150 to 159 mmol/L, change baseline IV to 0.45% saline
      (2) If sodium level is at or higher than 160 mmol/L, change baseline IV to 0.25% saline
4. Transfuse if hematocrit is lower than 24%.

5. Adjust fraction of inspired oxygen and positive end-expiratory pressure to maintain oxygen saturation at or higher than 90%.
6. Insert a Foley catheter. Measure fluid input and urine output and monitor urine specific gravity every 2 hours.
   a. If the urine output over 2 hours is greater than 500 ml with specific gravity of 1.005 or lower:
      (1) Administer **aqueous Pitressin 10 U IVP every 6 hours.**
      (2) Replace hourly urine output milliliter for milliliter with D5W
   b. If the urine output persistently remains higher than 200 ml/hour:
      (1) Stop the aqueous Pitressin IVP
      (2) Start **Pitressin 200 U/500 ml D5W; begin at 10 ml/hour (4 U/hour) and titrate to maintain urine output to less than 200 ml/hour**
7. Check the finger stick glucose level every 4 hours.
   If finger stick glucose level is higher than 350 mg/dl over 8 hours, begin **insulin drip (100 U regular insulin in 1000 ml 0.9% saline), starting at 20 ml/hour (2 U/hour).**

SELECTED NEUROLOGIC DISORDERS

chapter 20 | Nerve and Muscle Diseases

LOUIS H. WEIMER

Patients with neuromuscular disease generally present with weakness, sensory loss, or both of these conditions. Your approach should initially focus on localizing the problem to a specific component of the peripheral nervous system that is involved (e.g., neuropathy or myopathy) and then be directed toward identifying a specific disease process. The major anatomic components of the peripheral nervous system are listed in Table 20–1.

■ APPROACH TO THE PATIENT WITH SUSPECTED NEUROMUSCULAR DISEASE

History

1. **Clarify the pattern of weakness.** Proximal weakness suggests myopathy; distal weakness suggests neuropathy.
2. **Characterize any sensory symptoms.** Have the patient identify the exact regions involved and symptom character (sensory loss or unpleasant sensation).
3. **Ask about cramps and muscle twitches (fasciculations).** These symptoms point to disease of the motor neuron (amyotrophic lateral sclerosis [ALS]) or muscle (myopathy).
4. **Ask about pain.** Pain may be related to a musculoskeletal structure (e.g., herniated disk), or it may be neuropathic or muscular.
5. **Is there any autonomic involvement?** Ask about orthostatic dizziness, anhidrosis, visual blurring, urinary hesitancy or incontinence, constipation, and impotence.

Examination

1. **Determine whether the patient has true weakness.** Decreased strength needs to be differentiated from limitation arising from pain, and from submaximal effort. Effort-limited weakness is inconsistent and tends to "give way" suddenly.
2. **Map out any sensory deficits.** Think in terms of identifying *diffuse, distal sensory loss* (stocking-glove pattern), as seen in polyneuropathy; *focal sensory loss* restricted to a single root dermatome or peripheral nerve; or *multifocal sensory loss*,

Table 20-1 □ BASIC ANATOMIC SUBTYPES OF NEUROMUSCULAR DISEASE

Anatomic Site	Typical Pattern of Motor and Sensory Deficit	Examples
Motor neuron disease	Weakness, wasting, fasciculations; no sensory deficits; hyperreflexia with ALS	Amyotrophic lateral sclerosis, spinal muscular atrophy, polio
Monoradiculopathy	Distribution of a single nerve root (dermatomal pattern)	L5 or S1 root compression from herniated disk
Polyradiculopathy	Distribution of multiple nerve roots	Cauda equina syndrome; carcinomatous meningitis
Plexopathy	Distribution of a nerve plexus	Acute brachial neuritis
Mononeuropathy	Distribution of a single peripheral nerve	Carpal tunnel syndrome
Mononeuropathy multiplex	Multifocal process affecting several discrete peripheral nerves	Vasculitis, leprosy
Polyneuropathy	Diffuse, symmetric, distal stocking-glove pattern; distal hyporeflexia	Diabetic polyneuropathy
Neuromuscular junction disease	Fluctuating weakness with fatigability; no sensory deficits; reflexes preserved	Myasthenia gravis
Myopathy	Diffuse proximal muscle weakness; no sensory deficits; preserved reflexes until late	Polymyositis; muscular dystrophy

which suggests mononeuropathy multiplex or a plexus lesion (Fig. 20–1).
3. **Test the reflexes.** Loss of deep tendon reflexes suggests peripheral nerve involvement.
4. **Undress the patient to check for wasting and fasciculations** (irregular individual muscle twitches). These findings indicate lower motor neuron disease.

■ MOTOR NEURON DISEASE

The clinical hallmarks of anterior horn cell disease are the lower motor neuron signs of **weakness, wasting (atrophy), and fasciculations.** These signs may be seen alone or in combination with upper motor neuron signs (hyperreflexia, upgoing toes) in the case of ALS. Sensory disturbances are absent. There are several distinct forms of motor neuron disease:
1. **Amyotrophic lateral sclerosis**
    Also known as Lou Gehrig's disease, ALS is the most common form of motor neuron disease. It is easily recog-

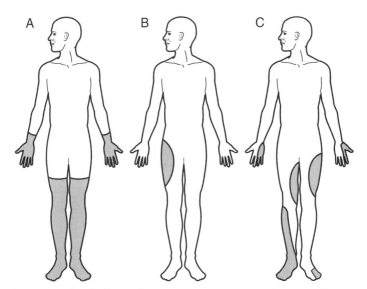

Figure 20–1 □ Patterns of sensory loss in patients with neuropathy. *A*, Polyneuropathy: diffuse stocking-glove pattern. *B*, Mononeuropathy: focal involvement corresponding to a single peripheral nerve. *C*, Mononeuritis multiplex: pattern of multiple, asymmetric regions of sensory loss, corresponding to multiple peripheral nerves.

nized on the basis of progressive weakness, wasting, fasciculations, and upper motor neuron signs. It is familial in 5 to 10% of cases. The presence of bulbar involvement (dysarthria, dysphagia) carries a worse prognosis. Median survival after diagnosis is 3 years. Approximately 5% of patients have a circulating paraprotein, and in these cases an underlying lymphoma or plasma cell dyscrasia may be detected. ALS is a clinical diagnosis, which is supported by the finding of diffuse, chronic partial denervation in at least three limbs on electromyography (EMG).

2. Spinal muscular atrophy

This condition resembles ALS but is limited to pure lower motor neuron degeneration (e.g., no upper motor neuron signs are seen). Spinal muscular atrophy typically has infantile or childhood onset, but adult forms also occur. Adult onset progression is slower than ALS and is more often hereditary. Genetic confirmation of some forms is available.

3. Multifocal motor neuropathy

This is an immune-mediated motor neuropathy, differentiated by the presence of **conduction block** on nerve conduction studies. The course is protracted over many years, and the weakness is asymmetric. Some patients have anti-GM1 antibodies. The disorder is important to recognize because it is treatable with intravenous immune globulin (IVIG).

4. Other motor neuron diseases

These diseases include poliomyelitis, hereditary neurodegenerative diseases, and metabolic systemic storage disorders.

Diagnosis

Diagnostic testing for suspected motor neuron disease should include the following: EMG/nerve conduction studies (NCS), serum and urine electrophoresis, serum immunoelectrophoresis, quantitative immunoglobulins, and anti-GM1 antibody levels. Cervical spine magnetic resonance imaging (MRI) and lumbar puncture should be considered. In patients with a paraprotein, bone marrow biopsy may be indicated.

Treatment

ALS is incurable, but **riluzole 50 mg PO twice per day**, a glutamate antagonist, may slow the progression of the disease. Clinical trials of additional agents are ongoing. Patients with multifocal motor neuropathy may improve with treatment with **IVIG 0.4 g/kg given every 6 to 12 weeks.**

■ MONORADICULOPATHY AND POLYRADICULOPATHY

Monoradiculopathies typically result from disk herniation and nerve root compression. They present with a radicular distribution of pain and are discussed in Chapter 17. *Polyradiculopathy* involving multiple lumbosacral nerve roots (cauda equina syndrome) presents with low back pain, urinary disturbances, and gait failure.

■ PLEXOPATHY

Diseases that cause diffuse injury to either the brachial or the lumbosacral plexus lead to **regional motor, sensory, and reflex disturbances in one limb**. The key to identifying the syndrome is to find a pattern of deficits that cannot be explained by involvement of one nerve root or a single peripheral nerve. EMG and NCS are helpful in confirming and defining the syndrome; complex repetitive discharges on EMG are characteristic. See Appendices A–3 and A–4 for the anatomy of the brachial and lumbosacral plexus.

Brachial Plexopathy

Upper brachial plexus injury (arising from C5 to C7) results in weakness and atrophy of the shoulder and upper arm muscles (Erb's palsy). Lower brachial plexus injury (arising from C8 and T1) leads to weakness, atrophy, and sensory deficits in the forearm and hand (Klumpke's palsy). The main causes of brachial plexopathy include the following:

- **Trauma**
- **Idiopathic brachial neuritis (Parsonage-Turner syndrome)**
  This underrecognized syndrome presents with the sudden onset of pain in the shoulder and arm; as the pain resolves over 2 to 4 weeks, weakness and muscle wasting become evident.
- **Tumor infiltration**
  Metastatic disease and neurofibroma are most common.
- **Radiation plexopathy**
  High-dose irradiation for lymphoma or breast cancer can lead to painless progressive brachial plexopathy 1 to 5 years later. *Myokymia* (irregular worm-like muscle movement) may be a distinguishing feature.
- **Cervical rib or bands (thoracic outlet syndrome)**
  This rare condition is caused by compression of the lower trunk of the brachial plexus as it passes over an abnormal first cervical rib or fibrous band. Patients complain of pain and paresthesias in the C8–T1 distribution of the hand and

medial forearm when carrying heavy objects or when raising the arm above shoulder level. Surgical decompression may be helpful in rare cases.

Diagnosis

In many cases, the cause of brachial plexopathy is readily apparent (e.g., trauma or radiation). If not, chest and cervical spine radiographs, lumbar puncture (LP), and MRI of the plexus should be considered.

Treatment

Physical therapy can help speed recovery, minimize muscle wasting, and prevent contractures.

Lumbosacral Plexopathy

Unilateral lumbosacral plexopathy is rare. The main diagnostic considerations include idiopathic neuritis, diabetic infarction, and compression from a retroperitoneal abscess, hemorrhage, or neoplasm. MRI or CT of the pelvis should be performed to exclude a compressive mass lesion.

■ MONONEUROPATHIES

Mononeuropathies result from injury, compression, or entrapment of a single nerve, usually at a specific site. There are multiple different syndromes.

Carpal Tunnel Syndrome

Carpal tunnel syndrome is by far the most common cause of mononeuropathy; it results from compression of the median nerve at the wrist and usually presents with wrist pain and tingling of the first three digits. The pain may radiate proximally to the elbow and is almost always worse at night. Examination may reveal Tinel's sign (radiation of pain into the first three digits when the wrist is tapped with a hammer). Thenar muscle wasting and persistent sensory deficits in the distal median nerve distribution are advanced findings (Fig. 20–2). Risk factors include repetitive "overuse" injury, thyroid disease, pregnancy, acromegaly, diabetes, and amyloidosis.

Diagnosis

EMG and NCS show focal sensory and/or motor slowing across the wrist in the median nerve. Check thyroid function tests (TFTs) and fasting glucose level to screen for hypothyroidism and diabetes.

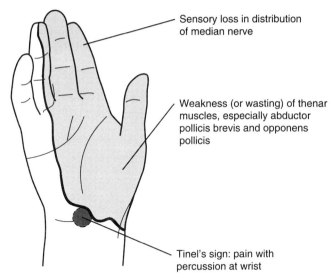

Figure 20–2 □ Sensory and motor involvement in carpal tunnel syndrome.

Treatment

Mild disease can be treated with a neutral position wrist splint; more severe disease may require surgical decompression. Repetitive stress to the wrist can be minimized with special occupational devices.

Facial Palsy (Bell's Palsy)

Facial palsy (Bell's palsy) is the most common cranial mononeuropathy. Patients present with acute unilateral facial paralysis, with equal involvement of the forehead and lower half of the face. The disorder is thought to result from inflammation of CN7 within the facial canal. In some patients, an antecedent viral infection is identified, and approximately 25% of cases are associated with pain in the ipsilateral ear. If the injury to the facial nerve is proximal to the chorda tympani in the facial canal, loss of taste occurs on the anterior two thirds of the tongue ipsilaterally. Complete or near-complete recovery occurs in 85% of cases.

Diagnosis

The majority of cases are idiopathic (Bell's palsy). Examination should focus on searching for signs of other treatable diseases that can present with facial paralysis:

- Decreased hearing or a decreased afferent corneal reflex is suggestive of a cerebellopontine angle tumor (e.g., acoustic neuroma), which should be excluded by MRI with gadolinium.
- Vesicles in the external auditory canal are indicative of the Ramsay Hunt syndrome, which results from herpes zoster infection of the ipsilateral geniculate ganglion.
- An antecedent annular rash or tick bite is suggestive of Lyme disease. Serum Lyme antibody titers and LP with testing for cerebrospinal fluid (CSF) Lyme antibodies are required to establish the diagnosis.
- Interstitial lung disease with hilar adenopathy, uveitis, or parotitis may be clues to neurosarcoidosis. CSF examination may reveal a lymphocytic pleocytosis; biopsy of involved tissue is required to establish the diagnosis.

Treatment

Recovery from idiopathic Bell's palsy can be accelerated by treatment with **prednisone 80 mg PO daily for 5 days,** followed by a 7-day taper. Ramsay Hunt syndrome is treated with **acyclovir 800 mg PO five times daily for 7 days** in addition to prednisone. The likelihood of complete recovery is increased when treatment is started within 7 days of onset. Treatment for Lyme disease (see Chapter 21) and neurosarcoidosis (see Chapter 22) is discussed elsewhere. Patients with incomplete eye closure should use an ophthalmic ointment (e.g., Lacri-Lube) and a protective eye shield at night to prevent corneal abrasions.

Other Common Nerve Entrapment Syndromes

The nerves implicated in additional selected entrapment syndromes are the following:
- Ulnar nerve at the medial epicondyle of the humerus (cubital tunnel syndrome)
- Median nerve at the pronator teres (pronator syndrome)
- Radial nerve at the spiral groove of the humerus (Saturday night palsy)
- Obturator nerve at the obturator foramen (childbirth)
- Peroneal nerve at the fibular head (leg crossers and surgical malpositioning)
- Lateral femoral cutaneous nerve (meralgia paresthetica)
- Posterior tibial nerve at the tarsal tunnel (tarsal tunnel syndrome).

■ MONONEUROPATHY MULTIPLEX

Diseases that affect multiple peripheral nerves at different sites result in the syndrome of *mononeuropathy multiplex*. The presence of **asymmetric and multifocal motor, sensory, and reflex deficits** is the key to identifying the syndrome. The patient's history may reveal a stepwise progression of deficits. The differential diagnosis of mononeuropathy multiplex includes the following:

- *Vasculitis*
    Polyarteritis nodosa is the most common vasculitis associated with this condition. Systemic lupus erythematosus, rheumatoid arthritis, and cryoglobulinemia may occasionally produce the condition.
- *Diabetes mellitus*
- *Leprosy*
- *Sarcoidosis*
- *Human immunodeficiency virus (HIV) infection*
- *Lymphoma*
- *Lyme disease*
- *Hereditary liability to pressure palsies*
- *Multifocal motor neuropathy (pure motor)*
- *Chronic inflammatory demyelinating polyneuropathy (CIDP)*

Diagnosis

Initial blood tests should include fasting glucose level with chem-20 screen, complete blood count (CBC), erythrocyte sedimentation rate (ESR), antinuclear antibody (ANA), rheumatoid factor (RF), antineurotrophil cytoplasmic antibody (ANCA), HIV testing, hepatitis serologies, cryoglobulins, and serum angiotensin-converting enzyme (ACE) activity. LP should be considered to rule out inflammatory conditions (e.g., chronic inflammatory demyelinating polyneuropathy, neurosarcoidosis) and carcinomatous meningitis. A comprehensive EMG and NCS examination is often needed to prove multifocal involvement. Muscle or nerve biopsy is usually necessary to rule out vasculitis, sarcoidosis, leprosy, and lymphoma.

Treatment

Therapy is directed toward treating the underlying disease.

■ POLYNEUROPATHY

The prototypical polyneuropathy patient presents with gradual **distal, symmetric sensorimotor deficits and hyporeflexia.** Typically, the longest nerves in the body are affected first, resulting in a stocking-glove distribution of symptoms and signs (see Fig. 20–1). Dysesthetic sensory changes are often the first symptom, with weakness developing later.

The number of entities that can cause peripheral neuropathy is vast (Table 20–2), and pinpointing a precise cause can be difficult.

Table 20-2 □ CAUSES OF PERIPHERAL POLYNEUROPATHY

Metabolic and endocrine diseases
  Diabetes mellitus*
  Renal failure*
  Hepatic failure
  Porphyria
  Hypothyroidism
  Critical illness polyneuropathy*
Vitamin deficiency states
  Beriberi (thiamine deficiency)
  Vitamin B_6 (pyridoxine) deficiency
  Vitamin B_{12} deficiency
  Vitamin B complex deficiency
  Pellagra (niacin deficiency)
  Vitamin E deficiency
Toxins and poisons
  Alcohol
  Heavy metals: arsenic, lead, mercury, thallium
  Organic and industrial solvents: carbon disulfide, *n*-hexane, acrylamide, methyl-*N*-butyl ketone
  Pyridoxine (vitamin B_6) overdose
  Nitrous oxide (also causes myelopathy)
Medications
  Antibiotics: dapsone, nitrofurantoin, isoniazid, ethambutol, metronidazole, stavudine (d4T), 3TC, didanosine (ddI), dideoxycytidine (ddC)
  Antiarrhythmics: amiodarone, procainamide, propafenone
  Chemotherapeutic agents*: vincristine, vinblastine, cisplatin, paclitaxel (Taxol), adriamycin, suramin, tacrolimus
  Cimetidine
  Chloroquine (also causes myopathy)
  Colchicine (also causes myopathy)
  D-Penicillamine
  Disulfiram

An organized and stepwise approach is essential. **Consideration of the following points can help narrow the possibilities and allow screening for the most common and important (i.e., treatable) causes.**

Clinical Approach to the Patient with Polyneuropathy

1. History
   - **Is the neuropathy acute or chronic?** Acute polyneuropathy (Guillain-Barré syndrome) is discussed in Chapter 15.
   - **Ask a carefully directed set of questions to identify an**

Table 20-2 □ **CAUSES OF PERIPHERAL POLYNEUROPATHY** Continued

Medications Continued
 Gold salts
 Hydralazine
 Podophyllin
 Pyridoxine
 Phenytoin
 Thalidomide
Immunologic or paraprotein-mediated diseases
 Acute inflammatory polyneuropathy (Guillain-Barré syndrome)*
 Chronic inflammatory polyneuropathy (chronic inflammatory demyelinating polyneuropathy)*
 Paraneoplastic disease (sensorimotor or pure sensory)*
 Multiple myeloma
 Anti–myelin-associated glycoprotein antibody-mediated disease
 Amyloidosis
 Lymphoma with paraprotein
 Monoclonal gammopathy
 Cryoglobulinemia
 Collagen vascular disease (systemic lupus erythematosus, rheumatoid arthritis, etc.)
 Sarcoidosis
 Waldentröm's macroglobulinemia
Genetic/hereditary diseases
 Charcot-Marie-Tooth disease*
 Refsum's disease
 Storage diseases (metachromatic leukodystrophy, adrenomyeloneuropathy, etc.)
 Inherited metabolic enzyme defects
Infectious diseases
 Human immunodeficiency virus infection*
 Cytomegalovirus infection*
 Leprosy
 Lyme disease
 Human T-cell leukemia virus type I (HTLV-1) infection (also causes myelopathy)

*Common.

obvious cause. Ask about diabetes, renal disease, HIV infection, current medications, alcohol use, potential exposure to toxins, and family history. *The majority of polyneuropathies are complications of previously evident medical disorders, medications, or alcohol.*

- **Do the symptoms fluctuate?** Fluctuations suggest a relapsing demyelinating neuropathy (CIDP) or repeated exposures to toxins.

2. **Examination**
   - **Determine the predominant systems involved.** Most neuropathies are sensorimotor, with the sensory component predominant. Identifying a predominantly motor, pure sensory, or particularly painful neuropathy helps to limit the differential diagnosis considerably (Table 20–3).
   - **Determine whether the findings are asymmetric.** Patchy and asymmetric motor, sensory, and reflex deficits suggest *mononeuropathy multiplex* or *polyradiculopathy* (see earlier discussion).
   - **Check for palpably enlarged nerves.** Although it is unusual, a finding of enlarged nerves can help pinpoint the diagnosis (see Table 20–3).
3. **EMG and NCS**
   - **Determine whether the neuropathy is axonal or demyelinating.** Electrodiagnosis is critical for making this distinction, which can help to narrow your differential diagnosis. *Distal axonal sensorimotor neuropathies* are the most common. *Demyelinating neuropathies* have a much smaller differential diagnosis (see Table 20–3).

Management

Laboratory Testing for Evaluation of Polyneuropathy

1. If an obvious cause for the neuropathy exists (e.g., post–vincristine chemotherapy), no further workup may be needed. Otherwise proceed with the next steps.
2. The following initial laboratory tests should be performed: fasting glucose with full chemistry panel including liver function tests (LFTs), CBC, TFTs, initial rheumatologic screen (ESR, ANA, RF), serum protein electrophoresis, vitamin B_{12} level.
3. Other tests to consider include LP, testing of urine for paraproteins, serum immunofixation electrophoresis, quantitative immunoglobulins, testing urine for heavy metals, tests for HIV, CMV, human T-cell leukemia virus type I (HTLV-1), Lyme antibody, other vitamin levels (vitamins B and E), ANCA, ACE level, homocysteine/methionine levels (vitamin B_{12} deficiency), genetic testing (Charcot-Marie-Tooth disease), special antibody assays (anti-Hu, anti-GM1, anti-MAG, anti-sulfatide), and bone marrow biopsy.
4. Nerve and muscle biopsy is helpful for confirming several diagnoses (Table 20–4), but it is most useful in evaluating *mononeuropathy multiplex*.

Table 20–3 ◻ FEATURES HELPFUL IN NARROWING THE CAUSE OF PERIPHERAL NEUROPATHY: SYNDROMES OTHER THAN DISTAL AXONAL NEUROPATHIES

Pure (or predominantly) motor neuropathy	Lymphoma, multifocal motor neuropathy (with or without anti-GM1 antibodies) *Toxic:* dapsone, lead, organophosphates Porphyria Guillain-Barré syndrome Tick paralysis Diphtheria
Pure (or predominantly) sensory neuropathy*	Acute idiopathic sensory neuropathy Primary biliary cirrhosis Sjögren's syndrome Diabetes mellitus Human immunodeficiency virus infection Leprosy Hereditary sensory and autonomic neuropathies Uremia Paraneoplastic sensory ganglioneuritis (anti-Hu, ANNA-I antibodies) *Toxic:* thallium, pyridoxine (vitamin B_6) intoxication
Palpably enlarged nerves	*Genetic:* Charcot-Marie-Tooth disease, Dejerine-Sottas disease, Refsum's disease, neurofibromatosis, hereditary liability to pressure palsies Leprosy Chronic inflammatory demyelinating polyneuropathy
Demyelinating neuropathies	*Immunologic:* Guillain-Barré syndrome, chronic inflammatory demyelinating polyneuropathy, paraproteinemia, anti-MAG (myelin-associated glycoprotein) antibodies *Toxic:* diphtheria, buckthorn toxin, amiodarone, perhexiline *Genetic:* Charcot-Marie-Tooth type I disease, storage diseases, hereditary liability to pressure palsies *Paraneoplastic:* osteosclerotic multiple myeloma

*Usually small-fiber sensory loss (pain, temperature) with prominent autonomic dysfunction.

Table 20-4 □ CAUSES OF PERIPHERAL NEUROPATHY THAT CAN BE DIAGNOSED BY NERVE BIOPSY

Vasculitis
Leprosy
Lymphoma
Cytomegalovirus (causes polyradiculopathy or mononeuropathy multiplex)
Storage diseases (metachromatic leukodystrophy [MLD], adrenomyeloneuropathy [AMN], Krabbe's disease)
Sarcoidosis
Amyloidosis
Immune-mediated diseases (IgM and complement deposition)

Selected Causes of Neuropathy

- **Diabetes mellitus**

  Diabetes is the most common cause of neuropathy in the United States. Several different forms of neuropathy may occur, and an individual may have more than one type:

  1. **Distal axonal sensorimotor neuropathy** is most common. Sensory symptoms (small fiber) usually predominate, including painful dysesthesias.
  2. **Autonomic neuropathy** is commonly seen in combination with axonal small-fiber sensory neuropathy. Symptoms may include anhidrosis, orthostatic hypotension, impotence, gastroparesis, and bowel and bladder disturbances.
  3. **Mononeuropathy** may occur from either nerve infarction or entrapment (e.g., carpal tunnel syndrome).
  4. **Mononeuropathy multiplex**
  5. **Diabetic amyotrophy (asymmetric proximal motor neuropathy)** presents with dull, aching proximal pain, followed by asymmetric proximal leg weakness and wasting not limited to a root, plexus, or nerve territory.

- **Ethanol**

  Ethanol is a very common cause of axonal sensorimotor neuropathy with prominent distal paresthesias and numbness. Vitamin B complex supplements and alcohol cessation can lead to improvement.

- **Uremia**

  Renal failure often leads to a distal, axonal, sensorimotor neuropathy with prominent cramps and unpleasant dysesthesias. Improvement may occur with dialysis or kidney transplantation.

- **Chronic inflammatory demyelinating polyneuropathy**

  CIDP presents as a chronic relapsing sensorimotor polyneuropathy or, rarely, as mononeuropathy multiplex. The diagnosis is confirmed by *elevated CSF protein* and *a demyelinating pattern on EMG/NCS*. In some cases, a plasma cell dyscrasia or paraprotein may be identified. **Prednisone, starting at 60 mg/day,** is the treatment of first choice. Long-term daily maintenance doses of 5 to 20 mg may be required in responders. **Plasmapheresis, IVIG (0.4 g/kg per treatment),** and **azathioprine 150 mg per day** are other treatment options.

- **Paraprotein-associated neuropathy**
  These neuropathies can result in a demyelinating or axonal sensorimotor neuropathy. CSF protein is elevated in 80% of demyelinating cases. The protein can be identified by either serum or urine protein electrophoresis or immunofixation electrophoresis. Bone marrow biopsy may be helpful in the two thirds of cases with plasma cell dyscrasia; in the remaining patients, multiple myeloma (in 12%), amyloidosis (in 9%), lymphoma (in 5%), leukemia (in 3%), or Waldenström's macroglobulinemia (in 2%) may be identified. **Prednisone 40 to 100 mg per day** or **azathioprine 150 mg per day** may benefit some patients; **plasmapheresis** and **IVIG** are other treatment options.

- **Critical illness polyneuropathy**
  This polyneuropathy is associated with sepsis and multisystem organ failure. It often presents as failure to wean from mechanical ventilation. EMG/NCS is consistent with severe sensorimotor axonal neuropathy. There is no specific treatment, but if the patient survives, recovery is the rule.

- **Paraneoplastic neuropathy**
  Paraneoplastic neuropathy most often manifests as an *axonal sensorimotor neuropathy,* but it can also take the form of a *large-fiber pure sensory neuropathy,* a *demyelinating sensorimotor neuropathy,* or a *pure motor neuronopathy* (usually seen with lymphoma). These and other paraneoplastic syndromes (see Chapter 23) are mediated by autoimmune responses against peripheral nerve.

- **Genetic (hereditary) neuropathies**
  These neuropathies are unusual except for **Charcot-Marie-Tooth disease,** which comes in two forms: type I (demyelinating) and the less common type II (axonal). The disease is autosomal dominant, with variable expression from one generation to the next. Patients present with insidious distal lower extremity weakness and wasting ("stork leg deformity"), high arches, pes cavus, and minimal sensory symptoms.

General Care of the Patient with Neuropathy

1. **Remove any potential neurotoxic medications,** even if these are not the primary cause (see Table 20–2 for a list).

2. **Treat neuropathic pain** with **gabapentin (Neurontin) 300 to 3600 mg daily,** tricyclic antidepressants **(amitriptyline 25 to 100 mg daily or nortriptyline 10 to 25 mg daily),** or carbamazepine 200 mg three to four times a day.
3. **Initiate occupational and physical therapy** in patients with moderate to severe disability for gait training, prevention of contractures, orthoses, and assistive devices.
4. **Skin care** is important in patients with severe sensory neuropathy to prevent trophic ulcers, infections, and neuropathic (Charcot) joints.
5. **Autonomic neuropathy** may require treatment for orthostatic hypotension **(fludrocortisone 0.1 to 0.3 mg a day or midodrine 5 to 10 mg two to three times a day)** and gastroparesis **(metoclopramide 5 to 10 mg three times a day).**

■ NEUROMUSCULAR JUNCTION DISEASE

Myasthenia gravis and **botulism,** both of which can lead to respiratory failure, are discussed in Chapter 15.

■ LAMBERT-EATON MYASTHENIC SYNDROME

Lambert-Eaton Myasthenic Syndrome (LEMS) is an autoimmune disease caused by antibodies directed against voltage-gated calcium channels of the presynaptic nerve terminals, causing impaired neuromuscular transmission. Most cases are paraneoplastic; LEMS occurs in up to 60% of patients with small cell lung carcinoma. The disease is initially identified with proximal limb weakness. Lower extremity areflexia, myalgias, dry mouth, and impotence may also occur, but diplopia, dysphagia, and dyspnea do not occur. The disease is diagnosed by the presence of an incremental response on repetitive nerve stimulation (>10 Hz). LEMS is treated with drugs that facilitate the release of acetylcholine: **guanidine 20 to 30 mg/kg daily** or **3,4-diaminopyridine 20 mg tid.** Pyridostigmine, plasmapheresis, and IVIG may also be tried.

■ MYOPATHY

Diseases of muscle typically lead to **proximal, symmetric weakness** without sensory deficits or bowel or bladder symptoms. The patient may complain of difficulty reaching above the head, getting out of a chair, or climbing stairs.

Questions to Ask the Patient with Suspected Myopathic Disease

1. Does the patient have muscle aches or tenderness, suggestive of muscle inflammation or necrosis?
2. Has the patient noticed darkened, cola-colored urine *(myoglobinuria)*?
3. Does the weakness fluctuate or worsen with exercise, suggestive of myasthenia gravis or periodic paralysis?
4. Are there any sensory or bowel or bladder symptoms? (Such symptoms would make a myopathic disease unlikely.)
5. Have there been any new cardiac symptoms? (Many entities affect both skeletal and cardiac muscle.)

Examination

1. Map out the pattern of weakness (proximal versus distal). Most myopathies cause proximal weakness; exceptions include myotonic dystrophy, inclusion body myositis, and rare genetic causes.
2. Check for *myotonia* (prolonged muscle contraction after voluntary contraction or percussion), which can be tested by handgrip, forced eye closure, or muscle percussion.
3. Palpate for muscle tenderness.
4. Undress the patient to evaluate for a pattern of muscle wasting.

Management

Diagnostic Testing

1. **Initial laboratory tests.** Creatine kinase (CK) level, chem-20 screen, TFTs, sedimentation rate, ECG
2. **EMG/NCS.** Needle electromyography in patients with myopathy shows abnormal, short-duration, low-amplitude, polyphasic motor unit potentials and overly rapid recruitment of motor units with an excessively low amplitude interference pattern (see Chapter 3).
3. **Muscle biopsy** is often needed to establish a diagnosis.
4. **Other tests to consider** include ACE level, serum cortisol level, serum and CSF lactate (mitochondrial myopathy), genetic testing (for muscular and myotonic dystrophy), and toxicology screen.

Causes of Myopathy

Causes of myopathy can be categorized into five main groups: **inflammatory, endocrine, toxic, hereditary, and infectious.**

1. **Inflammatory myopathies**
   a. **Polymyositis**
      This inflammatory autoimmune muscle disease is characterized by chronic and relapsing proximal limb weakness. Although the eyes and face are almost never affected, pharyngeal and neck weakness is common (in approximately 50% of patients). Cardiomyopathy, interstitial lung disease, and other systemic autoimmune diseases (e.g., systemic lupus erythematosus, Crohn's disease) are also found in a significant proportion of patients.
      (1) Diagnosis: CK levels are elevated in almost all cases, and EMG shows myopathic findings with denervation secondary to segmental muscle necrosis. Muscle biopsy reveals endomesial lymphocytic infiltrates, necrotic and atrophic muscle fibers, and connective tissue deposition.
      (2) Treatment: **Prednisone 60 to 100 mg daily** leads to improvement in most patients within 2 to 3 months and is most effective early in the disease course. **Azathioprine 1 to 3 mg/kg per day** or **methotrexate 25 to 50 mg per week** can be used for disease suppression in steroid nonresponders.
   b. **Dermatomyositis**
      Dermatomyositis is similar to polymyositis but is accompanied by a characteristic rash that precedes or accompanies muscle weakness. Skin manifestations include a heliotrope (bluish) rash on the upper eyelids, erythematous rash on the face and trunk, violaceous scaly eruptions on the knuckles (Gottron's papules), and subcutaneous calcifications.
      (1) Diagnosis: Muscle biopsy findings differ from polymyositis in showing perivascular inflammation and *perifascicular atrophy*. A malignancy screen is prudent with a later age of onset.
      (2) Treatment: Treatment is the same as for polymyositis.
   c. **Inclusion body myositis**
      This entity differs from polymyositis in that it tends to produce distal and asymmetric weakness, it occurs primarily at an older age, and it responds poorly to steroids. Muscle biopsy reveals rimmed vacuoles and eosinophilic cytoplasmic inclusions with amyloid. **IVIG (0.4 mg/kg per treatment)** may improve strength in isolated cases. Finger flexor and quadriceps weakness is a hallmark.
   d. **Sarcoidosis**
      Patients with sarcoidosis can develop focal or generalized myopathy. Biopsy shows noncaseating granulomas. Steroids usually produce clinical improvement.
2. **Endocrine myopathies**
   Patients with endocrine myopathy usually show systemic signs of endocrine disease before the onset of weakness, but in

some instances, myopathy is the presenting feature. CK levels are usually normal or only mildly elevated. In all cases, weakness is reversed by treating the underlying endocrinopathy, which includes **thyroid disease, Cushing's disease (hyperadrenalism),** or **parathyroid disease.**

3. **Toxic myopathies**
   a. **Medications**
      Drugs and medications produce subacute, generalized proximal muscle weakness through a variety of mechanisms. Table 20–5 lists some medications and toxins commonly associated with myopathy.
   b. **Critical illness myopathy**
      This myopathy presents as a failure to wean from mechanical ventilation in ICU patients treated with steroids and nondepolarizing paralyzing agents (e.g., vecuronium); however, neither precipitant is necessary for disease development. Muscle biopsy shows selective loss of thick myosin filaments. This condition is much more common than typically diagnosed.
   c. **Neuroleptic malignant syndrome**
      Dopamine blockers (e.g., haloperidol, chlorpromazine [Thorazine]) can produce this rare, idiosyncratic response characterized by generalized muscle rigidity with rhabdomyolysis, fever, altered mental status, tremor, and autonomic instability (especially hypertension). CK levels are always elevated; white blood cell counts are usually increased. Treatment includes discontinuation of the offending agent, surface cooling, **dantrolene 1 to 10 mg/kg**

Table 20–5 □ DRUGS THAT CAN CAUSE MYOPATHY

Rhabdomyolysis	**Myopathy (weakness and myalgia)**
Amphotericin B	Colchicine
ε-Aminocaproic acid	Zidovudine
Fenfluramine	Steroids
Heroin	Clofibrate
Phencyclidine	Chloroquine
Alcohol	Emetine
Barbiturates	Labetalol
Cocaine	Statin class anti-cholesterol
Hypokalemic myopathy	Steroids
Diuretics	Vincristine
Azathioprine	
Myositis (inflammatory)	
Penicillamine	
Procainamide	
Cimetidine	

per day IV every 4 to 6 hours as needed to attain muscle relaxation, and **bromocriptine 2.5 to 5 mg three times a day.**
    d. **Malignant hyperthermia**
       This autosomal dominant condition predisposes to severe muscle rigidity, rhabdomyolysis, fever, and metabolic acidosis following exposure to inhalation anesthetics or succinylcholine. Treatment is with **dantrolene 2.5 to 10 mg/kg IV in repeated doses.**
4. **Hereditary myopathies**
    a. **Muscular dystrophy**
       Muscular dystrophy is a progressively degenerative genetic myopathy. Weakness is usually present in early life, gets worse over time, and often leads to early death.
       (1) **Duchenne's muscular dystrophy** (X-linked). The onset is by age 5 with inability to walk occurring by age 10 and with eventual respiratory failure. Features include calf pseudohypertrophy, cardiomyopathy, and occasional mental impairment. *Becker's muscular dystrophy* is a later-onset form of the disease with less severe manifestations. **Prednisone 20 to 40 mg per day** can increase strength and function, but it does not alter the overall course. Diagnosis is confirmed by abnormal dystrophin staining on biopsy.
       (2) **Myotonic dystrophy** (autosomal dominant). This most common form of muscular dystrophy leads to progressive *distal* myopathy. The disease occurs earlier and is more severe with successive generations (genetic anticipation). Besides myotonia, features include a distinctive facies with ptosis and frontal balding, cataracts, cardiac conduction defects, gonadal atrophy, and mental impairment. **Phenytoin 300 mg per day PO** and **procainamide 20 to 50 mg/kg per day three times a day** occasionally are used to treat the myotonia, if clinically necessary. ECGs performed at least yearly are prudent to assess for evolving heart block. Definitive genetic triple repeat analysis is available for diagnosis confirmation.
       (3) **Other myopathies.** These entities include facioscapulohumeral (autosomal dominant), limb girdle (autosomal recessive), oculopharyngeal (autosomal recessive), and Emery-Dreifuss (X-linked) myopathies. Many of these myopathies now have precise genetic diagnoses.
    b. **Metabolic myopathies**
       Seen mostly in the pediatric population, these diseases result from deficiencies of specific enzymes involved in utilization of glucose or lipid (the two main sources of skeletal muscle energy). Besides muscle weakness, patients with metabolic myopathies often experience *rhabdomyolysis*

and *myoglobinuria*. Muscle biopsy is necessary to establish the diagnosis. The most common metabolic myopathy is **McArdle's disease,** an autosomal recessive disorder resulting from myophosphorylase deficiency. It presents in childhood with painful muscle cramps and myoglobinuria after intense exercise. A lack of increase in lactate levels with ischemic forearm testing is characteristic. Laboratory confirmation of urinary or serum myoglobin in an acute phase is key.

c. **Periodic paralysis**

These rare disorders are caused by genetic abnormalities of membrane ion channels. The majority are inherited in autosomal dominant fashion. Patients are usually normal between attacks of severe weakness. **Hypokalemic** and **hyperkalemic** forms have been described.

d. **Congenital myopathies**

This group of rare disorders presents mostly at birth with floppy infant syndrome, and the disorders are usually nonprogressive. Examples include nemaline (rod) body myopathy, myotubular (centronuclear) myopathy, and central core disease. Adult onset cases may be seen.

e. **Mitochondrial myopathy**

These diseases result from defects in the mitochondrial genome and hence are maternally inherited. Muscle biopsy shows "ragged red fibers." Suspicious signs for mitochondrial diseases include ptosis, ophthalmoparesis, and high serum lactate levels. Variants include myoclonic epilepsy with ragged red fibers, MELAS (mitochondrial encephalomyopathy, encephalopathy, lactic acidosis, and stroke-like episodes), and Kearns-Sayre syndrome (pigmentary retinopathy, cardiac conduction defects, high CSF protein). Genetic analysis is available for many types of mitochondrial myopathies.

5. **Infectious myopathies**

Muscle infiltration with the organisms that cause *trichinosis*, *toxoplasmosis*, and *cysticercosis* can lead to a widespread or a localized inflammatory myopathy. Acute rhabdomyolsis and myoglobinuria can occur as a result of infection with influenza virus, rubella virus, coxsackievirus, echoviruses, and mycoplasma. HIV myopathy is not uncommon and must be distinguished from zidovudine toxicity.

chapter 21
Demyelinating and Inflammatory Disorders of the Central Nervous System

Demyelinating and inflammatory diseases of the central nervous system (CNS) are varied and often enigmatic. *Multiple sclerosis (MS)*, the prototype inflammatory demyelinating disease, is a chronic autoimmune disorder characterized by loss of myelin and relative preservation of axons. *Acute disseminated encephalomyelitis (ADEM)* is a monophasic illness that is pathologically similar to MS, but typically triggered by an antecedent viral infection. *Central pontine myelinolysis (CPM)* refers to osmotic demyelination in the setting of rapid correction of hyponatremia. *Sarcoidosis* and *Behçet's disease* are idiopathic systemic inflammatory diseases that may involve the CNS. Dysmyelinating diseases, such as Alexander's and Canavan's diseases, are genetic disorders in which there is an intrinsic abnormality of myelin; they present in childhood and will not be discussed in this chapter.

■ MULTIPLE SCLEROSIS

MS typically occurs in young adulthood and is characterized by episodic focal demyelination that occurs throughout the CNS. **The clinical hallmark of the disease is recurrent neurologic deficits that are disseminated in space and time.** There are 250,000 to 350,000 patients with MS in the United States. Relatives of MS patients have 5% risk of developing the disease, which is 20 to 40 times the risk in the general population, and the risk in monozygotic twins is 30%. Although MS has a variable prognosis, outcomes are often poor: 50% of patients need help walking within 15 years of onset, and the mortality rate is approximately twice that of the general population.

Clinical Features

When symptoms appear, they often develop steadily over a period of days. The most common manifestations are sensory disturbances, unilateral optic neuritis, diplopia (internuclear ophthalmoplegia), Lhermitte's sign (trunk and limb paresthesias evoked by neck flexion), limb weakness, clumsiness, gait ataxia, dysarthria, and neurogenic bowel and bladder symptoms. Many patients suffer from fatigue, which is often worst in the afternoon, and symptomatic worsening is often precipitated by elevations in temperature (Uhthoff's phenomenon). Some patients have paroxysmal neuropathic pain involving the trunk or face. Hemispheric involvement can result in cortical deficits (aphasia, apraxia, seizures, visual field loss, dementia), basal ganglia demyelination can lead to extrapyramidal signs (chorea and rigidity), and spinal cord involvement results in progressive spastic paraparesis. Depression and emotional lability are particularly common in the late stages of MS. Clinical signs to check for on examination are shown in Box 21–1.

Clinical variants of MS include the *Marburg variant* (stupor or coma and acute fulminant disseminated demyelination) and *Devic's disease* (optic neuritis and necrotizing transverse myelitis). In rare cases, large MS plaques can take on the appearance of an enhancing mass lesion that resembles a brain tumor.

Four standard categories are used to describe the clinical course of MS (Fig. 21–1). Eighty percent of patients present with *relapsing-remitting* MS, in which symptoms and signs evolve over several days and then improve over weeks, with full or incomplete recovery following a stable course between relapses. Onset of relapsing-remitting MS is typically between the ages of 10 and 30, and females predominate by 2:1. Half of patients with relapsing-remitting disease eventually develop *secondary progressive* MS, in which persistent and progressive neurologic deficits develop between relapses. Ten to 20% of patients have *primary progressive* MS, which presents as gradual, nearly continuous deterioration from the onset of symptoms. These patients tend to be older at onset (ages 30 to 50), men are affected as often as women, and many have progressive myelopathy. *Progressive-relapsing* MS, the least common subtype, refers to gradual neurologic deterioration with superimposed relapses that occur later in the course of the disease. As a rule, relapsing-remitting MS responds best to

---

Box 21–1. CHARACTERISTIC NEUROLOGIC SIGNS IN MULTIPLE SCLEROSIS

Mental status	Dementia, emotional lability, dysarthria
Cranial nerves	Optic atrophy, papillitis, afferent pupillary defect, internuclear ophthalmoplegia, nystagmus, myokymia
Motor	Spastic hemiparesis, paraparesis, or quadraparesis
Sensory	Variable
Coordination	Intention tremor, dysdiadokinesis
Reflexes	Hyperreflexia, clonus
Gait	Truncal ataxia, titubation

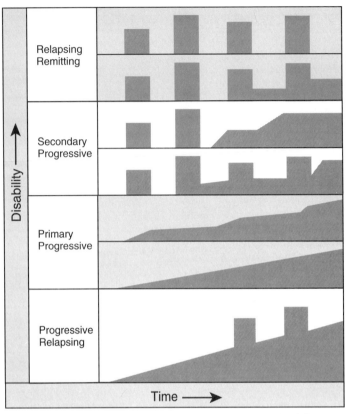

Figure 21-1 □ Clinical patterns of multiple sclerosis (MS). Relapsing-remitting MS is characterized by complete or incomplete recovery after attacks, with a stable course between attacks. Secondary progressive MS begins with a relapsing-remitting course, and later evolves into a progressive deteriorating course, with or without superimposed relapses. Primary progressive MS begins with continual or stepwise progressive deterioration. Progressive-relapsing MS, which is rare, starts as progressive deterioration, with later superimposed relapses.

treatment, and primary progressive MS is the least responsive subtype.

Pathogenesis

MS is generally believed to be an immune-mediated disorder that develops in genetically susceptible people. The name "multiple sclerosis" is derived from the multiplicity of lesions with a sclerotic appearance on cut sections. The patches of demyelination occur solely in the white matter of the brain and spinal cord. Clinical manifestations result from disruption of central nerve transmission. Remyelination is sometimes incomplete, and secondary axonal damage can occur, so neurologic deficits may accumulate steadily over the course of the disease.

There is considerable evidence to suggest that both genetic susceptibility and environmental factors contribute to the clinical expression of MS. The disease is rare in tropical climates and more common in temperate zones. There is a genetic association with certain HLA (human leukocyte antigen) class II molecules on chromosome 6; the most important at-risk allele is HLA-DR2.

Although the cause of multiple sclerosis is unknown, the possibility that infection interacts with or stimulates an altered immunologic mechanism is suggested by the unusual epidemiology, genetic susceptibility, alterations in the immune cell reactivity, and presence of increased IgG and oligoclonal IgG in spinal fluid and within the plaques themselves. There is evidence for a T cell immunopathology with activated T cells in plaques, supporting the concept of T cell–mediated autoimmune response directed at myelin antigens.

Diagnosis

Multiple sclerosis is a *clinical diagnosis*. For clinically definite MS, there must be a minimum of two clinical episodes separated in time, characteristic of an MS attack. The term "multiple sclerosis" should not be used until the diagnosis is certain. Table 21–1 includes the criteria for clinically definite and clinically probable MS.

In addition to the clinical picture, laboratory data can support the diagnosis. Characteristic white matter lesions on MRI, prolonged P100 responses on visual evoked potentials, and positive oligoclonal bands (OCBs) from the cerebrospinal fluid (CSF) should be sought. A diagnosis of laboratory-supported definite or laboratory-supported probable MS may be made if there was only one characteristic MS attack, but supporting laboratory data are positive (see Table 21–1). When there is diagnostic uncertainty, repeat MRI after several months may demonstrate that the lesions are disseminated in time. Other disorders to consider in the differential diagnosis of MS are listed in Box 21–2.

Laboratory Investigations

1. **Lumbar puncture**
    The spinal fluid is abnormal in 90% of patients. The white blood cell count may be increased up to $50/mm^3$ in 50% of patients. CSF pleocytosis is a measure of disease activity and tends to be more marked during acute exacerbations. In 40%

Table 21-1 □ **CRITERIA FOR THE CLINICAL AND LABORATORY DIAGNOSIS OF MULTIPLE SCLEROSIS**

Clinically definite:
- At least two attacks separated by at least 1 month (relapsing-remitting), or a gradual or stepwise progressive course for at least 6 months (primary progressive)
- Documented neurologic signs of lesions in two or more sites, or neurologic signs of one lesion, and evidence of other lesions on laboratory testing (MRI or evoked potentials)
- Onset of symptoms usually between ages 10 and 50 years
- No better neurologic explanation

Laboratory-supported definite:
- History of one attack, and neurologic signs of two lesions, or neurologic signs of one lesion and evidence of other lesions on laboratory testing

  or
- History of two attacks, and evidence of one lesion on examination or laboratory testing (but not both)

  and
- Abnormal CSF IgG or oligoclonal band (OCB) studies

Clinically probable:
- History of one attack, and neurologic signs of two lesions, or neurologic signs of one lesion and evidence of other lesions on laboratory testing

  or
- History of two attacks, and evidence of one lesion on examination or laboratory testing (but not both)

  and
- Normal CSF IgG and OCB studies

Laboratory-supported probable:
- History of two attacks, with no evidence of lesions on clinical examination or laboratory testing
- Abnormal CSF IgG or OCB studies

---

of patients there is an increase in total protein, usually less than 100 mg/dl. Elevation of the gamma globulin subfraction above 12% of total protein is found in 60 to 75% of patients. The OCB pattern is more specific and occurs in 90% of established cases but is not specific to MS. Elevated CSF myelin basic protein has been demonstrated in 70% cases of acute MS, but this finding is also nonspecific.

2. **Neuroimaging**

Computed tomography (CT) can detect abnormalities in one third of MS patients, but magnetic resonance imaging (MRI), which is abnormal in over 95% of patients with MS, is vastly more sensitive. MRI can be used to predict whether a patient with a single episode of demyelination is likely to develop clinically definite MS: patients with >3 cm^3 of

> **Box 21–2. DIFFERENTIAL DIAGNOSIS OF MULTIPLE SCLEROSIS**
>
> The **VITAMINS** mnemonic may be helpful in remembering a differential diagnosis for multiple sclerosis:
>
> **V (vascular):** multiple lacunar infarcts, cerebral autosomal dominant arteriopathy with subcortical infarcts and leukoencephalopathy (CADASIL), spinal arteriovenous malformations*
> **I (infectious):** HIV myelopathy,* progressive multifocal leukoencephalopathy (PML), Lyme disease, syphilis, HTLV-I myelopathy*
> **T (traumatic):** spondylytic myelopathy*
> **A (autoimmune):** acute disseminated encephalomyelitis (ADEM), CNS vasculitis, Behçet's disease, sarcoidosis
> **M (metabolic/toxic):** central pontine myelinolysis, hypoxia (Grinker's encephalopathy), hexachlorophene poisoning, Marchiafava-Bignami disease, vitamin B_{12} deficiency (subacute combined degeneration), vitamin B_6 deficiency (optic neuritis), radiation
> **I (idiopathic/genetic):** Friedreich's ataxia, spinocerebellar degeneration, Arnold-Chiari malformation, adrenal leukodystrophy, metachromatic leukodystrophy
> **N (neoplastic):** CNS lymphoma, glioma, paraneoplastic encephalomyelitis, metastatic cord compression*
> **S (psychiatric):** conversion disorder, malingering
>
> *Note:* Relevant to progressive myelopathy.

plaque at initial presentation have nearly a 100% chance of developing MS within 10 years. By contrast, patients with an initial demyelinating episode and a normal MRI at presentation have only a 6% chance of developing MS over 5 years. T2-weighted images demonstrate demyelination and edema, and gadolinium (T1 images) indicates the presence of acute inflammation in most new MS lesions. The enhancement disappears in two thirds of the lesions by 4 to 6 weeks. Most gadolinium-enhancing lesions are clinically silent, but clinical changes tend to be associated with bursts of gadolinium enhancement. MRI has demonstrated that MS is much more dramatic and dynamic than was previously thought and that the disease is a continuous process and is active in most patients long before diagnosis.

3. **Evoked potentials**

    Evoked potentials are useful for demonstrating disseminated CNS involvement and are used to support the diagnosis of MS in patients who present with a single isolated neurologic deficit such as spastic paraparesis or an internuclear ophthalmoplegia. Visual evoked potentials (VEPs) can support optic nerve involvement by demonstrating abnormal conduction of a chessboard pattern presented to the eyes. VEPs are positive in 90% of patients with clinically obvious MS, in 50% with probable MS, and in 25% with possible MS. Brain stem auditory evoked potentials (BAERs) are abnormal in 50% of those with definite MS and 20% of those with probable MS. Somatosensory evoked potentials (SSEPs) are abnormal in 70% of cases of probable or definite MS (see Chapter 3, Diagnostic Tests).

Management

Significant advances in the treatment of MS have been made over the past 10 years, and new treatments are being developed at a rapid pace. Treatments for MS can be categorized as **disease-modifying therapy** (Table 21–2) and **symptomatic therapy**. Psychologic support, physical therapy, and occupational therapy are essential throughout the illness.

Disease-Modifying Therapy

Treatment of Disease Progression

Interferon beta-1b (Betaseron) was the first therapeutic intervention shown to be effective in altering the natural history of relapsing-remitting MS, and it has also been shown to reduce the rate of relapse and progression of disability in secondary-progressive MS. Two double-blind multicenter studies demonstrated that interferon beta-1b decreases the number and severity of exacerbations in relapsing-remitting MS, and one study demonstrated slowing of disease progression. In addition, the number of gadolinium-enhancing MRI lesions is decreased. It is proposed to work by modifying the effects of endogenous interferon on the immune system.

Interferon beta-1a (Avonex) and **glatiramer acetate (Copaxone)** have also been shown to reduce the frequency of relapse in relapsing-remitting MS and to reduce the development of new enhancing lesions on MRI. Both drugs reduce the 2-year rate of clinical relapse by approximately 30%. Interferon beta-1a has also been shown to delay the development of a second, disease-defining episode of demyelination in patients who present with a first clinical episode of possible MS. Both drugs may induce the formation of neutralizing antibodies, especially within the first 18 months of treatment, and both cause flu-like symptoms in approximately half of patients. Although **intravenous immune**

Table 21-2 □ DISEASE-MODIFYING THERAPY FOR MULTIPLE SCLEROSIS

Type of MS or Relapse	Agent	Dose	Possible Benefits of Treatment*	
			Reduces Relapses	*Delays Disability*
Relapsing-remitting	Interferon beta-1b (Betaseron)	8 million IU SC every other day	++	0
	Interferon beta-1a (Avonex)	30 μg IM once a week	++	+
	Glatiramer acetate (Copaxone)	20 μg SC daily	++	0
	Immune globulin	0.15–0.2 g/kg IV monthly for 2 years	++	+
Secondary progressive	Interferon beta-1b (Betaseron)	8 million IU SC every other day	++	+
	Mitoxantrone hydrochloride	5 or 12 mg/m² of body surface area every 3 months for 2 years	++	++
Primary progressive	None			
Acute relapses	Methylprednisolone	1 g IV daily for 3–5 days	Hastens clinical recovery	
	Prednisone	60–100 mg daily followed by gradual taper	Hastens clinical recovery	
	Plasmapheresis	Seven exchanges of one plasma volume every other day	Hastens recovery in patients unresponsive to steroids	

Key: ++ indicates strong evidence in clinical trials; + indicates partial evidence.
Adapted from Noseworthy J, et al: Multiple sclerosis. N Engl J Med 343:938–952, 2000.

globulin has been shown to reduce the rate of clinical relapses in relapsing-remitting MS, it is more expensive than interferon therapy and is not widely used for this indication in the United States.

Mitoxantrone (Novantrone), a chemotherapeutic agent, has been recently approved for the treatment of secondary progressive MS. The most common side effects are nausea, hair loss, mouth sores, menstrual abnormalities, and diarrhea. Because of the risk of myocardial toxicity, patients should regularly undergo echocardiography and should not be treated for longer than 2 to 3 years.

Treatment of Acute Relapses

Corticosteroids are most commonly used to treat acute exacerbations of MS. Although there is no consensus about the optimal form, dose, route, or duration of steroid therapy, it is generally believed that steroids hasten recovery from acute relapses. High-dose **methylprednisolone** is most often used to treat major relapses, whereas **prednisone** is used to treat minor recurrences (Table 21–2). Both are generally followed by a tapering course of prednisone over 2 to 4 weeks. A recent clinical trial showed that seven alternate-day **plasma exchanges** produced substantial clinical improvement in 40% of patients who were unresponsive to steroids. Other immunosuppressive agents that have been used to treat MS include ACTH, azathioprine, cyclophosphamide, cyclosporine, levamisole, methotrexate, cladribine, and total lymphoid irradiation. These agents have been used with variable but generally limited success, and many have significant side effects.

Symptomatic Therapy

1. Spasticity/pain

    Exercise, physical therapy, and occupational therapy with pharmacologic support are the main approaches. Medications used for spasticity and painful flexor spasms include oral **baclofen 10 mg PO three times a day, tizanidine (Zanaflex) 2 to 12 mg three times a day, diazepam 5 to 10 mg PO three times a day**, and **dantrolene 25 to 50 mg two to four times a day.** When rehabilitation and medications fail, severe spasticity can be treated with an implantable spinal cord stimulator or with intrathecal baclofen via continuous pump infusion.

2. Bladder dysfunction

    Urodynamic (cystometric) studies are important to clarify the cause of incontinence. For the 30% of patients with incontinence due to involuntary bladder contractions (spastic bladder), parasympatholytic agents such as **propantheline (Pro-Banthine) 15 mg PO three times a day** or **oxybutynin (Ditropan) 5 mg PO two or three times a day** can aid in the retention of urine. For the 20% who have difficulty emptying the bladder (atonic bladder), **bethanecol chloride 10 to 50 mg PO two to four times per day** (a cholinergic agonist) or **phenoxybenzamine 20 to 40 mg three times a day** (an alpha blocker that relaxes the urethral sphincter) may be of benefit, in addition to Credé's or Valsalva's maneuver. The remaining 50% have a combination of the two problems (detrussor dysynergia), and in these cases, if combination pharmacotherapy does not work, regular intermittent self-catheterization or permanent catheterization may be required. Because asymptomatic bacterial colonization of the bladder is common, antibiotics should be reserved for active infection to prevent the selection of highly resistant organisms.

3. **Tremor**

    Coarse cerebellar and rubral tremor is common in patients with MS. Medical therapy with **clonazepam 0.5 to 2 mg three times a day, propranolol 10 to 40 mg four times a day, glutethimide 250 mg two or three times a day,** and **isoniazid 100 to 300 mg one to three times a day** may provide partial relief. Ventrolateral thalamic ablation may have to be considered in severe cases. Subthalamic electrical stimulation is a novel promising therapy.

4. **Psychiatric complications**

    Depression, euphoria, emotional lability, and psychosis may require psychiatric management. **Fluoxetine 20 mg per day** may be particularly helpful for treating emotional lability.

5. **Fatigue**

    The fatigue associated with MS may respond to **amantadine 100 mg twice a day, pemoline 37.5 mg taken in the morning,** or **modafinil (Provigil) 200 mg PO once daily.**

6. **Neuropathic pain**

    Neuropathic pain can be treated with **gabapentin 100 to 900 mg three times a day** or **carbamazepine 100 to 600 mg three times a day.**

Prognosis

The course of MS in an individual patient is largely unpredictable. Roughly 10% of patients do well for 20 years and thus are considered to have benign MS. Approximately 70% will develop secondary progression of neurologic deficits. Frequent relapses in the first 2 years, primary progressive onset, male sex, multiple MRI lesions on presentation, and early motor or cerebellar findings are associated with a more severe course, whereas women with predominantly sensory symptoms and optic neuritis have a more favorable prognosis.

■ OPTIC NEURITIS

Optic neuritis produces unilateral impairment of vision in young and middle-aged adults. Although this condition may appear as part of MS (see preceding discussion) or other generalized demyelinating diseases, it may occur in isolation. The onset is usually rapid, with blindness, blurred vision, or achromatopsia in the affected eye. Painful retrobulbar neuritis occurs in 50% of patients, and some will have papillitis on fundoscopy. In optic neuritis, the visual acuity is diminished in 40% of patients, and there is typically an afferent pupillary defect (Marcus Gunn pupil) on the affected side. In severe cases, there may be no direct light reflex with preservation of the consensual reflex. Half of patients have only unilateral optic neuritis. Functional vision is restored within 2 weeks in 25% of cases and within 2 months in 75%, but recovery may require up to 1 year for the remainder of cases. Recurrence occurs in approximately 10 to 15% of patients within the first year.

Differential Diagnosis

V (vascular): ischemia, e.g., retinal ischemia, central retinal artery occlusion, ischemic optic neuropathy

I (infectious): local (retinitis, periostitis, meningitis) or systemic (syphilis, toxoplasmosis, typhoid fever, leptospirosis). These infections rarely cause such rapid visual loss without other symptoms.

T (trauma): rare

A (autoimmune): giant cell (temporal) arteritis, multiple sclerosis

M (metabolic/toxic): diabetes mellitus, vitamin B_{12} and B_1 deficiency, tropical ataxic neuropathy (cassava diet), methyl alcohol, lead, benzene, tobacco use associated with a defect in cyanide detoxification

I (idiopathic/hereditary): Friedreich's ataxia, Leber's optic atrophy (suspicion is raised when new vessel formation is noted on fundoscopy or when the visual acuity fails to improve after 3 months; the condition goes on to affect the second eye following an interval of weeks to months.)

N (neoplastic): orbital tumor—usually slower progression to visual loss

S (psychiatric): conversion reaction

Diagnosis and Management

The CSF in optic neuritis, as in MS, may show pleocytosis and increased IgG production. **Intravenous methylprednisolone 250 mg every 6 hours for 3 days** followed by **oral prednisone 1 mg/kg each day for 11 days** speeds the recovery of visual loss in severe optic neuritis, but it results in similar vision as with placebo or oral steroids alone at 1 year. In addition, the combination reduces the rate of development of MS, especially in those patients with an abnormal MRI scan, over a 2-year period.

■ OTHER DEMYELINATING DISORDERS

Devic's Disease (Neuromyelitis Optica)

Considered by some to be an MS variant, this condition is characterized by *acute bilateral optic neuritis* and *transverse myelitis*. The eye and spinal involvement may occur together or may be separated by days or weeks. Devic's disease may occur as a phase in a typical MS case or it may be a manifestation of postinfectious encephalomyelitis. The pathology demonstrates severe necrosis of axons as well as myelin, and the clinical outcomes are accordingly poor. The prognosis is poor. It is more common in Asia and India.

Acute Disseminated Encephalomyelitis (Postvaccinal Encephalomyelitis, Postinfectious Encephalomyelitis)

ADEM is an acute demyelinative disorder with diffuse involvement of the brain, spinal cord, and meninges. The onset is acute with confusion, somnolence, seizures, headache, fever, meningismus, and complete or partial para/quadriplegia with bladder and bowel involvement. Ataxia, myoclonus, chorea, and decerebrate posturing can occur. It can occur following measles, rubella, chickenpox, mumps, influenza, or *Mycoplasma pneumoniae* infection or following flu vaccination. Foci of demyelination surrounding small and medium-sized vessels are scattered throughout the brain and spinal cord. It is thought that an immune-mediated complication of infection is responsible, possibly via a delayed hypersensitivity mechanism. The laboratory model of demyelinating disease (experimental allergic encephalomyelitis) supports this concept. The mortality rate is high, and significant neurologic deficits commonly persist. **Methylprednisolone IV 1 g each day** or **plasmapheresis** can be used to modify the severity of ADEM, but experience is limited.

Acute Necrotizing Hemorrhagic Encephalomyelitis

This most fulminant demyelinative disease affects children and young adults and is probably a variant of acute disseminated encephalomyelitis. The onset is abrupt following a respiratory illness. The presentation is similar to that with acute disseminated encephalomyelitis, but the CSF, under increased pressure, has marked pleocytosis (approximately 3000 to 30,000 cells/mm^3), red blood cells, normal glucose levels, and high protein concentration. The erythrocyte sedimentation rate (ESR) is high, and neuroimaging demonstrates extensive white matter destruction. It is important to consider herpes simplex, brain abscess, and subdural empyema in the differential diagnosis. The prognosis is poor.

Central Pontine Myelinolysis

This condition is characterized by symmetric destruction of the pontine white matter. Rapid correction of hyponatremia is associated with the onset of CPM in most cases. CPM occurs more frequently in patients with a history of alcoholism, malnutrition, and multiorgan failure. The lesion destroys the myelin sheath, sparing neurons and axons. It presents as a rapidly progressing spastic quadriplegia with facial, glottal, and pharyngeal paralysis in a debilitated patient suffering from an acute illness. When the pons alone is involved, the patient may become "locked-in," mute and paralyzed. In more severe cases, demyelination also involves white matter tracts in the basal ganglia, a condition termed *extrapontine myelinolysis*. MRI is the imaging modality of choice. Recovery from even the most severe cases is possible but may take 4 to 12 months. The disease is rarely directly fatal, but the mortality rate can be high due to secondary complications.

CPM is best avoided in severely hyponatremic patients by slowly correcting the serum sodium no faster than 0.5 mEq/L per hour (12 mEq/L per day), to a maximum level of 130 mEq/L (Table 21–3).

Table 21–3 □ FORMULA FOR CORRECTING HYPONATREMIA*

$$\text{Change in serum Na}^+ = \frac{\text{infusate Na}^+ - \text{serum Na}^+}{\text{total body water} + 1}$$

Infusates
- 3% saline — 513 mEq/L
- 0.9% saline — 154 mEq/L
- Ringer's lactate — 130 mEq/L
- 0.45% saline — 77 mEq/L

*Equation yields the effect of 1 L of infusate on serum Na$^+$ concentration in milliequivalents per liter. The rate of the infusion should be adjusted to correct the serum Na$^+$ no faster than 8 to 12 mEq/L per day. The suggested target Na$^+$ concentration is 130 mmol/L. Total body water in liters is estimated as a fraction of body weight in kilograms; the fraction is 0.6 in men and 0.5 in women.

Adapted from Adrogue HJ, Madias NE: Hyponatremia. N Engl J Med 342: 1581–1589, 2000.

■ CNS INFLAMMATORY DISORDERS

Sarcoidosis

Sarcoidosis is a generalized disease characterized by a granulomatous reaction to an unknown stimulus involving any organ. The cause remains unknown but may be infectious. It most commonly affects the lungs, mediastinal lymph nodes, and skin. Systemic features include fever, malaise, lassitude, erythema nodosa, polyarthralgia, mediastinal hilar lymphadenopathy, uveoparotid fever (Heerfordt's syndrome: parotitis, uveitis, and facial palsy), keratoconjunctivitis sicca, hepatosplenomegaly, anemia, cardiac conduction defects, phalangeal bone cysts, and hypercalcemia.

Sarcoidosis affects the nervous system in 5% of patients, primarily the leptomeninges, especially at the base of the brain. The clinical presentation relates to the site of involvement, and may include headache, vertigo, impaired vision, isolated cranial nerve lesions (e.g., bilateral facial palsy), intracranial mass lesions, hemiparesis, ataxia, paresthesias, diabetes insipidus or hypotestosteronism (from pituitary and hypothalamic dysfunction), seizures, encephalopathy, psychosis, dementia, hydrocephalus, peripheral neuropathy, or myopathy. Rarely the spinal cord is involved. Sarcoidosis is five times more common in women and is found worldwide with a prevalence of 3 to 50 per 100,000. The median age of onset of sarcoidosis is 27 to 30 years; however, the range is broad.

Diagnosis

Laboratory investigations in sarcoidosis may reveal hypercalcemia, hyperuricemia, a raised serum globulin level, and increased serum angiotensin-converting enzyme (ACE). The CSF ACE is positive in 55% of patients with neurosarcoidosis but normal in those without CNS involvement. The CSF may be abnormal, with raised pressure, a slight pleocytosis, an absence of organisms, markedly raised protein, and hypoglycorrhachia in 20 to 30% of patients. An elevated IgG index is found in 33% of patients. An association with HLA-B8 has been reported. MRI with gadolinium classically shows nodular leptomeningeal enhancement and parenchymal lesions. The diagnosis is made clinically and confirmed by a biopsy of a suitable granuloma revealing a focal collection of epithelioid histiocytes surrounded by a rim of lymphocytes, endothelial cells, and giant cells (Langhans' type) without organisms or caseation. Isolated neurosarcoidosis, seen in only 2 to 3% of patients with CNS involvement, is a difficult diagnosis to make. Its differential diagnosis includes leprosy, cryptococcosis, syphilis, and tuberculosis.

Management

Corticosteroids **(Prednisone 100 mg daily)** and azathioprine **(1–3 mg/kg/day)** are the first-line treatments for CNS sarcoidosis, but many patients do poorly despite therapy.

Behçet's Disease

Behçet's disease is an inflammatory disorder of unknown etiology characterized by a relapsing iritis and uveitis associated with oral (100%) and genital (75%) aphthous ulceration. Systemic features include recurrent fevers, keratoconjunctivitis, hypopyon, migrating superficial thrombophlebitis (25%) that may present as deep venous thrombosis, erythema nodosum (65%), furunculosis, intestinal ulceration, epididymitis, systemic and pulmonary arterial aneurysms, and arthralgia of large joints (60%).

Neurologic manifestations, including abrupt onset of recurrent meningoencephalitis and cranial nerve palsies, occur in 5 to 30% of patients with Behçet's Disease. Papilledema (intracranial hypertension due to venous sinus occlusion), hemiparesis, quadriparesis, pseudobulbar palsy, and involvement of the basal ganglia, cerebellum, or spinal cord involvement can occur. Its cause is presumed to be viral or immunologic. It is more common and more severe in men, and the peak age of onset is in the 20s.

Diagnosis

The diagnosis is chiefly clinical and is based on the occurrence of a meningoencephalitis in combination with the characteristic cutaneous and ocular lesions. It may mimic MS or strokes, with transient or persistent multifocal involvement of the nervous system. There is no single confirmatory test, but an ESR over 50 mm/hour is common. CSF studies show a mild pleocytosis with a moderate increase in protein. Brain imaging may show infarction (25%), hypodense/hypointense enhancing lesions, and leptomeningeal enhancement. Pathologically, inflammatory changes are found in the iris, choroid, retina, optic nerve, and meninges and in the perivascular spaces (vasculitis) of the cortex, basal ganglia, brain stem, and cerebellum. Focal areas of necrosis may also be seen.

Management

Treatment may include analgesia, anticoagulants, colchicine, dapsone, levamisole, thalidomide, steroids, and immunosuppression (azathioprine, chlorambucil, cyclophosphamide). Posterior uveal tract and neurologic lesions, if untreated, may lead to blindness or death.

Chapter 22 | Infections of the Central Nervous System

Most infections of the central nervous system (CNS) are life-threatening. For this reason, prompt diagnosis and treatment are essential to prevent death or permanent neurologic disability. **The possibility of CNS infection is usually raised by the combination of fever, headache, and neurologic signs or symptoms.** After your initial history and examination, the goal is to identify the possible causative organisms and treat them empirically. Definitive treatment will later be based on the results of cultures or other diagnostic tests.

■ APPROACH TO THE PATIENT WITH SUSPECTED CNS INFECTION

History and Examination

1. **Check for the following symptoms:** fever, headache, change in mental status, focal weakness, or back pain.
2. **Identify any predisposing causes of immunosuppression:** diabetes, alcoholism, malignancy, steroids, chemotherapy, human immunodeficiency virus (HIV) infection, or acquired immunodeficiency syndrome (AIDS).
3. **Check for evidence of infection elsewhere in the body:** endocarditis, pneumonia, osteomyelitis, or tick bite.
4. **Always be sure to check for the following:** papilledema, meningismus, skin rash, sinus tenderness, otitis media, or spine tenderness.

Lumbar Puncture

Lumbar puncture (LP) is the single most important test for establishing the presence of a CNS infection and for identifying the causative organism. The technique for performing LP is covered in Chapter 3. Herniation is a serious but rare complication of LP. **If CNS infection is suspected, when deciding whether to perform an LP, the following clinical rule may be helpful:**

1. Fever
2. Headache   } Any 2 of these 3 require LP
3. Change in mental status

Computed tomography (CT) scan is required prior to LP if ANY of the following are present:
1. Papilledema
2. Depressed level of consciousness (lethargy, stupor, or coma)
3. Focal neurologic deficit
4. Known intracranial mass lesion
5. AIDS

■ ACUTE MENINGITIS

Bacterial Meningitis

Bacterial meningitis typically presents as the classic triad of *fever, headache, and stiff neck*. The presentation is usually dramatic but may be less obvious at the extremes of age (in infants and in the elderly), in whom change in mental status is often the only symptom. Seeding of the leptomeninges usually results from hematogenous spread of the infecting organism (e.g., pneumococcal pneumonia complicated by meningitis), but it can also result from a parameningeal infection (e.g., otitis media) or following trauma or neurosurgery (e.g., cerebrospinal fluid [CSF] leak).

Diagnosis

The diagnosis is established by LP, which demonstrates polymorphonuclear pleocytosis, elevated protein level, and reduced glucose level (Table 22–1). The organism is identified on the basis of CSF cultures.

Treatment

The prognosis in bacterial meningitis depends on the interval between onset of disease and initiation of therapy. Selection of antibiotics for empirical coverage depends on age and risk factors, as shown in Table 22–2. Most adults should be treated with **ampicillin and ceftriaxone** pending the results of CSF cultures (see Table 22–2). **Dexamethasone 6 mg IV every 6 hours for 4 days** may also be given in severe cases to reduce the severity of residual neurologic and cranial nerve damage.

Viral (Aseptic) Meningitis

Viral meningitis is a self-limited illness seen most frequently in children and young adults. The presentation is similar to bacterial meningitis, except that neurologic dysfunction (e.g., change in mental status, neurologic focality) does not occur, and the overall prognosis is excellent. The diagnosis is suggested by lymphocytic pleocytosis with a normal glucose level in the CSF (see Table 22–1) and is confirmed by negative bacterial cultures. In some

Infections of the CNS 287

Table 22-1 □ CEREBROSPINAL FLUID FINDINGS IN SELECTED INFECTIONS OF THE CENTRAL NERVOUS SYSTEM

	No. of White Blood Cells (per mm³)	Cell Type	Concentration of Protein (mg/dl)	Concentration of Glucose (mg/dl)	CSF Pressure (cm H₂O)
Normal	≤5	Lymphocytes and monocytes only	15 to 45	45 to 80	80 to 180
Bacterial meningitis	5 to 10,000	Polymorphonuclear leukocytes	Increased	Decreased	Increased
Viral meningitis	5 to 1000	Lymphocytes	Increased	Normal	Normal, occasionally increased
Tubercular meningitis	5 to 500	Lymphocytes	Increased	Decreased	Increased
Cryptococcal meningitis	5 to 100	Lymphocytes	Increased	Normal, occasionally decreased	Increased
Active neurosyphilis	5 to 500	Lymphocytes	Increased	Normal, occasionally decreased	Normal

Table 22-2 □ EMPIRICAL ANTIBIOTIC THERAPY FOR BACTERIAL MENINGITIS

Risk Group	Etiologies	Antibiotic Coverage
Neonates (less than 1 month)	Group B or group D streptococci Gram-negative rods (e.g., *Escherichia coli*) *Listeria monocytogenes*	Ampicillin 50 mg/kg IV every 6–8 hours Cefotaxime 50 mg/kg IV every 8 hours
Children (3 months to 7 years)	*Haemophilus influenzae* *Streptococcus pneumoniae* *Neisseria meningitides*	Ceftriaxone 50 mg/kg IV every 12 hours
Young adults (7 to 50 years)	*S. pneumoniae* *N. meningitides*	Vancomycin 1 g IV every 12 hours Ceftriaxone 2 g IV every 12 hours
Adults older than 50 yrs; alcoholics; patients with a debilitating medical condition	*S. pneumoniae* Gram-negative rods *Listeria monocytogenes*	Ampicillin 2 g IV every 4 hours Ceftriaxone 2 g IV every 12 hours
Patients with postneurosurgical procedure or head trauma	*Staphylococcus aureus* Gram-negative rods *S. pneumoniae*	Vancomycin 1 g IV every 12 hours Ceftazidime 2 g every 8 hours

instances, the virus can be cultured from CSF, from blood, or from nasal, pharyngeal, or rectal swabs. Causes include enteroviruses, lymphocytic choriomeningitis virus, and a variety of other viruses, as well as infection with HIV. Medications that can cause aseptic meningitis include NSAIDs, metronidazole, carbamazepine, trimethoprim/sulfamethoxazole, and IVIG. Treatment is supportive.

■ CHRONIC MENINGITIS

Tuberculosis

Meningitis caused by *Mycobacterium tuberculosis* is a severe infection that carries high morbidity and mortality rates. *Cranial nerve palsies* and *vasculitic small-vessel infarctions* occur frequently and result from severe granulomatous inflammation of the basal meninges. Tuberculosis can also produce a *miliary encephalitis* or *focal tuberculoma*, with or without meningitis. Although immunosuppressed patients (patients with AIDS or alcoholic patients) are particularly at risk, the disease can strike anyone. Evidence of active pulmonary disease is found in only 30% of the cases, and only 50% of the cases are purified protein derivative (PPD)–positive. *Hydrocephalus* is a frequent late complication.

Diagnosis

The CSF shows lymphocytic pleocytosis, elevated protein level, and reduced glucose level (see Table 22–1). The diagnosis is established by observing *acid-fast* mycobacteria in the CSF; the yield exceeds 50% when multiple large-volume taps (10 to 25 ml) are examined. *M. tuberculosis* can also be *cultured* from the CSF, but the yield is low, and 4 to 6 weeks are needed for the organism to grow. *Polymerase chain reaction (PCR)* testing can establish the diagnosis by amplifying small amounts of tubercle bacillus DNA.

Treatment

Until antibiotic sensitivity is known, treatment with four drugs is recommended for the first 2 months. A full course of treatment requires 9 to 12 months. Options include **isoniazid 300 mg per day** (also give **pyridoxine 50 mg per day), rifampin 600 mg per day, pyrazinamide 15 to 30 mg/kg per day, ethambutol 15 to 20 mg/kg per day, streptomycin 15 mg/kg per day IM,** and **ciprofloxacin 750 mg two times a day.**

Cotreatment with **dexamethasone 6 mg IV every 6 hours** may also be used in severe cases (with depressed level of consciousness, focal deficits, or multiple cranial nerve palsies) to inhibit the inflammatory response and limit damage.

Neurosyphilis

Syphilis is a chronic systemic infection caused by the spirochete *Treponema pallidum*. **Primary infection** is characterized by a chancre (firm, painless genital ulcer). A **secondary bacteremic stage** may occur 2 to 12 weeks later, and this results in generalized mucocutaneous lesions (palmar and plantar rash) and lymphadenopathy. In 40% of the cases, the CNS is asymptomatically seeded at this point, and mild CSF changes (elevation of cells and protein) can be detected. Two percent of patients with secondary infection experience acute *meningovascular syphilis*.

Following a latent period of 15 to 20 years, **tertiary syphilis** manifests as a slowly progressive systemic inflammatory disease of the skin (gummas), heart (aortitis), eyes (chorioretinitis), or CNS. *Tertiary neurosyphilis* develops in 7% of patients with untreated primary syphilis and results from chronic meningeal and parenchymal inflammation. The classic manifestations include the following:

1. **General paresis**
   This condition results from diffuse infection of brain parenchyma and manifests as dementia with prominent psychiatric features and bilateral upper motor neuron signs.
2. **Tabes dorsalis**
   Tabes dorsalis results from chronic spinal polyradiculitis with secondary dorsal root and column degeneration. Symptoms may include neuropathic shooting pains in the lower extremities, loss of posterior column sensation, and areflexia.
3. **Argyll Robertson pupils**
   These are small irregular pupils that react to accommodation but not to light and reflect chronic optic neuritis. Optic atrophy and blindness may also occur.

Diagnosis

Neurosyphilis is defined by a positive serologic test (Venereal Disease Research Laboratory [VDRL] test) in the CSF and may be latent (normal CSF) or active (elevation of white blood cell count and protein level). Patients with active neurosyphilis are often asymptomatic. **LP is required to rule out neurosyphilis in patients with a serum nontreponemal antibody titer (RPR or VDRL) at 1:32 or higher, or in any patient with a positive serologic test and neurologic symptoms, treatment failure, no prior treatment, concurrent systemic tertiary syphilis, or HIV infection.** Note that in late syphilis, serum VDRL and rapid plasmin reagin (RPR) reactivity (nontreponemal tests) often falls to 70%, whereas fluorescent treponemal antibody absorption (FTA-ABS) reactivity remains positive in 90 to 95% of patients.

Treatment

Primary and secondary syphilis can be treated with **benzathine penicillin, 2.4 million units IM weekly for 3 weeks.** Neurosyphilis, whether latent or active, is treated with **penicillin G 2 to 4 million units IV every 4 hours for 10 days.**

Lyme Disease

Lyme disease is caused by the spirochete *Borrelia burgdorferi*, which is inoculated into humans by the bite of an infected deer tick *(Ixodes dammini)*. A characteristic expanding erythematous "target" lesion, erythema chronicum migrans, develops at the site of the tick bite, and this is often accompanied by fever, fatigue, arthralgias, and headache. Chronic infection can lead to arthritis, carditis, and CNS involvement (Table 22–3).

Diagnosis

The CSF shows a mononuclear pleocytosis with elevated protein levels, and the diagnosis is confirmed by detecting intrathecal production of IgG antibodies to *Borrelia* (CSF titer is higher than the serum titer) using an ELISA assay or Western blot. A PCR test for *Borrelia* DNA in CSF is also available. *Positive serologic blood testing alone is not enough to confirm the diagnosis in patients with suspected neurologic Lyme disease.*

Treatment

For patients with Lyme meningoradiculitis, treat with **ceftriaxone 2 g IV per day** or **penicillin G 4 million units IV every 4 hours for 2 to 4 weeks.** Early Lyme disease (less than 30 days) without neurologic manifestations or isolated facial palsy can be

---

Table 22–3 □ NEUROLOGIC MANIFESTATIONS OF LYME DISEASE

Stage 1 (less than 1 month after infection)
  Headache, neck stiffness (CSF normal)
Stage 2 (occurs in 15% of patients 1 to 6 months after infection)
  Meningitis
  Cranial neuritis, single (e.g., facial) or multiple nerves
  Polyradiculopathy
  Plexopathy
  Mononeuritis multiplex
  Acute polyneuropathy (resembles Guillain-Barré syndrome)
Stage 3 (months to years after infection)
  Chronic encephalopathy
  Demyelinating syndrome (multiple sclerosis–like)
  Chronic myelitis

treated with **doxycycline 100 mg PO two times a day** or **amoxicillin 50 mg PO three times a day for 7 to 21 days.**

Fungal Meningitis

Fungal infection of the CNS typically occurs in immunocompromised hosts (patients with AIDS, malignancy, diabetes, or alcoholism), but exceptions may occur. The vast majority of cases in the United States result from *Cryptococcus neoformans*; other causes include *Coccidioides immitis* (southwestern United States), *Candida albicans, Histoplasma capsulatum,* and *Blastomyces* species. *Aspergillus* and *Mucor* species are unique in their tendency to invade local tissues and cause vasculitic infarction.

Diagnosis

The CSF shows mononuclear pleocytosis, elevated protein level, and normal or reduced glucose level. Diagnosis is based on demonstrating the organism by wet smear or culture. *Cryptococcus* infection can also be diagnosed using the India ink stain or by detecting capsular antigen in the CSF with latex agglutination.

Treatment

All forms of fungal meningitis are treated with **amphotericin B 0.5 to 1.5 mg/kg per day IV for 4 to 6 weeks.** Severe cryptococcal meningitis is treated with the combination of **amphotericin B** and **flucytosine (5-FC) 25 mg/kg PO every 6 hours;** milder cases can be treated with **fluconazole 400 mg PO each day for 8 to 10 weeks** (HIV-positive patients need suppressive therapy with **fluconazole 200 mg PO every day indefinitely**). **Dexamethasone 6 mg IV every 6 hours** can be used to limit cranial nerve damage or reduce intracranial pressure (ICP) in severe infections.

Leptospirosis

Leptospirosis is caused by a group of closely related spirochetes, most often *Leptospira interrogans*. Humans are incidental hosts for these spirochetes, which typically infect and colonize wild and domestic animals, including cats, dogs, rodents, and cattle. Humans become infected by coming in contact with infected animal tissue or urine or contaminated water or soil; the spirochete is thought to enter via mucocutaneous abrasions.

Constitutional symptoms, including fever, chills, myalgia, nausea, and diarrhea, usually appear 1 to 2 weeks after exposure. Conjunctivitis, pharyngitis, rash, hepatitis, and renal failure may also occur. Clinical meningitis (headache, neck stiffness) may occur during the acute stage of infection, during which the organism can be isolated from the CSF, or several weeks later because of an immune-mediated reaction, at which time the CSF is sterile.

Diagnosis

Although neutrophils may be present early, the CSF usually shows a mononuclear pleocytosis with elevated protein levels. The diagnosis is confirmed via blood or CSF cultures or acute and convalescent serologic studies.

Treatment

Treatment is most effective when given in the first few days of illness. Leptospiral meningitis can be treated with **doxycycline 100 mg IV every 12 hours,** or **penicillin G 5 million units IV every 6 hours,** for 7 days.

■ BRAIN ABSCESS AND PARAMENINGEAL INFECTIONS

Bacterial Abscess

Brain abscess most commonly presents with subacute progression of headache (in 75% of patients), altered mental status (in 50% of patients), focal neurologic signs (in 50% of patients), and fever (in 50% of patients). The infection usually begins as a focus of cerebritis, which develops into a localized collection of pus with a surrounding fibrovascular capsule. Most abscesses are formed by contiguous spread from a parameningeal infection (otitis media, osteomyelitis, sinusitis) or by hematogenous spread in patients with endocarditis, bronchiectasis, or congenital cyanotic heart disease. The most common organisms encountered are streptococci, *Staphylococcus aureus*, gram-negative bacilli, and anaerobes such as *Bacteroides fragilis*. Polymicrobial infections are common.

Diagnosis

The diagnosis is suggested by a ring-enhancing lesion (Fig. 22–1) in the brain on CT or MRI. The CSF may be normal or may show a mild pleocytosis; a pathogen can be isolated from CSF cultures in less than 10% of cases. Blood cultures, echocardiography, chest x-ray, HIV testing, and a skull CT scan (to rule out sinusitis, otitis, or tooth abscess) should be performed in addition to LP in all patients with brain abscess of unknown etiology. Culture of pus obtained from a surgical drainage procedure is often the only way to establish the diagnosis, but even these cultures are negative in 20% of cases.

Treatment

For broad-spectrum empirical coverage of suspected bacterial abscess, treat with (1) **oxacillin 2 g IV every 4 hours or penicillin G 4 million units IV every 4 hours;** (2) **metronidazole 500 mg**

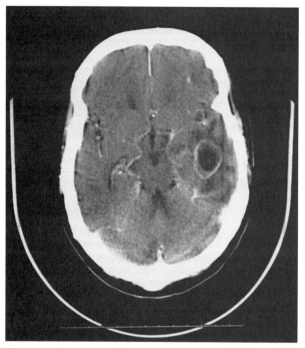

Figure 22–1 □ Ring-enhancing lesion on CT scan, characteristic of bacterial abscess.

IV every 6 hours, and (3) **ceftriaxone 2 to 4 g IV every 12 hours.** If the patient fails to respond, consideration should be given to administering **amphotericin B** to treat a possible fungal infection. Complete treatment takes 4 to 8 weeks; the duration of therapy should be guided by the results of serial CT or MRI scans. **Surgical options** include stereotactic needle aspiration, abscess drainage, and abscess excision (e.g., removal of capsule). Patients with depressed level of consciousness should also be treated with **dexamethasone 4 to 10 mg IV every 6 hours for 4 to 6 days** to reduce edema.

Subdural Empyema

Subdural empyema is a closed-space infection between the dura and arachnoid, usually over the hemispheric convexity. In adults, spread of infection from a contiguous source (e.g., sinusitis or otitis) is the cause in most cases, whereas in children, subdural empyema often occurs as a complication of meningitis. The organisms most often cultured are similar to those for brain abscess, and empirical antibiotic coverage is the same. Surgical drainage at the earliest opportunity is essential for successful treatment.

Cranial and Spinal Epidural Abscess

Epidural CNS infection almost always results from infection from a contiguous source and is often seen in combination with osteomyelitis. The CSF often shows mild signs of inflammation (elevated WBC and protein levels) but is sterile.

Cranial epidural abscess usually presents with localized pain and tenderness and can lead to cranial nerve deficits. For example, infection of the petrous temporal bone (Gradenigo's syndrome) often results in CN 5 and CN 6 deficits. Common infecting organisms are the same as for brain abscess, and empirical antibiotic treatment is the same.

Spinal epidural abscess is most common in the thoracic region and often occurs in diabetics and intravenous drug users. Symptoms may include intense local pain and tenderness, local root irritation with referred pain, and cord compression, which is a neurologic emergency. *S. aureus* and streptococci account for 75% of the infections, and gram-negative organisms account for 20%; unusual causes include *M. tuberculosis* (Pott's disease) and fungi. MRI of the spine is the diagnostic technique of choice. Treatment with high-dose steroids **(dexamethasone 60 to 100 mg IVP, followed by 10 to 20 mg IV every 6 hours)** and **surgical drainage** should be performed immediately to prevent cord compression. **Vancomycin** and **ceftriaxone** usually provide adequate empirical antibiotic coverage for bacterial infection (see Table 22–2).

Toxoplasmosis

Toxoplasmosis is the most common opportunistic infection affecting the CNS in patients with AIDS. *Toxoplasma gondii* is an intracellular protozoan; infection usually results in necrotic abscess formation, but disseminated meningoencephalitis can develop in some cases.

Diagnosis

The diagnosis is suggested by one or more ring-enhancing lesions in the brain on CT or MRI. The CSF may show mild elevation of the WBC count or protein level. The presence of serum antibodies to *Toxoplasma* is evidence of prior exposure to the organism, but it does not prove active infection. Demonstration of the organism by biopsy is required for definitive diagnosis and differentiation from CNS lymphoma but is generally required only in patients who fail a 7- to 10-day trial of empirical treatment.

Treatment

Patients with suspected toxoplasmosis should be treated empirically with **sulfadiazine 25 mg/kg PO every 6 hours** and **pyrimethamine 200 mg PO on day 1, followed by 75 to 100 mg per day for 6 to 8 weeks.** Folinic acid 10 to 20 mg PO every day should also be given to minimize hematologic toxicity. **Clindamycin 600 mg IV or PO four times a day** can be used instead of sulfadiazine in patients who are allergic to sulfa drugs. **Dexamethasone 6 mg IV every 6 hours** should be restricted to patients with large mass lesions and reduced level of consciousness, because it increases the rate of false-negative results for lymphoma, should biopsy be performed at a later date.

Cysticercosis

Cysticercosis is the most common parasitic CNS disease. Ova shed by the intestinal tapeworm *Taenia solium* in human feces can contaminate food ingested by the host or others, which leads to hematogenous dissemination of encysted larvae throughout the body, including the CNS. Most cases occur in Latin America (e.g., Mexico) and Southeast Asia.

Diagnosis

CT and MRI scans are usually highly characteristic: *Uninflamed cysts* appear as small (less than 1 cm), fluid-filled cysts. *Active, inflamed cysts* occur when the larvae are dying, and are identified by the presence of contrast enhancement. *Inactive cysts* result once the inflammatory reaction to a dying larval cyst has resolved; they appear as small, punctate calcified lesions. In the *racemic form*, cystic membranes fill the ventricles and the subarachnoid space, resulting in hydrocephalus. Detection of *serum antibody titers* to *Cysticercus* can confirm the diagnosis, but sensitivity is less than 100% in patients with inactive disease or with a single enhancing lesion. Patients and family members should undergo stool examinations for ova and parasites, because treatment can prevent reinfection.

Treatment

Patients with inactive (calcified) neurocysticercosis or with a single enhancing lesion and minimal symptoms (e.g., seizures controlled with anticonvulsants and a nonfocal examination) do not require treatment. In the latter case, follow-up neuroimaging 6 to 10 weeks later usually shows progression of the enhancing lesion to a small, calcified nodule. **Praziquantel 50 mg/kg per day** or **albendazole 15 mg/kg per day, split into three divided doses for 14 days,** will kill surviving larvae in patients with active infestation. Treatment results in active inflammation from dying organisms, which can be limited by a brief course of **dexamethasone (4 to 6 mg every 6 hours for 5 days)** in patients with severe disease. Surgical resection is often more effective than ventriculoperitoneal shunting for treating intraventricular cysticercosis resulting in hydrocephalus.

■ VIRAL ENCEPHALITIS

Herpes Simplex Encephalitis

Herpes simplex virus type 1 (HSV-1) encephalitis is the most common cause of viral encephalitis (approximately 15% of all cases) and is fatal in up to 40% of untreated patients. Patients present with fever, altered mental status, headache, and seizures. The disease results from reactivation of dormant HSV-1 within the trigeminal ganglion, with viral spread via sensory pathways into the brain, rather than the more common picture of retrograde viral expression leading to perioral herpetic lesions.

Diagnosis

The CSF may show mild lymphocytic pleocytosis, increased red blood cells, and increased protein, but it may be normal, particularly early in the disease. CSF cultures usually do not yield the virus. Focal necrotizing lesions of the inferior frontal and temporal lobes are highly characteristic and are best seen with contrast MRI. An electroencephalogram (EEG) often shows periodic lateralized epileptiform discharges, consistent with structural temporal lobe lesions. CSF polymerase chain reaction (PCR) testing has become the favored method for establishing the diagnosis, but false-positive results are common. Definitive diagnosis is made by brain biopsy, which demonstrates eosinophilic intracellular (Cowdry type I) inclusions. Biopsy may not be necessary if the clinical, radiologic, and EEG findings are highly characteristic.

Treatment

All patients with suspected viral encephalitis should be treated empirically with **acyclovir 10 to 12.5 mg/kg IV every 8 hours for 14 to 21 days.** *Because efficacy depends on early treatment, acyclovir should be started as soon as possible and should never be withheld pending the results of diagnostic studies.* Steroids should not be used unless signs of herniation are present. Anticonvulsants (e.g., **phenytoin**) should be given to all patients and discontinued after 2 weeks if no seizures occur. An ICP monitor is recommended in patients who are comatose (Glasgow Coma scale score less than 8).

Other Causes of Encephalitis

Causes of viral encephalitis other than HSV-1 are listed here. Serologic testing for these agents, as well as viral cultures of the CSF, pharynx, urine, and stool, may be helpful in establishing the diagnosis, but CSF PCR testing is rapidly becoming the diagnostic procedure of choice. With the exception of HSV and cytomegalovirus (CMV), no specific treatment is available.

1. **Mumps virus**
    Infection with mumps virus is unusual now since most children are vaccinated.
2. **Enteroviruses**
    This group includes **coxsackievirus, echovirus,** and **poliovirus**. Encephalitis occurs during summertime epidemics of gastroenteritis.
3. **Arboviruses (arthropod-borne viruses)**
    These viruses are spread by mosquitoes. They can also infect horses and birds, and they are most prevalent in the late summer and early fall.
    - **Equine encephalomyelitis viruses.** Eastern equine encephalomyelitis virus (Atlantic and Gulf coasts) is the most severe form and infection carries a mortality rate of 50%. Others include western equine encephalomyelitis virus (in the western United States and the Midwest) and Venezuelan equine encephalomyelitis virus.
    - **St. Louis encephalitis virus.** This disease occurs in epidemics in the rural Midwest.
    - **California encephalitis virus**
    - **Colorado tick fever virus**
    - **Japanese encephalitis virus**
    - **West Nile virus.** This potentially fatal form of encephalitis has occurred in recent summer epidemics in the northeastern United States; it can also manifest as acute inflammatory demyelinating polyneuropathy.
4. **Measles virus**
    Besides causing acute encephalitis 1 to 14 days after a viral exanthem (rubeola), measles virus can cause (1) a relentlessly progressive subacute encephalitis in immunosuppressed patients, (2) postinfectious immune-mediated demyelinating encephalomyelitis, and (3) **subacute sclerosing panencephalitis (SSPE),** a "slow" viral infection characterized by progressive dementia, ataxia, myoclonus, periodic sharp waves on EEG, elevated titers of anti-measles virus antibodies in the CSF, and pathologic intracellular viral inclusion bodies.
5. **Rabies virus**
    Rabies is spread by the bite of an infected (rabid) animal. After a variable incubation period (1 to 3 months), rabies encephalomyelitis invariably leads to delirium, seizures, pa-

ralysis, and death. After inoculation, the virus travels to the CNS via retrograde axonal transport. Negri bodies, dark intracellular viral inclusions, are the characteristic pathologic lesion.
6. **Lymphocytic choriomeningitis (LCM) virus**
   This usually causes viral (aseptic) meningitis. Infection comes from exposure to mice and hamster feces.
7. **Epstein-Barr virus (EBV)**
   EBV produces a systemic viral infection known as *mononucleosis* (pharyngitis, malaise, fever, adenopathy, liver function test abnormalities, splenomegaly, and atypical lymphocytes on blood smear), which may be complicated by encephalitis.
8. **Cytomegalovirus**
   CMV causes a systemic infection similar to EBV that can be complicated by encephalitis but that more often manifests as ventriculitis or encephalitis in immunosuppressed patients (see following section).
9. **Human herpesvirus 6**

■ NEUROLOGIC COMPLICATIONS OF AIDS

Opportunistic Infections

Patients with AIDS are at risk for the following opportunistic infections of the CNS, particularly when CD4$^+$ T helper lymphocyte counts are less than 200/mm^3. The approximate percentage of AIDS patients affected is shown in parentheses. *Patients with AIDS are at risk for multiple, simultaneous opportunistic infections.*
1. **Toxoplasmosis (10%)**
   Toxoplasmosis usually presents as single or multiple brain abscesses or as meningoencephalitis.
2. **Cryptococcus (10%)**
   Cryptococcus presents as acute or chronic meningitis. In contrast to patients without AIDS, CSF WBC counts may be normal or minimally elevated in up to 50% of patients. After 2 weeks of treatment with **Amphotericin B 0.5 to 1.5 mg/kg/day,** maintenance therapy with **fluconazole 200 mg/day** is required indefinitely.
3. **Progressive multifocal leukoencephalopathy (PML) (5%)**
   PML presents with multiple, relentlessly progressive demyelinating lesions within the CNS. It is caused by papovaviruses (JC and SV-40 viruses), which can be demonstrated by biopsy or detected by CSF PCR testing; median survival after diagnosis is 6 months. There is no effective treatment, although highly active antiretroviral therapy (HAART), with two nucleotide inhibitors and a protease inhibitor, may prolong survival in some patients.

4. **CMV infection (5% excluding retinitis)**
   CMV infection most often presents as *ventriculitis* but can also manifest as *encephalitis, myelitis*, and *lumbosacral polyradiculitis*. CMV retinitis is extremely common (it occurs in 20% of all AIDS patients). The diagnosis of ventriculitis is suggested by ependymal enhancement on MRI. All forms of infection may be treated with **gancyclovir 5 mg/kg IV every 12 hours for 14 to 28 days,** but efficacy has been shown only with retinitis and polyradiculopathy. **Foscarnet 60 mg/kg IV every 8 hours for 14 days** can be used as a second-line agent. Because CMV infection is difficult to diagnose in the setting of an acute illness, therapy should be started empirically prior to culture results.
5. **Herpes zoster (5%)**
   Herpes zoster radiculitis can be treated topically with acyclovir cream. **IV treatment (acyclovir 10 to 12.5 mg/kg every 8 hours)** is necessary only if multiple dermatomal levels are involved.
6. **Syphilis (less than 5%)**
   The course of syphilis is often accelerated in HIV-infected patients, and the early symptomatic forms of secondary syphilis (meningitis and meningovasculitis) predominate. The CSF VDRL test may be negative, and treatment may require a prolonged course of penicillin G (>10 days).

Nonopportunistic Nervous System Complications of AIDS

Besides opportunistic infections, patients with AIDS are subject to peripheral neuropathy, dementia or myelopathy from the direct effects of HIV infection, and CNS lymphoma. The frequency among AIDS patients is shown in parentheses.
1. **HIV sensory neuropathy (30%)**
   A small-fiber sensory neuropathy is seen frequently in advanced AIDS. Common findings include painful dysesthesias, hyperesthesia of the feet, and loss of ankle reflexes. Treatment of the neuropathic pain is symptomatic (see Chapter 7). Antiretroviral therapy (AZT, ddI, and ddC) may also cause small-fiber painful peripheral neuropathy. Treatment is symptomatic (see Chapter 17).
2. **HIV-associated dementia (15%)**
   Progressive dementia occurs frequently in HIV-infected patients, and it is an AIDS-defining illness. In addition to cognitive deficits and psychomotor slowing, pyramidal and extrapyramidal signs (rigidity, tremor, cogwheeling) may be seen. MRI shows diffuse atrophy, and the CSF is usually normal. With multidrug therapy using protease inhibitors and reverse-transcriptase inhibitors (HAART), the incidence

of AIDS dementia complex has been significantly reduced in recent years (see Chapter 18, Amnesia and Dementia).
3. **HIV myelopathy (5%)**
A progressive vacuolar myelopathy resulting in spastic paraparesis, sensory ataxia, and bowel or bladder incontinence is seen frequently in combination with AIDS dementia. A spinal cord compressive lesion, vitamin B_{12} deficiency, human T cell lymphotropic virus type I (HTLV-1) infection (tropical spastic paraparesis), and CMV or HSV myeloradiculitis should be excluded. MRI is normal, but somatosensory-evoked potentials are typically prolonged. There is no treatment.
4. **Primary CNS lymphoma (5%)**
CNS lymphoma presents as one or more enhancing mass lesions in the CNS and can be impossible to differentiate from toxoplasmosis with radiographic findings. Most patients have CD4$^+$ counts <50/mm^3, and many have ocular involvement, which can be diagnosed by slit-lamp examination. In most patients, the diagnosis is established by biopsy after failure to respond to empirical treatment for toxoplasmosis. Thallium SPECT showing increased local uptake is 88% specific for PCNSL, and, if positive, the patient should be referred directly for brain biopsy. Steroids cause tumor necrosis and reduce the diagnostic yield of biopsy tissue; hence, if biopsy is being considered, **dexamethasone should be withheld** unless absolutely necessary. Most lymphomas respond radiographically and clinically to whole-brain radiation; however, the effects are palliative, and survival rarely exceeds 3 to 6 months.
5. **HIV-associated myopathy (2%)**
A myopathy characterized by slowly progressive proximal muscle weakness, CK elevation (90%), and painful myalgias (30%) may occur in association with HIV infection. Both an inflammatory autoimmune mechanism and AZT exposure have been implicated in the pathogenesis. Steroids may be helpful if muscle biopsy reveals an inflammatory process.
6. **HIV (aseptic) meningitis (1 to 2%)**
Acutely infected patients occasionally develop a self-limited aseptic meningitis, in combination with constitutional symptoms of viral infection (fever, malaise, adenopathy).
7. **Acute demyelinating polyneuropathy (less than 1%)**
This complication is clinically indistinguishable from Guillain-Barré syndrome (see Chapter 15).

chapter 23 | Neuro-oncology

J. TORRES-GLUCK
C. BALMACEDA

Most brain tumors are diagnosed when computed tomography (CT) or magnetic resonance imaging (MRI) shows an enhancing intracranial mass lesion in a patient with new progressive neurologic symptoms that have developed over weeks to months. Many brain tumors are known to arise in particular locations within the central nervous system (CNS), and the differential diagnosis of a suspected brain tumor is greatly influenced by considering age and location. Figure 23–1 lists the most common primary CNS neoplasms in adults by location. Except in patients with known systemic cancer and presumed metastases, tissue biopsy is mandatory for establishing the diagnosis.

Dexamethasone, 4 to 10 mg IV or PO every 6 hours, is a potent glucocorticoid that can dramatically reduce vasogenic peritumoral edema associated with CNS neoplasms. It is indicated in all patients who are symptomatic from mass effect related to a brain tumor, but it should be withheld prior to biopsy if possible if primary CNS lymphoma is a consideration because of its tendency to produce nondiagnostic results. Apart from dexamethasone, which is a mainstay of treatment for CNS neoplasms, diagnostic and management considerations for specific tumors are provided here.

■ GLIOMAS

Gliomas are the most common type of primary brain tumor, secondary in incidence only to metastases. In the United States approximately 13,000 new gliomas are diagnosed each year, and their incidence seems to be on the rise. These tumors arise from glial cells and are classified according to their oncogenic precursors as astrocytoma, oligodendroglioma, and ependymoma.

Astrocytoma

Astrocytomas are the most common type of glioma (about 80% of all gliomas). They are highly infiltrative tumors; in their early stages, astrocytomas can infiltrate between neurons without affecting their function. They are heterogeneous, with different

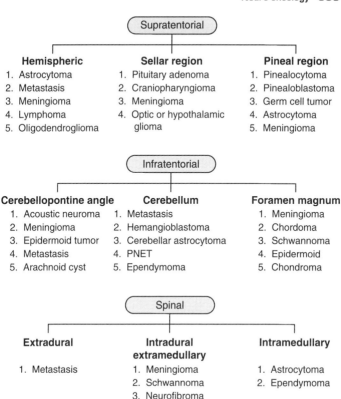

Figure 23-1 □ Radiographic differential diagnosis of solitary CNS neoplasms in the adult patient, by location. PNET, primitive neuroectodermal tumor.

areas of the tumor harboring cells of different histologic and malignant characteristics. Astrocytoma cells also have the potential to mutate, becoming more malignant as time passes.

Glioblastoma Multiforme

Glioblastoma multiforme tumors (GBMs) (grade IV astrocytoma) are the most malignant and common form of astrocytoma. They are rapidly growing and infiltrative, with cells reaching several centimeters beyond the gross margins of the tumor.

Epidemiology. GBMs represent about 50% of all gliomas. The peak incidence of GBM is between ages 50 and 60, and the incidence is slightly higher in men than women.

Pathology. The main histologic features of GBM are hypercellularity, nuclear atypia with multiple mitotic figures, endothelial proliferation, and necrosis. This development leads to a pattern of necrotic tissue surrounded by ribbons of hypercellularity, a phenomenon termed "pseudopalisading."

Presentation. Patients present most often with headache (80%), mental status changes (50%), and focal motor deficits (40%). Seizures are less common, occurring at presentation in fewer than 30% of patients.

Diagnosis. The imaging test of choice is gadolinium-enhanced MRI, which typically reveals a mass of irregularly enhancing tissue surrounding a nonenhancing necrotic center. This appearance has been described as a "ring-enhancing lesion." GBMs can also be seen to grow along white matter tracts, such as the corpus callosum, giving rise to the pathognomonic *butterfly glioma*. The tumor mass is poorly demarcated and is surrounded by variable amounts of cerebral edema that shows as areas of hypointensity on T1 and hyperintensity on T2-weighted or flare images.

Treatment. *Surgical resection* is the most effective means to achieve substantial tumor load reduction (debulking) and should be performed whenever feasible. Extent of resection has been shown to positively correlate with survival. Biopsy or subtotal resection is reserved for cases in which the tumor is inaccessible or in which more complete removal is deemed likely to result in severe neurologic deficit. *External beam radiation* directed with wide margins is effective in temporarily curbing tumor growth. A dose of up to 6000 cGy is administered. *Chemotherapy* may be used in conjunction with radiation or in patients in whom tumor recurs after initial therapy. The most commonly used agents are the nitrosoureas (BCNU, CCNU) and a regimen called PCV (procarbazine, CCNU, vincristine). Even after gross total resection, the tumor will invariably recur, and two thirds of the time it recurs within the margin of the previous resection. In patients with good neurologic performance status, reoperation should always be considered. Experimental treatments are in various stages of development and include brachytherapy (placement of radioactive seeds within the tumor), local delivery of chemotherapy by placing BCNU-impregnated wafers into the resection cavity at the time of surgery, gene therapy, therapy with immune modulators, and high-dose chemotherapy with bone marrow rescue.

Prognosis. Theprognosis for this tumor is poor, with approximately one half of the patients dying within a year and fewer than 10% surviving more than 2 years. Poor prognosis is associated with advanced age, poor performance status, and tumor

> **Box 23–1. PROGNOSIS FOR GBM WITH MULTIPLE THERAPIES**
>
> | Therapy | Survival Time |
> |---|---|
> | Corticosteroids alone | <3 months |
> | Surgery | 16–20 weeks |
> | Surgery plus radiation | 45–50 weeks |
> | Surgery plus radiation plus chemotherapy | 55–60 weeks |

location within eloquent brain, precluding aggressive surgical resection. With multimodality therapy the median survival improves incrementally (Box 23–1).

Anaplastic Astrocytoma

Anaplastic astrocytomas (grade III astrocytoma) are gliomas of intermediate malignancy between GBM and low-grade astrocytoma.

Epidemiology. Anaplastic astrocytoma accounts for about 30% of gliomas. The peak incidence is between ages 40 and 50.

Pathology. These are hypercellular tumors, with variable amounts of nuclear pleomorphism and mitoses. As in GBM, there may be neovascular proliferation, but endothelial proliferation is rare, and necrosis is distinctly absent.

Presentation. The average duration of symptoms at the time of diagnosis is 15 months, compared with 5 months for GBM. Seizures are the most common presentation, occurring in at least 50% of cases. Headache and focal neurologic deficit are also common.

Diagnosis. Gadolinium-enhanced MRI is the imaging test of choice. The tumor may or may not enhance with contrast material, and the borders of the tumor are generally poorly defined. Biopsy is required to make the diagnosis.

Treatment. Treatment strategy is identical to that for its more malignant counterpart, the GBM.

Prognosis. Median survival time with multimodality treatment is approximately 2 years.

Low-Grade Astrocytoma

Low-grade astrocytomas (grades I to II astrocytoma) are slow-growing tumors. These cells often infiltrate areas of brain without destroying them or interfering with their normal function. Over time, these tumors have the potential to dedifferentiate into more malignant forms of glioma; approximately 85% of low-grade astrocytomas will eventually degenerate into a GBM. This change usually occurs within 8 to 10 years from the time of diagnosis.

Incidence. Low-grade astrocytomas constitute about 20% of all gliomas. They occur primarily in young adults.

Pathology. These tumors have mild hypercellularity but completely lack mitotic figures, nuclear atypia, endothelial proliferation, and necrosis. Astrocytoma cells may resemble reactive astrocytes. This benign histologic feature has caused these tumors on occasion to be confused with simple glial scars.

Presentation. The presentation is typically indolent and of long duration. The most common presentation is seizures (65%), which in many cases may be present years prior to the diagnosis. Headache occurs in nearly half of patients. Focal deficits are rare.

Diagnosis. MRI is the imaging test of choice. The tumor does not enhance with gadolinium. It appears as areas of hypointensity on T1-weighted images and hyperintensity on T2-weighted images. There is no surrounding edema, and despite the occasionally large size of these lesions there is remarkably little mass effect. Biopsy is required for confirmation.

Treatment. Because of the lack of good prospective data, the treatment of low-grade astrocytomas is a topic of intense controversy. Some authorities advocate aggressive surgical resection and radiation, while others advise mere follow-up. Several retrospective studies suggest that aggressive treatment may ameliorate symptoms (particularly seizures) and lower the incidence of malignant transformation. Because as many as 75% of these tumors may include areas of perfectly functioning brain within them, surgery is an option only when the tumor is located within noneloquent areas of brain.

Prognosis. Median survival is 8 to 10 years. Older age, change in mental status, and focality on neurologic examination are poor prognostic factors.

Oligodendroglioma

These uncommon tumors arise from oligodendrocytes, the cells that form axonal myelin sheaths within the CNS.

Epidemiology. Oligodendrogliomas represent about 5% of all gliomas and occur with peak incidence from ages 40 to 50.

Pathology. The tumor cells have a characteristic "fried egg" appearance, with an area of clear cytoplasm surrounding the nucleus. They are frequently observed histologically to invade the cerebral cortex. Anaplastic features such as hypercellularity, nuclear pleomorphism, and abundant mitoses may or may not be present. Depending on the degree of histologic anaplasia they can be classified as low-grade or anaplastic oligodendrogliomas, but their histologic appearance does not correlate with the degree of biologic malignancy.

Presentation. Seizures are the most common presenting problem (~60%); headaches are also common (~20%). Because these tumors are highly infiltrative they often cause subtle behavioral or cognitive problems that can be detected only with formal neuropsychological testing. Focal neurologic deficits are uncommon even when the tumor has attained a large size.

Diagnosis. MRI reveals a tumor with indistinct margins and variable amounts of contrast enhancement. Calcification is present in nearly 75% of these tumors.

Treatment. Low-grade oligodendrogliomas may simply be followed unless they are highly symptomatic or until there is evidence of clinical or radiographic progression of the tumor. Traditionally anaplastic oligodendrogliomas have been treated with surgical resection, followed by radiation. The latter is done with or without chemotherapy. These tumors are generally exquisitely sensitive to chemotherapy; the most effective regimen combines procarbazine, CCNU, and vincristine (PCV).

Prognosis. As with all gliomas, this tumor tends to become increasingly malignant over time. Median survival is about 3 years.

Ependymoma

These rare neoplasms arise from ependymal cells and can arise anywhere within the neuraxis.

Epidemiology. Ependymomas account for less than 5% of all gliomas. They are most common in children and young adults, with two peak ages of incidence at 5 and 25 years. They comprise about 3% of intracranial gliomas and about 60% of spinal cord gliomas.

Pathology. *Papillary ependymomas* are most common, with well-differentiated cuboidal cells that form "rosettes" (around a central blood vessel) or perivascular "pseudorosettes." *Myxopapillary ependymomas* are more benign and occur exclusively in the sacral filum terminale. *Ependymoblastomas* are more malignant and tend to occur in children. *Drop metastases*, which result from seeding via the CSF, occur in approximately 10% of patients.

Presentation. Presentation depends on the location of origin and on the presence of drop metastases. In children, in whom the most common site of origin is the floor of the fourth ventricle, they tend to cause noncommunicating hydrocephalus, giving rise to increased intracranial pressure with headache (~80%), vomiting (~70%), or ataxia (~50%). Less commonly, they present with signs of brain stem dysfunction such as vertigo or cranial nerve deficits.

Diagnosis. MRI is the imaging test of choice. The tumor enhances irregularly with gadolinium, and some degree of calcification is present in over half of cases. When the tumor arises in the fourth ventricle it tends to grow to fill and dilate this structure, sometimes extruding itself into the subarachnoid space through the foramina of Luschka and Magendie. Spinal MRI and lumbar puncture for cerebrospinal fluid (CSF) cytologic examination are mandatory for the detection of drop metastases.

Treatment. Surgical resection is indicated to confirm the diagnosis and debulk the tumor. Surgery by itself may relieve hydrocephalus by removing the obstruction to CSF flow at the level of the fourth ventricle; in some cases ventriculoperitoneal shunting may also be considered. Ependymomas are very radiosensitive. Focal irradiation (4000–6000 cGy) should be directed postoperatively to the tumor bed. If drop metastases are detected, they are treated with low-dose radiation to the entire neuraxis, with boosts to the lesions themselves.

Prognosis. The five-year survival rate is approximately 40%, and the prognosis tends to be worse in children.

■ NONGLIAL BRAIN TUMORS

Primitive Neuroectodermal Tumor

This category encompasses several different tumors that seem to have common origin from embryonic remnants of neuroectodermal cells. They are highly malignant and have the propensity to disseminate through the CSF (drop metastases).

Epidemiology. Primitive neuroectodermal tumors (PNETs) occur almost exclusively in children and adolescents.

Pathology. PNETs arise from primitive neuroectodermal cells. They are cellular tumors that often exhibit signs of frank malignancy such as nuclear pleomorphism and abundant mitotic figures. Individual cells are small and darkly staining and often show evidence of neuronal differentiation on immunocytochemistry. Subtypes of PNETs include:
- **Medulloblastoma**
    The most common malignant brain tumor in children

(~20% of all pediatric brain tumors) is usually localized to the cerebellar vermis, where on MRI it appears as a bulky and uniformly enhancing mass. Because of their tendency to grow, obstructing the fourth ventricle, they most frequently present with hydrocephalus and signs of raised intracranial pressure. Nearly one third of these tumors have given rise to detectable drop metastases by the time they are diagnosed.

- **Pineoblastoma**
  These tumors occur in the pineal region and are highly responsive to radiation and chemotherapy. They present with hydrocephalus and Parinaud syndrome (impaired upward gaze, loss of accommodation, retraction nystagmus).
- **Neuroblastoma**
  Neuroblastomas may arise in the cerebral hemispheres or be intrathoracic (sympathetic ganglia), and sometimes they present with paraneoplastic opsoclonus.
- **Retinoblastoma**
  This tumor presents as an intraocular mass in infants. It is often bilateral, involving both eyes, and it is associated with an abnormality in the 13th chromosome.
- **Esthesioneuroblastoma**
  These tumors arise from the olfactory neuroepithelial tissue in the nasal passages and extend through the cribriform plate into the base of the skull and brain.

Presentation. Symptoms depend on tumor location. Extraneural metastases (to bone, lymph nodes, liver, and lung) occur more often with PNETs than any other CNS neoplasm.

Treatment. Complete *surgical resection* should be performed in all patients, as limited by the eloquence of surrounding brain structures. Most PNETs are responsive to *radiation* (5000+ cGy), but recurrence is common. Even if seeding of the CSF is not documented, many practitioners advocate prophylactic craniospinal irradiation. *Chemotherapy* is indicated in widely disseminated disease but is rarely successful.

Prognosis. The overall prognosis is poor. Even with surgery, radiation, and chemotherapy, average survival time is 2 years. Surgery and radiation are sometimes curative with highly localized tumors; patients surviving for a period of time equal to age at diagnosis plus 9 months can be considered cured.

Primary CNS Lymphoma

Epidemiology. Primary CNS lymphoma (PCNSL) accounts for 1 to 2% of all primary brain tumors, but the incidence is rising. Patients who are immunocompromised (e.g., patients with AIDS, organ transplant recipients) are at particularly high risk.

Pathology. PCNSLs are non-Hodgkin's lymphomas, usually of B cell origin, occurring in the absence of systemic lymphoma.

Presentation. There are four distinct clinical presentations of primary CNS lymphoma.
- **Solitary or multiple discrete tumors** are the most common form of presentation; ~50% are multifocal.
- **Diffuse infiltrative PCNSL** presents as a widespread infiltrative process throughout the brain, or as carcinomatous meningitis.
- **Ocular PCNSL** demonstrates retinal or vitreous infiltration that antedates or follows the development of CNS lesions in 10% of patients.
- **Spinal PCNSL** is an isolated intramedullary spinal cord lesion and is rare.

Diagnosis. *MRI* is the imaging test of choice, because PSNSL may appear isointense on CT. The tumor is often periventricular and usually enhances uniformly with gadolinium, although ring enhancement may occur with larger tumors. The diagnosis is established by biopsy. Because steroids have a strong tumoricidal effect and greatly increase the likelihood of a nondiagnostic biopsy, every attempt should be made to prevent treatment with dexamethasone prior to tissue diagnosis. *Spinal tap* should be performed unless significant mass effect is present; positive CSF cytologic findings may confirm the diagnosis and obviate the need for a biopsy. Spinal tap may also help in detecting CSF dissemination, which occurs in up to 35% of patients. *Slit-lamp examination* is required in all patients to detect ocular involvement. In patients with ocular symptoms, a vitreous biopsy should be performed.

Treatment. The role of surgery is limited to tissue diagnosis, and a complete surgical resection should not be attempted. **Dexamethasone 10 mg four times a day** leads to temporary tumor regression in many patients, but *radiation* is the mainstay of treatment. Radiotherapy (up to 5000 cGy) may be whole-brain or craniospinal, depending on the extent of dissemination. *Chemotherapy* has been used in lieu of radiation to prevent the long-term sequelae of this modality of treatment. Methotrexate or cytosine arabinoside (ara-C) may be given after irradiation, and intrathecal methotrexate via an Ommaya reservoir is sometimes used to treat patients with diffuse meningeal disease.

Prognosis. Mean survival time with corticosteroids and irradiation is 1 to 2 years in immunocompetent patients, and much less in immunosuppressed patients. Neuraxis dissemination ultimately occurs in 60% and systemic lymphoma in 10% of patients who survive 1 year, suggesting that systemic chemotherapy should be used as a primary treatment for this disease.

Meningioma

Epidemiology. Meningiomas account for 20% of all intracranial tumors and, after gliomas, are the second most common type of brain tumor in adults. They are twice as common in females than in males; peak incidence is between ages 40 and 60.

Pathology. Meningiomas are usually histologically benign tumors that arise from arachnoid cap cells. They do not invade cerebral tissue, and they cause symptoms by compressing surrounding structures. The more benign histologic subtypes (meningothelial, fibroblastic, transitional, psammomatous) are indolent and slowly growing; because of this they can often attain a very large size before becoming symptomatic. The more malignant subtypes (sarcomatous, angioblastic, and hemangiopericytoma) grow more rapidly and have a high tendency to recur even after gross total resection.

Presentation. The most frequent sites of meningioma in decreasing order are as follows:

- **Hemispheric (parasagittal or convexity)** tumors account for 50% of meningiomas; they usually present with headache, focal symptoms, and seizures.
- **Sphenoid wing** tumors present with headache, diplopia (especially when the cavernous sinus is involved), or visual loss. Proptosis may occur if significant hyperostosis of the bony orbit is present.
- **Olfactory groove** tumors classically present with dementia, or ipsilateral optic atrophy and contralateral papilledema (Foster-Kennedy syndrome).
- **Suprasellar** tumors present with headache, bitemporal hemianopia, and less frequently hypothalamic dysfunction.
- **Posterior fossa (clivus, foramen magnum, cerebellopontine angle)** tumors typically present with cranial nerve deficits (dysphagia, dysarthria, diplopia, tinnitus, vertigo). When large, they can lead to symptoms of brain stem compression (ataxia, hemiparesis).

Diagnosis. MRI and CT reveal a homogeneous, sharply demarcated tumor that enhances uniformly with contrast material and has a broad-based dural attachment. Enhanced-enhanced MRI may show a classic enhancing "dural tail." CT or plain x-rays of the skull may often show overlying areas of calvarial thickening and sclerosis (hyperostosis), which may be helpful for differentiating meningiomas from other durabased tumors.

Treatment. Tumors that are asymptomatic may simply be followed with serial MRI, definitive treatment being withheld until symptoms arise or the tumor is seen to enlarge. Definitive treatment for these tumors is *surgical resection* of the tumor along with its dural attachment. When planning surgery it should be noted that these tumors cause symptoms only because of their sheer bulk and that they grow slowly. In many cases, as in the elderly and the infirm, it is not necessary to achieve a total removal, which would add to the surgical morbidity. The rate of symptomatic recurrence directly correlates with the degree of resection and can range from 9% to over 30% in 10 years. Meningioma cells may have estrogen or progesterone receptors on their surface. For this reason, when recurrent or unresectable, these tumors have been treated with hormonal manipulation (tamoxifen, RU-486), although results with this type of therapy have been generally disappointing.

Prognosis. Prolonged survival after surgical resection is the rule. The rate of symptomatic resection directly correlates with the degree of resection and can range from 9% to over 30% in 10 years.

Acoustic Neuroma

This tumor arises from the Schwann cells of the vestibular division of the eighth cranial nerve; hence, a more appropriate name is "vestibular schwannoma." This benign tumor arises within the internal acoustic canal and follows the path of least resistance, growing into the cerebellopontine angle.

Epidemiology. These tumors account for 8% of all brain tumors and occur mainly in middle-aged adults. About 5 to 10% of patients have neurofibromatosis type 2 and may harbor bilateral acoustic neuromas, cranial or spinal meningiomas, schwannomas, and gliomas.

Presentation. The most common presenting symptom is unilateral tinnitus or hearing loss. As the tumor grows it compresses the adjacent cranial nerves, including the trigeminal (facial numbness, reduced corneal reflex), facial, and vestibular (vertigo) nerves. Ataxia from compression of the pons and cerebellum is a late sign.

Diagnosis. *Gadolinium-enhanced MRI* can reveal even small intracanalicular tumors. Both *audiography* and *brain stem auditory evoked potentials* are important for quantifying the extent of damage to the cochlear nerve.

Treatment. *Surgical resection* is curative in most cases, particularly when the tumor is small (<2 cm in diameter). The main difficulty of surgery is preservation of the cochlear and facial nerves, something that becomes progressively difficult with increasing tumor size. Conventionally administered radiation is not effective in the treatment of these tumors, but stereotactic radiosurgery (LINAC radiosurgery, gamma knife) shows promise in treating patients with small tumors, in which medical comorbidity precludes surgery.

Pituitary Adenoma

Epidemiology. Pituitary adenomas account for about 10% of all brain tumors and occur most frequently in young adults (20s and 30s). They arise from the adenohypophysis within the sella turcica, where they frequently remain. When large they can extend into the suprasellar region through an incompetent diaphragma sella.

Pathology. These histologically benign tumors tend to be slow growing and compress rather than invade surrounding neural tissue. Anatomically, pituitary adenomas can be divided into *microadenomas* (<10 mm in diameter), *diffuse adenomas* (surrounded by dura but with some suprasellar extension), and *invasive adenomas* (infiltrating dura, bone, or brain). Histologically, cells may appear chromophobic (most common), acidophilic, or basophilic (least common). However, the light microscopic appearance correlates poorly with secretory activity. The majority of pituitary adenomas are nonsecretory or prolactinomas.

Presentation. Pituitary adenomas may present via one of three mechanisms:
- **Pituitary hormone hypersecretion:** Functional or secretory pituitary adenomas may present as (1) Cushing's disease, from ACTH secretion, (2) amenorrhea/galactorrhea, from prolactin secretion, or (3) acromegalic gigantism, from growth hormone secretion. Production of sex hormones (LH, FSH) or TSH by a pituitary adenoma is extremely uncommon. Secreting tumors are most frequently diagnosed when quite small (<1 cm), as severe endocrinologic disturbances bring them to medical attention early.
- **Mass effect:** Nonsecreting tumors rarely cause symptoms until they have attained a large size. They can then cause panhypopituitarism by compressing the normal pituitary, visual disturbances (bitemporal hemianopia) by compressing the optic apparatus, and headache.
- **Pituitary apoplexy:** This syndrome results from acute infarction or hemorrhage into a large, highly vascular tumor and can be life-threatening. Patients present suddenly with headache, visual loss, ophthalmoparesis, and mental status changes. Emergency decompression may be required.

Diagnosis. *MRI* is more sensitive than CT for detecting microadenomas and is the imaging study of choice. Gadolinium normally causes enhancement of the pituitary gland, and tumor enhancement can be variable. Nonetheless, secretory adenomas are frequently too small to be seen, even on MRI. In these cases the diagnosis is made on careful endocrinologic evaluation, which should include the following: T_3, T_4, TSH, GH, prolactin, LH, FSH, fasting glucose, serum cortisol, and estradiol (women) or testosterone (men) levels. Formal ophthalmologic testing should be performed in all cases of macroadenoma.

Treatment. With the exception of prolactinomas, surgery is generally indicated if signs of mass effect on the optic chiasm or cranial nerves are present. *Transsphenoidal surgery* has the lowest morbidity and mortality rates and results in visual improvement in about 75% of cases. Adrenal insufficiency or diabetes insipidus may occur postoperatively, but is usually temporary. It is often impossible to completely remove a tumor with suprasellar extension, and in these cases the tumor usually recurs. Focused *radiation* (4000 to 6000 cGy over 4 to 6 weeks) reduces the postoperative recurrence rate, and is indicated if the tumor could not be completely resected.

Bromocriptine 2.5 to 5 mg three times a day, a synthetic dopamine agonist that inhibits pituitary secretion of prolactin, is the first line of treatment for prolactinomas regardless of size. Large prolactinomas may shrink dramatically with bromocriptine therapy, with resolution of visual field and endocrine disturbances. If significant deficits persist, surgery may then be performed with the added benefit of bromocriptine pretreatment.

Prognosis. The overall recurrence rate following surgical resection of pituitary adenoma is about 12%, with most tumors recurring after 4 years.

Craniopharyngioma

These tumors arise from squamous cell nests in the region of the pituitary stalk, and they present as suprasellar lesions.

Epidemiology. Craniopharyngiomas occur both in childhood and adulthood and represent 3% of all brain tumors. They are slightly more common in males.

Pathology. They are biologically and histologically benign but have the tendency to recur if incompletely resected.

Presentation. As with other suprasellar tumors, craniopharyngiomas cause symptoms by compressing the optic tracts, depressing hypothalamic or pituitary function, or increasing ICP.

Diagnosis. The tumor is often irregular and well demarcated from surrounding structures. Enhancement with contrast material is irregular, and many tumors are cystic. A common characteristic is of calcification (40 to 80%), which is best appreciated by CT.

Treatment. Most authorities advocate complete *surgical resection* whenever feasible. Subtotal resection carries a rate of recurrence of over 75% without adjuvant treatment. Postoperative *radiation* may substantially reduce or delay tumor recurrence.

Pineal Region Tumors

Epidemiology. Pinealomas represent 1% of intracranial tumors in adults and 3 to 8% of brain tumors in children. The average age at presentation is 13 years.

Pathology. Pinealomas may arise from germ cells or from pineal parenchymal cells.
- **Germ cell tumors:** The most common type of pineal tumor, these tumors are histologically indistinguishable from systemic germ cell tumors. There are two types: *germinomas* and *nongerminomatous germ cell tumors*. The latter secrete β-HCG and/or α-fetoprotein (AFP) in serum, CSF, or both. Elevation of these markers is associated with a more aggressive behavior; serial measurements are useful both for diagnosis and for monitoring response to therapy.
- **Pineal parenchymal tumors:** These tumors arise from the pineal gland and surrounding tissue. *Pinealoblastomas* are more aggressive and tend to seed the CSF. *Pineocytomas* are less aggressive and tend to present during adolescence.

Presentation. Common symptoms include nausea and vomiting caused by aqueductal compression, and headaches and mental status changes related to obstructive hydrocephalus. Compression of the superior colliculus can result in Parinaud syndrome (forced downgaze, impaired pupillary reactivity, and retractory nystagmus). Pseudoprecocious puberty caused by β-HCG can be observed with germ cell tumors.

Diagnosis. Evaluation of patients with a pineal-region tumor should include (1) MRI of the head and entire spine with gadolinium, (2) serum and CSF germ cell markers (β-HCG and AFP), (3) CSF cytologic examination, (4) evaluation of pituitary function if endocrine abnormalities are suspected, and (5) a visual field examination if suprasellar extension of tumor is noted on MRI.

Treatment. Initial management is directed at treating hydrocephalus and establishing a diagnosis. Further therapy is based on tumor pathology. *Surgery* is reserved for tumors with significant mass effect; small germinomas can often be successfully treated with chemotherapy and radiation alone. *Chemotherapy* with cisplatin is particularly useful for germinomas. *Radiation*

(400 to 6000 cGy) may be delivered to the whole brain, and the spinal axis if drop metastases are present. Prophylactic spinal irradiation is controversial.

Prognosis. Because germinomas are very sensitive to chemotherapy and radiation, the long-term survival rate is higher than 90%. Nongerminomatous germ cell tumors have a 30 to 40% 5-year survival rate with radiation therapy alone. Pineal region tumors can recur more than 5 years after diagnosis; lifelong follow-up is mandatory. MRI scans should be obtained periodically, as well as tumor markers for patients with germ cell tumors, even if these were normal at diagnosis.

■ METASTATIC DISEASE

Brain metastases occur in up to 25% of patients with cancer, and the incidence seems to be increasing. Metastases represent the most common form of intracranial neoplasms. Systemic cancers can spread to the CNS either hematogenously or by direct invasion. Systemic cancer can also affect the nervous system through the remote effects of cancer, which are known as paraneoplastic syndromes (Table 23–1).

Brain Metastases

Epidemiology. Approximately 40% of patients have a *solitary metastasis*. Gastrointestinal (e.g., colon) and gynecologic (e.g., ovarian, endometrial, and cervical) malignancies are the most common sources of a solitary metastasis. *Multiple metastases* are encountered radiographically in approximately 60% of cases, particularly with lung and breast cancer and, especially, with melanoma.

Pathology. Brain metastases are typically well demarcated and surrounded by extensive brain edema. Although they can occur anywhere in the brain, they are most commonly located at the *gray-white junction*. Because of their frequent occurrence near the cerebral surface, they are usually amenable to surgical resection.

Presentation. Symptoms usually develop over weeks to months. Headache (60%), motor weakness (60%), and mental status changes (35%) are the most common presenting complaints. *Seizures* occur in about 20% of patients and are most commonly seen with multiple lesions and with melanoma. An acute, stroke-like presentation can occur with sudden hemorrhage into the tumor. This is most common in highly vascular metastases, such as melanoma or renal cell carcinoma.

Table 23-1 □ PARANEOPLASTIC SYNDROMES

Syndrome	Common Tumors	Associated Antibody	Comments
Sensorimotor neuropathy	Lung (small cell), lymphoma	None	Most common syndrome; axonal or demyelinating
Motor neuron disease	Myeloma, lymphoma	Paraprotein (IgG, IgM)	May occur together with encephalomyelitis
Pure sensory neuropathy (ganglioneuritis)	Lung (small cell)	Anti-Hu (ANNA-1)	Neuropathy usually precedes tumor symptoms; painful paresthesias, severe sensory ataxia, areflexia, and CSF pleocytosis are characteristic
Limbic encephalitis	Lung (small cell), lymphoma	Anti-Hu	Agitation, confusion, amnesia, dementia; CSF pleocytosis and MRI abnormalities of limbic cortex may occur
Brain stem encephalitis	Testicular, ovarian, uterine, breast, lung (small cell)	Anti-Ta, anti-Yo, anti-Hu	Oculomotor disorders, hearing loss, dysarthria, dysphagia
Cerebellar degeneration	Ovarian, lung (small cell), breast	Anti-Yo, anti-Purkinje cell, anti-Ri	Ataxia, dysarthria, nystagmus; normal CSF
Opsoclonus, ataxia, myoclonus	Neuroblastoma, breast, lung	Anti-Ri	Constant irregular movements of the eyes; may be associated with ataxia
Necrotizing encephalomyelitis	Lung (small cell), lymphoma, breast	Anti-Hu	Poor prognosis
Dermatomyositis	Lung, breast, lymphoma, ovary	None	Treat with steroids; elevated CK level
Lambert-Eaton myasthenic syndrome	Lung (small cell), breast, prostate, ovary, stomach	Anti-VGCC	Proximal limb weakness; EMG shows incremental response at >10 Hz
Carcinoma-associated retinopathy	Lung (small cell), cervical tumors	Antiretinal	Loss of vision

VGCC, voltage-gated calcium channel.

Diagnosis. Contrast-enhanced CT and MRI with gadolinium can show metastases to the brain. Because of its higher sensitivity, however, MRI is the test of choice. These lesions show as uniform or ring-enhancing lesions surrounded by extensive peritumoral edema.

Treatment. *Surgical resection followed by whole brain radiation therapy (WBRT)* is the gold standard for the treatment of solitary brain metastases. Surgery is generally contraindicated in patients with multiple metastases, unless one of the lesions is imminently life-threatening because of its size or location. Surgery may also be necessary to obtain tissue for histologic diagnosis in cases of metastases from an unknown primary tumor or in cases in which the primary disease has been well controlled for a long period of time. Surgical resection may also be required in cases in which the cellular type of the tumor is known to be relatively radioresistant (e.g., melanoma, renal cell carcinoma).

Radiation is recommended for patients with multiple metastases and for patients with solitary metastases in whom the location of the tumor or medical comorbidity precludes craniotomy. A total dose of around 3000 cGy is typically divided in fractions over 10 to 14 days. Concomitant administration of corticosteroids lowers the cerebral toxicity of radiation. Radiation leads to neurologic improvement in about 60% of cases, with complete disappearance of the lesion in up to 25% and reduction in size in another 35% of patients.

Stereotaxic radiosurgery (e.g., linear accelerator, gamma knife) is a newer modality in the treatment of brain metastases. Current trials are comparing it to surgery for the treatment of solitary lesions. Its greatest advantage is that it is a noninvasive, ambulatory procedure that is able to eradicate or significantly shrink the lesion in over 75% of cases. Its main disadvantages compared to surgery are that it may take 3 to 6 months for the lesion to respond and that its rate of success inversely correlates with the size of the lesion. It is generally not recommended for lesions >3 cm in greatest diameter. *Chemotherapy* has generally yielded disappointing results. It has been used with limited success for patients who have asymptomatic brain disease and who are responding favorably to systemic drugs.

Leptomeningeal Metastases

Epidemiology. This condition is also known as *meningeal carcinomatosis* or *carcinomatous meningitis*. Leptomeningeal spread is most common with carcinoma from the breast or lung, non-Hodgkin's lymphoma, and malignant melanoma.

Pathology. Malignant cells reach the leptomeninges via hematogenous spread. Once established, tumor cells can be carried by the CSF throughout the neuraxis and can invade structures traversing the subarachnoid space, such as cranial nerves and nerve roots. Cells can also enter the Virchow-Robin perivascular spaces, causing venous thrombosis and widespread microinfarctions of the brain. Malignant cells can also obstruct CSF flow, causing hydrocephalus.

Presentation. Leptomeningeal metastases classically present with multiple cranial neuropathies or spinal radiculopathies. Numbness in the distribution of the mental nerve *(numb chin syndrome)* can be a hallmark. Headache is extremely common, and in advanced cases there can be changes in mental status and seizures.

Diagnosis. *Lumbar puncture* for analysis of the CSF is the mainstay of diagnosis. The CSF reveals pleocytosis (mostly lymphocytic), elevated protein, and low glucose. CSF cytologic examination reveals neoplastic cells and confirms the diagnosis. Because there is a high rate of false negative cytologic findings, up to three spinal taps may be necessary to confirm the diagnosis. *MRI* may reveal leptomeningeal enhancement or nodules of disease throughout the leptomeninges, particularly along the surface of the spinal cord. When MRI is unavailable or contraindicated, *myelography* may be helpful for identifying spinal deposits of tumor.

Treatment. The prognosis of patients with leptomeningeal metastasis is dismal, with median survival ranging from 3 to 6 months. *Chemotherapy* is given intrathecally via lumbar puncture or preferably via an Ommaya reservoir. The most commonly used agents are **methotrexate (12 mg biweekly)** and **ara-C (50 mg biweekly).** These drugs are given twice weekly at first, then less frequently as the CSF begins to clear. *Craniospinal radiation* (4000 cGy to brain, 3000 cGy to spine) may also be offered in an attempt to reduce the tumor burden but may not be feasible in patients who have already received whole-brain radiation or in patients receiving concurrent chemotherapy due to the high risk of pancytopenia from bone marrow suppression.

Skull Metastases

Epidemiology. Tumors arising from the paranasal sinuses and nasopharynx can involve the CNS. They can do so either by directly invading and eroding through the skull base or by insinuating themselves through one of its multiple foramina. Hematogenous spread of tumor to the skull is rare. The most common tumors to reach the skull in this fashion are carcinomas of the breast and prostate.

Pathology. Skull base metastases can cause symptoms via one or more of the following mechanisms: compression of cranial nerves, invasion and erosion of the meninges, and increased brain compression with intracranial pressure when the tumor grows into a large bulky mass.

Presentation. The most common symptoms are localized pain from direct invasion of the dura mater and cranial nerve deficits. Five typical clinical syndromes have been described. *Orbital syndrome* presents with dull supraorbital pain, blurred vision, and diplopia. Examination may reveal proptosis, ophthalmoplegia, and decreased sensation along V1. *Parasellar syndrome* presents with frontal headache and ophthalmoparesis, but usually not proptosis. *Middle cranial fossa syndrome* presents as numbness along the distribution of V2 and V3 (numb chin syndrome). *Jugular foramen syndrome* is caused by tumor compressing CN 9, CN 10, and CN 11 as they exit the skull through the jugular foramen. This entity presents with unilateral occipital or glossopharyngeal pain, followed by hoarseness and dysphagia. *Occipital condyle syndrome* presents with orbital pain that worsens with neck flexion. On examination, patients tend to hold the neck stiffly, have tenderness on palpation over the occiput, and may have a CN 12 palsy.

Diagnosis. Optimal workup should include gadolinium-enhanced MRI and noncontrast CT. The former can better visualize the extent of the tumor, while the CT gives better detail of bony erosion/invasion.

Treatment. Surgical resection followed by focal radiation is the preferred mode of treatment. Good patient selection, however, is key as some of the surgical procedures required involve major reconstructive work on the base of the skull and carry a significant morbidity rate. Patients who are not candidates for surgery should be treated with focal radiation.

Spinal Metastases

Pathology. Metastases may reach the vertebral spine and spinal cord via *Batson's vertebral venous plexus*, a preferred drainage site for pelvic, abdominal, and thoracic organs. Blood vessel concentration in the *vertebral body* exceeds other parts of the vertebra and makes it vulnerable. Epidural cord compression usually results from direct extension of tumor from the vertebral column or from paravertebral metastases that grow through the neural foramina.

Presentation. The thoracic spine is the most common site of involvement. Pain is the first symptom in 95% of patients with cord compression. Features that help differentiate metastatic from musculoskeletal back pain include thoracic level pain and aggravation by lying supine.

Diagnosis. *Radiographs* are abnormal in 85% of patients with cord compression; loss of the vertebral pedicles is the first sign. *Noncontrast MRI* is preferred for detecting epidural tumor. Twenty-five percent of patients with focal signs show *multiple sites* of compression, so MRI should include the entire spine.

Treatment. The goals of treatment are preservation of neurologic function and alleviation of pain. *Radiation* usually includes two vertebral bodies above and two below the lesion. *Surgery* is considered for cord compression, neurologic deterioration despite radiotherapy and steroids, spinal instability, and radioresistant tumors. Prognosis depends on the patient's condition at the time of treatment; up to 80% of ambulatory patients remain ambulatory, whereas only 10% of those with paralysis will walk again.

■ NEUROLOGIC COMPLICATIONS OF CANCER TREATMENT

Radiation Toxicity

Delayed injury to the brain or spinal cord may occur weeks to years after radiation therapy. Radiation can also affect peripheral and cranial nerves.

1. **Acute toxicity (1 to 6 weeks after radiation)** may include headache, nausea, and vomiting; this type of toxicity occurs more frequently when large doses are given per fraction or elevated intracranial pressure is present. MRI shows localized brain swelling without enhancement. Steroids may reduce symptoms. Otitis can follow radiation therapy to the posterior fossa.
2. **Early-delayed toxicity (3 weeks to several months)** presents as somnolence and headache; it is seen most commonly in children receiving prophylactic whole-brain radiation for leukemia. Spontaneous recovery is the rule. *Rhombencephalopathy* with ataxia, dysarthria, and nystagmus may follow radiation to the middle ear area or for glomus jugulare tumors. Radiation myelopathy takes the form of Lhermitte's sign.
3. **Late-delayed toxicity (months to years)** can take several forms.
    - *Radiation necrosis* occurs in about 5% of patients given total doses above 5000 cGy with daily fraction sizes over 200 cGy. Median time for development is 14 months after treatment. Radiation necrosis may simulate the original tumor and can be difficult to differentiate from tumor recurrence on MRI. An enhancing mass lesion and diffuse white matter changes are the most common MRI abnormalities. Positron emission tomography may help distin-

guish tumor recurrence from radiation necrosis, because the latter is hypometabolic. Biopsy is often needed to establish the diagnosis. Steroids can lead to clinical stabilization, but when there is marked mass effect, surgical resection may be needed.
- *Cognitive impairment* is common in long-term survivors. Children under 5 years old are particularly susceptible. Memory is typically most severely affected. A syndrome of ataxia, cognitive disturbances, and urinary incontinence, sometimes ameliorated by ventriculoperitoneal shunting, has been described in adults.
- *Radiation myelopathy* develops within 3 years; the average latency period is 12 months. It is observed in 5% of patients who receive >4500 cGy at fractions of over 180 cGy. Symptoms include painless subacute numbness and paresthesias, a spastic gait disorder, and sphincter symptoms. MRI may be normal or may show cord swelling or atrophy. The diagnosis is made by exclusion. Steroids may improve symptoms.
- *Radiation-Induced vasculopathy* can affect both the intracranial and extracranial vessels. Most patients have had neck irradiation for head and neck cancer or for optic nerve or suprasellar tumors. Clinically, stroke occurs in the setting of occlusive large artery disease.
- *Endocrine dysfunction* can take several forms. Growth hormone deficiency is the most common; growth arrest occurs in children, whereas adults have a decrease in muscle mass and an increase in adipose tissue. Gonadotropin deficiencies manifest in children as failure to enter puberty and amenorrhea; adults have infertility, sexual dysfunction, and decreased libido. Thyrotropin deficiency manifests as weight gain and lethargy. ACTH deficiency presents with lethargy and decreased stamina.
- *Radiation optic neuropathy* follows treatment to the orbit, sinuses, pituitary, or intracranial tumors. Painless visual loss occurs within 3 years of treatment. About half of the patients improve. Steroids are ineffective. Measures to shield the optic nerve from the radiation portals may reduce the incidence of this complication.
- *Brachial plexopathy* resulting from radiation is described in Chapter 20.

4. **Secondary tumors** are an uncommon late complication of radiation therapy. *Peripheral nerve tumors* occur within the port of radiation in up to 9% of patients, especially those treated for breast cancer or lymphoma. Clinical presentation is an enlarging painful mass with progressive neurologic deficits. Mean interval is 16 years. *Meningiomas* may follow radiation for CNS tumors or for tinea capitis. Mean latency

period is 37 years if low-dose irradiation is given, and 18 months for doses >2000 cGy. Compared to spontaneously arising meningiomas, radiation-induced meningiomas are more likely to recur and undergo malignant degeneration.

Cancer Chemotherapy Toxicity

Antitumor chemotherapy may be toxic to both the peripheral and central nervous systems. The incidence of neurotoxicity may depend on the dosage, route, and schedule of administration; the age of the patient; and whether additional chemotherapy or radiation was given.

Antineoplastic drugs can cause a wide variety of neurotoxic effects (Table 23–2). *Peripheral nervous system toxicity* is most common with vincristine and vinblastine. Cisplatin causes a sensory polyneuropathy. The taxanes paclitaxel (Taxol) and docetaxel (Taxotere) cause a sensorimotor neuropathy. *Autonomic neuropathy* predominantly affects the GI tract with abdominal pain and constipation. 5-Fluorouracil causes a rare (5%) but characteristic acute *cerebellar syndrome*. A delayed *leukoencephalopathy* is associated with IV high-dose or intrathecal methotrexate.

Bone Marrow Transplantation

Bone marrow transplantation (BMT) from an HLA-matched donor often results in *graft-versus-host disease* (GVHD). Neurologic disorders include polymyositis, myasthenia gravis, sensorimotor neuropathy, aseptic meningitis, and leukoencephalopathy. Remis-

Table 23–2 □ NEUROTOXICITY OF ANTINEOPLASTIC DRUGS

Neurologic Disorder	Drugs
Peripheral neuropathy	Carboplatin, cisplatin, cytarabine, etoposide, fludarabine, oxaliplatin, procarbazine, suramin, taxol, taxotere, vinblastine, vincristine, vinorelbine
Cranial neuropathy	Carmustine, cisplatin, 5-fluorouracil, ifosfamide, vinblastine, vincristine
Autonomic neuropathy	Cisplatin, procarbazine, taxol, vinblastine, vincristine, vinorelbine
Encephalopathy	L-Asparaginase, busulfan, carmustine, cisplatin, cytarabine, 5-fluorouracil, fludarabine, ifosfamide, methotrexate, procarbazine
Cerebellar syndrome	Cytarabine, 5-fluorouracil, procarbazine
Acute myelopathy	Cytarabine, methotrexate, thiotepa

sion of neurologic toxicity has been reported with successful treatment of GVHD. *Neurologic complications* in patients who undergo allogeneic or autologous bone marrow transplant are cerebral hemorrhage (4%), metabolic encephalopathy (3%), and CNS infections (2%). Hemorrhages are mostly subdural and correlate with platelet dysfunction. Post-BMT leukoencephalopathy and a rare acute parkinsonian syndrome have also been described. Progressive multifocal leukoencephalopathy may occur in immunocompromised patients after either autologous or allogeneic bone marrow transplantation for chronic myelogenous leukemia.

Immunosuppressant drugs are used for BMT. *Cyclosporine* neurotoxicity may include tremor, paresthesias, lethargy, ataxia, and a reversible leukoencephalopathy that can lead to seizures and coma. White matter lesions are seen on CT and MRI. *FK-506* toxicity presents as tremors, headache, and paresthesias. *OKT3* toxicity presents as confusion, seizures, and lethargy.

chapter 24 | Cerebrovascular Disease

Cerebrovascular disease includes a wide spectrum of disorders, all sharing an acquired or inherited pathology of the cerebral vasculature. Stroke syndromes range in scope from a minor hemisensory loss in a single limb to hemiplegia, cognitive changes, and coma. The onset of deficits usually occurs in seconds to minutes. The **physical examination** can give an impression of the size and a fair estimate of the location of the infarct and can thus guide the urgency of subsequent management steps. **Brain imaging** is necessary in almost all evaluations of stroke. Magnetic resonance imaging (MRI) should identify all but the smallest lesions and is superior to computed tomography (CT) for brain stem and small, deep infarcts. CT is the equal of MRI in detecting acute hemorrhage and is superior for assessing bony abnormalities. Whereas CT may miss an infarct within the first several hours of onset, MR diffusion-weighted imaging (DWI) can show ischemia within minutes of onset. The brain can tolerate only a few hours of ischemia before becoming irreversibly infarcted. The window of opportunity for acute intervention therefore is narrow. This chapter focuses on the presentation of acute stroke, with attention to the pathophysiologic mechanisms that drive the management decisions discussed in Chapter 6.

■ CLASSIFICATION

Acute stroke comprises three broad categories: **subarachnoid hemorrhage (SAH), ischemic stroke,** and **intracerebral hemorrhage (ICH).** The clinical presentations may be similar, yet the pathophysiology and consequent management algorithms are distinct.

Subarachnoid Hemorrhage
Clinical Presentation

Sudden, severe ("thunderclap") headache is the classic presentation of SAH from a ruptured cerebral aneurysm. When asked, patients usually classify the headache as the worst they have ever had or rate it a 10 on a scale of 1 to 10. Stiff neck and photophobia are often present, requiring a consideration of acute bacterial meningitis in the differential diagnosis. Preceding minor headache may occur from a "sentinel bleed" as a preamble to a major hemorrhage. Trauma is a more common cause of hemorrhage in the subarachnoid space, but the clinical presentation is then usually obvious. The most common neurologic finding in SAH is altered mental status. If focal signs or symptoms appear, it is often because of the presence of a local, intracerebral clot or because of direct compression of the aneurysm on a cranial nerve (causing, for example a CN 3 palsy). Missing the diagnosis of SAH can be disastrous. Untreated SAH may be fatal in up to 50% of patients. A large percentage of the deaths may be an immediate consequence of the hemorrhage, but secondary vasospasm, rerupture of the aneurysm, and obstructive hydrocephalus can add significantly to the morbidity and mortality. The rate of rerupture may be as high as 1 to 2% per day for the first 2 weeks. Early diagnosis and surgical clipping or endovascular embolization of the aneurysm are therefore essential.

Diagnosis

1. **A CT or MRI should be obtained as soon as possible.**

    Both CT and MRI are good at detecting acute hemorrhage. CT hyperdensity in the sulci, major fissures, or around the brain stem is diagnostic. Particular attention should be paid to the basal cisterns. Subarachnoid blood pooling in the quadrigeminal plate cistern, for example, may appear only as a subtle hyperdensity in this space and may even appear isodense with brain if the blood is 5 to 7 days old. Figure 6–1 shows an example of SAH on CT. Other causes of SAH that may be detectable on CT or MRI include vascular malformation, venous thrombosis, and tumor.

2. **A negative CT or MRI scan does not rule out the diagnosis of SAH.**

    If there is clinical suspicion, and if CT or MRI is negative, a lumbar puncture should be performed. Cerebrospinal fluid will show greater than 1000 red blood cells (RBCs) per mm^3 that do not clear in later tubes. Pathognomonic for SAH is **xanthochromia,** a straw-colored appearance of the CSF supernatant after centrifugation. Lumbar puncture can also rule out a diagnosis of bacterial meningitis.

3. **Patients should be classified according to the SAH grading scale of Hunt and Hess** (Table 24–1).

    Grading SAH patients not only will help monitor the clinical course but also will allow more accurate determination of prognosis and will guide management decisions. SAH of Hunt and Hess grades 1 and 2 has a good prognosis. Patients with grades 3 and 4 have a worse prognosis, and grade 5 patients are moribund. Aggressive, early intervention will usually yield good results only if the initial presentation is at grades 1 to 3.

Table 24–1 □ CLINICAL GRADING OF SUBARACHNOID HEMORRHAGE ACCORDING TO THE CLASSIFICATION OF HUNT AND HESS

Grade	Description
0	Unruptured aneurysm
1	Minor headache, mild nuchal rigidity
2	Severe headache, nuchal rigidity, no focal deficits other than cranial nerve palsy
3	Lethargy, confusion, or mild focal deficit
4	Stupor, moderate to severe hemiparesis
5	Deep coma, decerebrate rigidity, moribund

4. **Once a diagnosis of SAH is made, a four-vessel cerebral angiogram should be performed as soon as possible.**
   MR or CT angiography is not indicated because it has a lower sensitivity; whether or not it is positive, an angiogram will still be necessary. The most common sites for aneurysm formation are at vascular branching points around the circle of Willis (Fig. 24–1) (see Box 24–1 for management of unruptured aneurysms). Fifteen percent of patients have more than one aneurysm. Nonaneurysmal causes for SAH that may be detectable on angiogram include arteriovenous malformation (AVM), angiopathies such as vasculitis and fibromuscular dysplasia, and venous thrombosis.
5. **If both MRI and angiogram are negative, the SAH may have arisen from a venous rupture around the midbrain (perimesencephalic SAH).**
   A coagulation profile and toxicology screen for cocaine should also be obtained if the diagnosis is still unclear. Cervical MRI may reveal a dural AVM, but this is rare. All patients with a negative initial angiogram require follow-up angiography within 2 weeks unless the patient is grade 1 or 2 and the initial CT shows a classic perimesencephalic pattern.

Management

For patients with aneurysm identified by angiography, management is two-pronged. First, early operative intervention to clip the aneurysm will improve short- and long-term morbidity and mortality. Because the rerupture rate is as high as 20% in the first 2 weeks, clipping the aneurysm will remove a substantial secondary risk. Second, fluid management is crucial both preoperatively and postoperatively to maintain adequate cerebral blood flow in the presence of cerebral ischemia from vasospasm.

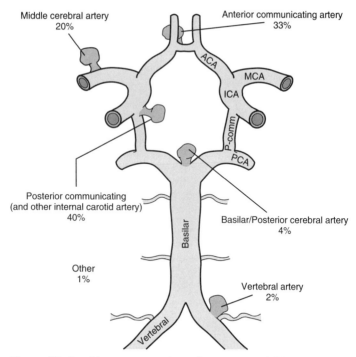

Figure 24–1 □ Most common sites of aneurysms. ACA = Anterior communicating artery; ICA = internal carotid artery; MCA = middle cerebral artery; PCA = posterior cerebral artery; P-comm = posterior communicating artery.

1. **Surgery**

    Surgical clipping of the aneurysm is generally done as early as possible after the hemorrhage, but it cannot be done without substantial risk if cerebral vasospasm is present. Vasospasm is rare in the first 3 days, and it peaks around day 7. If, within the first 5 days after hemorrhage, an angiogram shows the aneurysm clearly and shows no vasospasm, surgery should be done within the following 24 hours. Transcranial Doppler ultrasonography is an effective means of monitoring vasospasm both preoperatively and postoperatively, checking for increases in flow velocity in the major vessels around the circle of Willis.

2. **Endovascular embolization**

    An alternative to surgical clipping, packing the aneurysm with Guglielmi detachable coils (GDC) is an effective way to prevent active rebleeding, particularly when the aneurysm

> **Box 24–1. UNRUPTURED INTRACRANIAL ANEURYSMS**
>
> Intracranial aneurysms are uncommon in children but occur with a frequency of 2% in adults, suggesting that approximately 2 to 3 million Americans have an aneurysm. Unruptured intracranial aneurysms (IUAs) may be discovered incidentally or detected in SAH patients who present with another ruptured aneurysm, which was diagnosed because the aneurysm was symptomatic (e.g., cranial nerve compression, headache, seizure). Because surgical or endovascular aneurysm repair carries a 2% to 5% risk of stroke or death, the management of these aneurysms (which in most cases remain asymptomatic throughout life) is controversial. The annual risk of rupture of an IUA is approximately 0.7%, but this risk is higher in patients with large aneurysms (>10 mm), prior SAH, cigarette use, a family history of cerebral aneurysm, or a midline aneurysm (anterior communicating or basilar apex). Generally, treatment is strongly recommended for all patients with symptomatic IUAs or prior SAH and in young patients (<50) with large aneurysms. In light of their low risk of bleeding, incidental small IUAs (<10 mm) should be managed conservatively and followed with serial imaging, although treatment should be considered in younger patients wtih a larger (6–9 mm) midline aneurysm, a positive family history, or evidence of aneurysm growth. In addition, all patients should be counseled to avoid cigarette smoking.

presents a difficult surgical approach or the patient is a poor surgical candidate. In this procedure, the tiny coils are delivered to the aneurysm by superselective angiography catheterization. Thrombosis of the aneurysm is induced by the presence of the coils.
3. **Fluid management**
   Patients with SAH are best managed in an intensive care unit. Abnormalities of fluid and sodium homeostasis after SAH favor free-water retention and sodium loss. The emphasis on fluid management is therefore on maintaining normal or increased intravascular volume using isotonic fluids and on avoiding all potential sources of free water. A pulmonary artery catheter may be helpful in assessing volume status, particularly when there is symptomatic vasospasm (Table 24–2).

Table 24–2 □ FLUID MANAGEMENT IN SUBARACHNOID HEMORRHAGE

Preoperative:	Normal (0.9%) saline at 80 to 100 ml per hour
Postoperative:	Normal saline at 80 to 100 ml per hour and 250 ml of 5% albumin IV every 2 hours for central venous pressure equal to or less than 5 mm Hg
Postoperative, with symptomatic vasospasm:	500 ml 5% albumin IV over 30 minutes. Raise systolic blood pressure with IV pressors until deficit resolves (to maximum of 220 mm Hg)
	Normal saline at 80 to 100 ml per hour and 250 ml 5% albumin IV every 2 hours for pulmonary artery diastolic pressure equal to or less than 14 mm Hg

4. **Treatment of vasospasm**

In addition to fluid management, angioplasty of intracranial vessels that are narrowed by vasospasm is becoming an important treatment modality in centers with appropriate interventional neuroradiologic expertise.

Ischemic Stroke

Clinical Presentation and Diagnosis

Unlike SAH, both ischemic stroke and intracerebral hemorrhage (ICH) typically present with focal signs. The syndrome produced by infarction depends on the location of the lesion. Pain of any kind, including severe headache, is uncommon. One of the most difficult aspects of managing acute stroke patients is that focal symptoms, particularly minor ones, are often attributed by the patient to some nonneurologic cause and ignored. Visual changes may be interpreted as a need for new glasses. Sensory loss or weakness in an extremity may be brushed off as the result of lifting a heavy package or bumping into the door the day before. Transient symptoms (i.e., transient ischemic attack [TIA]) may portend stroke but may be identified as important only retrospectively (Box 24–2). Delay in treatment beyond the first several hours can result in a missed opportunity for acute intervention with a thrombolytic or neuroprotective agent. Despite an overlap in clinical syndromes among the various pathophysiologic stroke subtypes, one should try to identify the stroke subtype. The management algorithm for secondary prevention depends on the stroke mechanism. Four major categories of stroke mechanism are discussed.

> **Box 24–2. TRANSIENT ISCHEMIC ATTACKS**
>
> Transient ischemic attacks (TIAs) are defined as transient symptoms of vascular etiology that do not result in infarction. Although the standard clinical definition includes symptoms lasting up to 24 hours, most TIAs last from minutes to a few hours. Deficits lasting longer than 1 to 2 hours may show a lesion on MRI, even if the symptoms resolve completely by 24 hours. The definition of TIA and stroke is further complicated by recent advances in brain imaging, which may identify a small infarction even when the stroke symptoms resolve within a day. **The clinical importance of TIA is highlighted by the high incidence of subsequent strokes.** Up to 50% of patients with TIA proceed to have an infarction within 5 years, if they are untreated, 10% occurring in the first 90 days. Age greater than 60 years, diabetes mellitus, symptoms lasting longer than 10 minutes, and the symptoms of weakness or speech impairment all raise the likelihood of subsequent stroke. The most important etiology of TIA is high-grade carotid stenosis, producing hemodynamic failure or microemboli in the territory of the affected artery. Transient monocular blindness (TMB, amaurosis fugax) or a hemispheral syndrome such as unilateral weakness or sensory changes is a common presentation. Although TIAs may also arise from cardiac embolism or, rarely, from lacunar disease, the most important initial management step is to evaluate the internal carotid arteries, either with duplex Doppler ultrasonography or MR angiography. If stenosis greater than 70% is found, the patient should be considered for carotid endarterectomy. If no large-vessel stenosis is identified, the algorithm for investigating etiology of ischemic stroke should be followed. If no carotid stenosis or cardioembolic source is identified, **ASA 325 mg per day** is the first line of treatment.

Cardioembolic Stroke

Fifteen to 30% of strokes are embolic from a cardiac cause such as atrial fibrillation or valvular disease. The classic clinical presentation of cardioembolic stroke is of sudden deficit, maximal at onset. Syndromes more likely to be embolic include hemianopia without hemiparesis, pure Wernicke's aphasia, and ideomotor apraxia. Hemiparesis and forced gaze deviation suggest a large hemispheric (eyes look away from the side of weakness) or critical brain stem (eyes look toward the side of weakness) lesion, particularly if these signs are accompanied by decreased level of consciousness. Behavioral abnormalities such as aphasia or hemineglect without a gaze preference or altered level of consciousness suggest smaller hemispheric lesions. CT and MRI scans that show a single cortical branch territory infarct are also consistent with an embolic source, because atheroma rarely extends into the surface vessels. Main stem branch occlusions are also often embolic, but local atherostenosis is also a possibility in such a setting. A potentially misleading scenario is one in which the initial CT scan shows a deep-lying lucency involving the internal capsule and basal ganglia approximately 2 to 3 cm in size, apparently sparing cortex, which can be misidentified as a large lacune. Often such instances are of embolic origin, involving several lenticulostriate branches of the middle cerebral artery after temporary occlusion of the middle cerebral stem, followed by rapid collateralization from anterior or posterior cerebral branches or recanalization of the occlusion with distal migration of the embolus. A right-to-left shunt, usually a patent cardiac foramen ovale, can be inferred when transcranial Doppler ultrasonography shows microbubbles in the intracranial vessels after injection of 10 ml of agitated saline in the antecubital vein. Contrast transesophageal echocardiography can usually locate the defect in the cardiac atrial wall. If atrial fibrillation is suspected but is not apparent on routine electrocardiogram (ECG), Holter monitoring may be useful.

Large-Vessel Stenosis

In 15% of cases, severe large-vessel atherosclerosis is present and appears to be responsible for the stroke, particularly when there is severe extracranial internal carotid artery stenosis or occlusion and a "distal field" lesion is imaged on CT or MRI as an infarct high over the convexity, spreading caudally from the border zone between arterial territories. The most common clinical profile of this type of infarct is fractional arm weakness (the shoulder is different from the hand). Male gender, hypertension, and diabetes mellitus appear significantly more frequently in this group than in patients with cardioembolic stroke. Intracranial atherosclerosis is more prevalent in non-Caucasian populations, whereas extracranial disease is more prevalent in Caucasians. Duplex Doppler ultrasonography readily delineates the severity of the internal carotid stenosis and shows high-velocity, turbulent flow. Transcranial Doppler ultrasonography often shows dampened pulsatility in the ipsilateral middle cerebral artery. Focal stenoses in the intracranial internal carotid artery (ICA) or other major intracranial vessels may also be documented by transcranial Doppler ultrasonography or MR angiography. Duplex Doppler ultrasonography in combination with MR angiography has generally replaced the more invasive traditional angiogram for evaluating extracranial or intracranial vessels.

Artery-to-Artery Embolus

In another 15% of all stroke patients, large-vessel atherosclerosis with less than hemodynamic stenosis (less than 80% occluded or with an ulcerated plaque) is detected when, radiographically, the infarct appears embolic. In such a setting, embolic fragments may have arisen from atherosclerotic lesions in the ICA. Distinguishing interarterial embolism from a possible cardioembolic etiology may be difficult. The former usually produces a smaller cortical infarct, however, and the latter is more often associated with a decreased level of consciousness and an abnormal initial CT scan.

Lacunar Stroke (Small-Vessel Disease)

Small, deep lesions in the subcortical white matter, the thalamus, the basal ganglia, or the pons accompanied by an appropriate clinical syndrome suggest lacunar disease, accounting for 15 to 20% of all strokes. Arteriolar wall lipohyalinosis with fibrinoid necrosis is the most common pathologic finding, although microatheroma, or even microemboli, may produce small infarcts. Although more than 70 syndromes have been reported with small, deep infarcts, the classic lacunar syndromes are *clumsy hand dysarthria, pure motor hemiparesis, ataxic hemiparesis, sensorimotor syndrome,* and *pure hemisensory loss*. All are typically characterized by an absence of cortical signs. CT scanning is positive in only 50% of lacunar stroke patients, with MRI increasing the yield substantially, especially in the hyperacute period. Asymptomatic lacunes (silent strokes) occur in up to 20% of patients over age 65. Hypertension is the risk factor most associated with lacunar infarction.

Other Etiologies

Despite efforts to arrive at a diagnosis, the cause of infarction in up to 40% of cases remains undetermined after the standard workup is completed. This may result from an inability to perform appropriate laboratory studies because of the patient's advanced age or comorbidity or because of unwillingness on the part of the physician or patient. It may also result from improper timing of tests, such as an angiogram performed after an embolus has cleared or CT or MRI done before the infarction appears. In many cases, however, appropriate testing done at the proper time produces normal or ambiguous findings. Some of these cases may be explained by *hypercoagulable states* from protein C or protein S deficiency, abnormal fibrinogen levels, factor V Leiden abnormality, or lupus anticoagulant or anticardiolipin antibodies. Other patients may have had emboli from severe *aortic arch atherosclero-*

sis. Pain in the neck, side of face, teeth, jaw, or retro-orbital area may indicate *vertebral or carotid artery dissection*, even without a history of neck trauma. Migraine, meningitis, arteritis, or inherited metabolic abnormality may explain rare cases. For the purposes of management, cases that cannot be categorized under one of the first four etiologies should be called "cryptogenic stroke." Additional diagnostic studies may be needed to secure a final diagnosis. Because of its grave prognosis, vasculitis of the central nervous system should not be missed (Box 24–3).

Box 24–3. CEREBRAL VASCULITIS

Vasculitis is a rare cause of ischemic stroke. Infrequently appearing in the setting of a systemic collagen vascular disease such as polyarteritis nodosa, temporal arteritis, or Takayasu syndrome (aortic arch disease, pulseless disease), stroke may occasionally result from autoimmune disease restricted to the central nervous system. **Granulomatous angitis of the brain** is a rare condition that produces multiple small infarctions in the cortex and deep structures. The clinical presentation is usually one of fluctuating or stepwise progression of mental obtundation, with or without focal signs. CSF protein is elevated above 100 mg/dl and a pleocytosis of up to 500 mononuclear cells per mm^3 is common. The typical arteriographic appearance is of multiple segmental areas of arterial narrowing, often giving a "beaded" look. Clinical and radiographic data can be compelling in any given patient, but it is recommended that a brain and leptomeningeal biopsy specimen be obtained before embarking on the necessarily aggressive treatment regimen. The diagnosis is secured if there are multinucleated giant cells infiltrating arterial walls. Because of the multifocal nature of the disease, however, biopsy results may be negative in up to 50% of cases. Progression of encephalopathy or new focal signs in combination with new areas of arterial narrowing on angiography may be sufficient to begin treatment if the biopsy yields negative results initially. The usual treatment regimen includes high-dose steroids and pulse doses of an immunosuppressive agent such as cyclophosphamide for more than a year. The prognosis is poor overall, but occasionally there is functional restoration approximating previous levels.

Management

1. All patients with suspected stroke in which a deficit persists for more than 1 hour should undergo a CT or MRI head scan.
2. All patients with stroke symptoms of less than 3 hours' duration should be considered for acute treatment with intravenous recombinant tissue plasminogen activator (rt-PA). If CT scan shows no hemorrhage, mass effect, or edema and if the patient meets inclusion and exclusion criteria guidelines, **IV rt-PA 0.9 mg/kg** should be given according to protocol (see Box 24–4).
3. If the patient's stroke symptoms are of 3 to 6 hours' duration, intra-arterial thrombolysis my be performed, provided that interventional radiologic expertise and experience is available.
4. If the clinical picture and CT or MRI appearances are consistent with a small or moderate-sized ischemic stroke, and the suspected etiology is cardioembolic or large-vessel stenosis, intravenous **heparin may be administered** until the stroke subtype is confirmed, maintaining a partial thromboplastin time (PTT) of 1.5 to 2 times control. This treatment may also be given if there is hemorrhagic infarction on brain imaging, *but only if the infarction is minor.*
5. If the stroke is large and disabling, there is greater risk of *hemorrhagic transformation*; brain imaging should be repeated 48 to 72 hours after stroke onset, and anticoagulation should be started only if hemorrhagic conversion has not occurred. If the clinical and imaging diagnosis is of intracranial hemorrhage, anticoagulants and antiplatelet agents should not be given.
6. *Investigation of stroke etiology* should focus first on cardioembolic sources and large-vessel atherothrombosis. Transthoracic echocardiography, carotid duplex Doppler ultrasonography, and transcranial Doppler ultrasonography should be performed in nearly all cases. MR angiography and transesophageal echocardiography may deliver a diagnosis when the aforementioned studies are inconclusive.
7. Stroke patients with recent myocardial infarction, atrial fibrillation, valvular disease, or intracardiac thrombus should be given **oral anticoagulants such as warfarin** for at least 1 year. Patients with a patent foramen ovale or severe atherosclerosis of the aortic arch may be anticoagulated as well. The International Normalized Ratio (INR) of the prothrombin time (PT) should be targeted at 2.0 to 3.0. If there is atrial fibrillation, warfarin should be continued indefinitely, provided that reliable monitoring is available.
8. If the stroke is small, the heart is normal, and a duplex Doppler sonogram shows significant carotid stenosis

Box 24–4. AMERICAN HEART ASSOCIATION GUIDELINES FOR USE OF INTRAVENOUS rt-PA

Inclusion Criteria
1. Symptoms are consistent with acute ischemic stroke.
2. Timing of onset is clear; start rt-PA within 3 hours of symptom onset.
3. CT is negative or shows only early signs of ischemic stroke (blurring of gray-white junction, minor hypodensity). If sulcal effacement, mass effect, or edema is present, rt-PA should not be given. CT should be read by an experienced neurologist, neurosurgeon, or neuroradiologist.
4. Appropriate facilities must be available to handle bleeding complications should they occur (e.g., neurologic intensive care unit or stroke unit).

Exclusion Criteria
1. Current use of oral anticoagulants, PT >15 seconds or INR >1.7.
2. Use of IV heparin or IM low-molecular-weight heparin within 24 hours or prolonged partial thromboplastin time.
3. Platelet count <100,000/mm^3.
4. Large stroke or serious head injury within the past 3 months.
5. Major surgery within the past 14 days.
6. Pretreatment SBP >185 mm Hg or DBP >110 mm Hg.
7. Blood glucose <50 mg/dl or >400 mg/dl.
8. Gastrointestinal or urinary bleeding within the preceding 21 days.
9. Recent myocardial infarction.
10. Neurologic signs that are rapidly improving.
11. Isolated, minor neurologic deficits (e.g., pure sensory loss, isolated dysarthria, isolated ataxia).
12. Seizure at onset of stroke.

Administration of rt-PA
1. Intravenous rt-PA (0.9 mg/kg, maximum 90 mg) with 10% of the dose given as a bolus followed by an infusion lasting 60 minutes.
2. No anticoagulants or antiplatelet agents to be given within the first 24 hours after administration of rt-PA.
3. Blood pressure elevation to be treated by IV labetalol 10 to 150 mg (for SBP = 180 to 230 mm Hg or DBP = 105 to 120 mm Hg) or IV nitroprusside 0.5 to 10 μg/kg per minute (for SBP >230 mm Hg or DBP >120 mm Hg).

(greater than 70%), intravenous heparin should be continued until the exact degree of stenosis has been determined by MR angiography. Digital subtraction or cut film angiography may be used in instances in which MR angiography is unavailable or MR angiography results are equivocal. Prophylactic *endarterectomy* for patients with greater than 70% stenosis should be undertaken as soon as possible. For patients with lesser degrees of stenosis, Doppler monitoring should be undertaken at intervals of 3 to 12 months to document those patients whose stenosis increases to greater than 70% and who then qualify for surgery. Patients in whom asymptomatic carotid stenosis greater than 60% is identified should be considered for endarterectomy, provided the operation is done at a center at which the perioperative morbidity and mortality is less than 3%. The benefit from endarterectomy compared to medical therapy is a 6% versus an 11% chance of stroke in 5 years for the asymptomatic carotid stenosis group, and a 9% versus 26% chance of stroke in 2 years for the symptomatic group. Results are equivocal for female patients with asymptomatic stenosis.
9. If no cardioembolic source or operable carotid stenosis is identified, and if the patient is not considered at risk for hemorrhage, antiplatelet treatment with **aspirin 325 mg daily** should be given as chronic outpatient therapy. **Aspirin 25 mg/extended release dipyridamole 200 mg twice a day** or **clopidogrel 75 mg PO once a day** may also be used, particularly if aspirin therapy has failed.

Intracerebral Hemorrhage

Clinical Presentation

Primary intracerebral hemorrhage (ICH) is defined as nontraumatic bleeding into the parenchyma of the brain. ICH accounts for approximately 15% of all strokes. Except for a higher frequency of headache and severe hypertension, the presentation of ICH may be identical to that for ischemic stroke occurring in the same location. Coma occurs with greater frequency, particularly when the hemorrhage is of larger volume or involves the brain stem. Patients with hematoma volumes less than 20 ml have an excellent prognosis, whereas those with volumes greater than 80 ml are usually fatal. Chronic hypertension is the most common cause of ICH and is presumed to result from rupture of the smallest penetrating arteries that have undergone degenerative changes such as lipohyalinosis, fibrinoid necrosis, and microaneurysm formation. Acute hypertension is present in 90% of the cases. Hypertension from sympathomimetics such as pseudoephedrine, amphetamines, or cocaine may also be seen. Hypertensive bleeds occur most commonly in the territory of small penetrating arteries, in the basal ganglia or thalamus (70%), in the brain stem (13%), or in the cerebellum (9%). In the 10% of cerebral hemorrhages that occur in the hemispheres, other causes must be suspected. The differential diagnosis of lobar ICH includes cerebral amyloid angiopathy (Box 24–5), primary or metastatic tumors (melanoma, choriocarcinoma, bronchiogenic carcinoma, or renal cell carcinoma), coagulopathies (disseminated intravascular coagulation, hemophilia, leukemia, thrombocytopenia, overdose of anticoagulant therapy), and vascular malformations.

Diagnosis

The cornerstone for diagnosis of ICH is neuroimaging. Both CT and MRI can detect fresh parenchymal blood in the hyperacute stage. Because the clinical presentation may be indistinguishable from ischemic stroke but the treatment strategies are quite different, any patient presenting with suspected ICH must undergo CT or MRI as soon as possible. In a patient under 60 years of age with a lobar hemorrhage of unclear etiology, an MRI with and without contrast material may disclose tumor or the abnormal vessels of a vascular malformation. For an arteriovenous malformation, cut film angiography would then be necessary to make a definitive diagnosis and plan for treatment.

Distinguishing between ICH and ischemic infarction with hemorrhagic conversion may present a challenge. ICH tends to have a denser, homogeneous appearance, whereas the hemorrhagic infarction is usually spotted or mottled. The location of ICH is

---

Box 24–5. CEREBRAL AMYLOID ANGIOPATHY

Cerebral amyloid angiopathy (CAA) results from the pathologic deposition of an amorphous eosinophilic amyloid material (that stains with Congo red) in small blood vessels of the cerebral neocortex and adjacent leptomeninges. CAA causes lobar hemorrhage in elderly adults with a mean age of 72. Recurrent hemorrhages are common. The amyloid protein precursor is a gene product from chromosome 21, stimulating interest about the role of amyloid in Down syndrome and Alzheimer's disease. The disease may occur as a familial trait or sporadically. Over 40% of patients with CAA have some degree of dementia. Hemorrhages are most common in the frontal and parietal lobes. MRI, particularly gradient echo sequences, will usually demonstrate several old hemorrhages that may have been asymptomatic. No definitive treatment is currently available.

more often subcortical, often in the deep gray matter, whereas hemorrhagic infarction, most often occurring in the setting of embolic arterial occlusion, usually involves the cortex and follows a branch artery territory. Intraventricular blood may be seen with ICH, particularly if the hemorrhage is in the thalamus or basal ganglia. Ventricular hemorrhage from embolic infarction does not occur. Significant mass effect may be present from the outset in ICH, whereas the mass effect from hemorrhagic infarction results from secondary edema formation, which peaks after 48 hours. The appearance of the hematoma on MRI follows a characteristic course from the acute to the subacute to the chronic stage (see Chapter 3). Coagulation studies (PT/PTT, platelet count) should be obtained at the time of diagnosis to rule out coagulopathy as a cause for the hemorrhage. Liver function tests should be obtained.

Management

1. **Correction of a coagulopathy** with administration of fresh frozen plasma may be necessary to terminate active bleeding in a patient with a coagulation disorder.
2. **Active control of blood pressure** to systolic levels of 140 to 160 mm Hg should be attempted with oral or intravenous antihypertensives. Unlike in ischemic infarction in which reduction of blood pressure may result in decreased cerebral blood flow and consequent extension of infarction, reducing blood pressure in ICH may help prevent recurrent bleeding.
3. **Control of increased intracranial pressure** with pharmacologic measures and hyperventilation may allow the patient to pass through a critical phase until the hematoma begins to resolve. (See Chapter 12.)
4. **Placement of an intraventricular drain** may be necessary because intraventricular blood or direct compression of the cerebral aqueduct by a brain stem hematoma may cause obstructive hydrocephalus. If there is any clinical deterioration, a CT or MRI scan should be obtained to distinguish between hydrocephalus and worsening as a result of extension of the hemorrhage or edema.
5. Despite many surgical and medical series, indications for **surgical evacuation of a hematoma** have not been definitively established. When parenchymal hematoma threatens the life of a patient who was initially awake, surgical evacuation may be reasonable. The younger patient who is becoming progressively obtunded and has a large (greater than 30 ml) lobar hematoma may undergo CT-guided stereotactic or open evacuation of the clot. Cerebellar hematomas greater than 3 cm in diameter also appear to benefit from evacuation. For patients presenting in coma or for those with a stable neurologic deficit, surgery is unlikely to help.

chapter 25 | Movement Disorders

ELAN D. LOUIS

Movement disorders may be defined simply as *abnormal involuntary movements*. These movements are not the result of weakness or sensory deficits. Rather, they are the result of dysfunction of what may be defined anatomically as the basal ganglia or functionally as the extrapyramidal motor system.

The diversity of movement disorders can be overwhelming, with movements including those that are commonly known (tremors, tics) and those that are less familiar (dystonia, chorea, and hemiballismus). Despite this diversity, movement disorders may be conveniently categorized into two types:

1. *Hyperkinesias* are characterized by an excess of movement.
2. *Hypokinesias* are characterized by a paucity of movement.

Some basic principles should be kept in mind when first approaching a patient with a movement disorder.

■ BASIC PRINCIPLES

1. Take time to **observe** the patient. Some movements may be quite elaborate. At this point, do not make interpretations or think about treatment.
2. **Describe** what you see. Do not label anything yet. For example, note that "the eyes seem to be intermittently squeezing closed" or that "there are rapid jerking movements of the left arm every 5 seconds."
3. **Classify** the movement as a hyperkinesia or a hypokinesia, as defined earlier.
4. **Give the movement a name** (e.g., tremor, chorea). The list of different types of abnormal movements (see Step 4 in the following paragraphs) provides a glossary of terms. Read each term and its definition and try to decide which of these terms best describes what you have seen.
5. **Diagnose a specific disease** after naming the movement. For example, both tremor and bradykinesia are features of Parkinson's disease.
6. Finally, think about the appropriate **treatment**. Table 25–1 lists the medications and dosages for treatment of movement disorders.

Table 25-1 □ MOVEMENT DISORDER MEDICATIONS AND DOSAGES

Medication	Dose	Condition Treated
Amantadine (Symmetrel)	100 to 300 mg per day (two to three times a day)	Parkinson's disease
Baclofen (Lioresal)	10 to 80 mg per day (three times a day)	Dystonia
Bromocriptine (Parlodel)	7.5 to 30 mg per day (three to four times a day)	Parkinson's disease
Carbamazepine (Tegretol)	300 to 1200 mg per day (three to four times a day)	Dystonia
Clonazepam (Klonopin)	1 to 10 mg per day (two to three times a day)	Tics
Clonidine (Catapres)	0.2 to 1.0 mg per day, divided	Tics
Clozapine (Clozaril)	12.5 to 100 mg per day (two to three times a day)	Essential tremor
Diazepam (Valium)	2 to 10 mg per day, divided (two to three times a day)	Dystonia
Entacapone (Comtan)	200 to 600 mg per day divided	Parkinson's disease
Gabapentin (Neurontin)	900 to 1800 mg per day (three times a day)	Essential tremor
Haloperidol (Haldol)	1 to 10 mg per day (two to three times a day)	Tics, chorea
Levodopa/carbidopa (Sinemet)	100 to 2000 mg per day, divided	Parkinson's disease
Methazolamide (Neptazane)	50 to 100 mg per day (four times a day)	Essential tremor
Penicillamine (Cuprimine)	250 to 1000 mg per day	Wilson's disease
Pergolide (Permax)	0.75 to 3.0 mg per day (three to four times a day)	Parkinson's disease
Pimozide (Orap)	2 to 10 mg per day, divided	Tics, chorea
Pramipexole (Mirapex)	1.5 to 4.5 mg per day (three times a day)	Parkinson's disease
Primidone (Mysoline)	100 to 2000 mg per day (three to four times a day)	Essential tremor
Propranolol (Inderal)	40 to 240 mg per day (three to four times a day)	Essential tremor
Reserpine	0.5 to 8 mg per day (three to four times a day)	Tics, chorea
Ropinirole (Requip)	0.75 to 3.0 mg per day (three times a day)	Parkinson's disease
Selegiline (Eldepryl)	5 to 10 mg per day (two times a day)	Parkinson's disease
Tizanidine (Zanaflex)	8 to 24 mg per day (three times a day)	Dystonia
Tolcapone (Tasmar)	300 to 600 mg per day, divided	Parkinson's disease
Trientine (Syprine)	750 to 1250 mg per day (two to four times a day)	Wilson's disease
Trihexyphenidyl (Artane)	1 to 100 mg per day (three to four times a day)	Parkinson's disease

The most common error is for students to skip straight to diagnosis and treatment. It is important first to **observe, describe, classify, and name.**

The remainder of this chapter will follow the preceding six-step outline.

Step 1: Observe

Inform the patient that you are going to watch his or her movements and then *just observe the patient.* Some patients may be self-conscious and may try to inhibit their movements, particularly if these are embarrassing. If this is the case, ask the patient to allow the body to behave naturally and not stop any movements. Sometimes, you may need to ask the patient to perform certain maneuvers that will bring out the movement (e.g., writing may bring out a tremor, walking may bring out a dystonic foot movement). Some movements may be elaborate, and the period of observation may be lengthy before you get a sense of a pattern or before you can fully describe what you see.

Step 2: Describe

Try to describe the movements. This is not easy. In fact, neurologists find it easier to use gestures, rather than words, when describing a movement.

Some descriptions may be straightforward. For example, you might describe Mr. H.'s movements in the following way: "The right side of Mr. H.'s face twitches every 5 seconds." Other descriptions may be elaborate. For example, you might describe Mrs. R.'s movements as follows: "Mrs. R.'s neck remains completely hyperextended, and once every minute, there is a rapid, violent movement in the opposite direction, so that the head is completely anteroflexed for a brief moment."

Avoid describing Mr. H. as having hemifacial spasm and Mrs. R. as having torticollis. These statements are not descriptions; they are diagnoses.

Step 3: Classify

It is important to classify the movement as a hyperkinesia or a hypokinesia. This is the easiest step. One caveat is that some patients may simultaneously exhibit both types of movements. For example, a patient with Parkinson's disease may have a tremor (hyperkinesia) as well as bradykinesia (hypokinesia).

Step 4: Give the Movement a Name

The following is a list of different types of abnormal movements. Movements in **bold** letters are the hypokinesias; all others are hyperkinesias. The essential element of each movement is *italicized.*

Name of Movement	Definition or Description
Akathisia	A subjective *feeling of inner restlessness* that is relieved by movements. The movements are stereotypic and complex and convey restlessness (e.g., squirming, crossing and uncrossing legs, rocking back and forth, and pacing).
Asterixis	Sudden periods of *cessation of muscle contraction* best seen when the patient's arms are extended in front, as if stopping traffic.
Athetosis	Slow, *sinuous, writhing* movements, usually of the distal parts of the limbs.
Ballismus	Wild *flinging, flailing* movements that represent large-amplitude proximal choreiform movements. Ballismus is often unilateral (hemiballismus).
Bradykinesia	Movements that are either *slow* or of *diminished amplitude.*
Chorea	*Semipurposeful flowing* movements that flit from one part of the body to another in a continuous and random pattern.
Dyskinesia	A general term for any excessive movement. The term dyskinesia is often used as an abbreviation for "tardive dyskinesia" (repetitive oral movements often seen in patients taking certain psychiatric medications).
Dystonia	*Twisting* movements that are often *sustained* for variable periods of time.
Freezing	Brief episodes (usually lasting several seconds) during which a motor act is temporarily blocked or halted. Walking is the motor act that is most commonly affected.
Myoclonus	Sudden, brief shock-like *jerks.*
Myokymia	*Quivering* or rippling of muscle.
Rigidity	Muscle tone that is increased on passive motion. Distinct from spasticity, it is present equally in all directions of movement (i.e., both in flexors and in extensors).
Tachykinesia	Movements or speech characterized by *continuous acceleration* or loss of amplitude.

Tics *Repetitive, stereotypic* movements or sounds that are *suppressible* and that *relieve a feeling of inner tension.*

Tremor *Regular, oscillatory* movements that may be present at rest or with action.

Step 5: Diagnose a Specific Disease

Parkinson's Disease

Parkinson's disease was first described by James Parkinson in 1817.

Types of Movements

The types of movements involved in this disease are tremor, rigidity, bradykinesia, freezing, and tachykinesia. The *tremor* of Parkinson's disease is most commonly a *rest tremor*. This means that the tremor is present when the arms are resting in the patient's lap or when they are hanging at the patient's side. One way to bring out a rest tremor is to ask the patient to walk. The *rigidity* is often called *cogwheel* rigidity because it may have a ratchet-like quality. The *bradykinesia* is characterized by a decrease in the frequency of movements (diminished blink frequency, few facial expressions, or *masked facies*) and by slowness of movement, with loss of amplitude. *Postural reflexes*, lost later in the disease, may be tested by performing the *pull test*. Stand behind the patient and pull him or her backward. A normal response is for the patient to take one or two steps back without falling. Always stand behind the patient in the event that you need to catch him or her! *Freezing* is most commonly seen as *start hesitation* or *turning hesitation*. Walking in narrow, cramped quarters may bring on freezing. *Tachykinesia* may take the form of rapid accelerating speech *(tachyphemia)* or rapid accelerated walking *(festination)*.

Diagnostic Tests

Parkinson's disease is a clinical diagnosis. The cardinal features are tremor, rigidity, bradykinesia, and loss of postural reflexes. Lumbar puncture (LP), electroencephalogram (EEG), computed tomography (CT), and magnetic resonance imaging (MRI) are nonspecific. The deoxyglucose position emission tomography (PET) scan may show increased uptake in the region of the basal ganglia.

Treatment

Levodopa-carbidopa (Sinemet) 100 to 2000 mg per day of levodopa, with administration of individual doses ranging from every 2 to 3 hours to two times a day.

Bromocriptine (Parlodel) 7.5 to 30 mg per day, divided, three to four times a day.

Pergolide (Permax) 0.75 to 3.0 mg per day, divided, three to four times a day.
Pramipexole (Mirapex) 1.5 to 4.5 mg per day, divided, three times a day.
Ropinirole (Requip) 0.75 to 3.0 mg per day, divided, three times a day.
Amantadine (Symmetrel) 100 to 300 mg per day, divided, two to three times a day.
Trihexyphenidyl (Artane) 1 to 10 mg per day, divided, three to four times a day.
Tolcapone (Tasmar) 300 to 600 mg per day, divided, as an adjunct to levodopa-carbidopa.
Entacapone (Comtan) 200 to 600 mg per day, divided, as an adjunct to levodopa-carbidopa.
Selegiline (Eldepryl) 5 to 10 mg per day, divided, two times a day.
Stereotactic pallidotomy has been reported to improve bradykinesia, rigidity, rest tremor, impaired balance, and medication-induced dyskinesia in the limb contralateral to the pallidotomy.
Stereotactic thalamotomy has been shown to decrease the severity of parkinsonian tremor and allow for reductions in dosages of levodopa.
Fetal ventral mesencephalic tissue implantation into the striatum may improve parkinsonian symptoms and allow for a reduction in dosages of levodopa.
Electrical stimulation of the ventral intermediate nucleus of the thalamus following implantation of deep brain stimulation electrodes is beneficial in the treatment of contralateral parkinsonian tremor or essential tremor.

Benign Essential Tremor

Many cases of benign essential tremor are very mild, and the symptoms are often mistaken as part of normal aging.

Types of Movements

The movement involved is tremor. The tremor of benign essential tremor is most commonly an *action tremor*. It is present when the patient holds his or her arms extended in front of the body and is often present with tasks such as writing, pouring water, and touching the finger to the nose.

Diagnostic Tests

Essential tremor is diagnosed on the basis of the clinical features described above. Other causes of similar tremor, including hyperthyroidism and certain medications (e.g., lithium or valproate), should be ruled out. The diagnosis may be confirmed by computerized tremor analysis with accelerometry.

Treatment

> Propranolol (Inderal) 40 to 240 mg per day, divided, three to four times a day.
>
> Primidone (Mysoline) 100 to 2000 mg per day, divided, three to four times a day.
>
> Gabapentin (Neurontin) 900 to 1800 mg per day, divided, three times a day.
>
> Methazolamide (Neptazane) 50 to 100 mg per day, divided, two to four times a day.
>
> Clozapine (Clozaril) 12.5 to 100 mg per day, divided, two to three times a day.

Huntington's Disease

Huntington's disease was first described by George Huntington in 1872.

Types of Movements

Chorea and dystonia are common features of the disease. The *chorea* of Huntington's disease may involve the face, tongue, limbs, or trunk. It is often exacerbated by anxiety or stress and may be brought on by asking the patient to close the eyes, hold the arms extended in front of the body, and count backward or perform simple arithmetic. *Dystonia* and *tics* may also be present. The dystonia may take the form of fist clenching, shoulder elevation, or foot inversion during walking. Another feature of Huntington's disease is *motor impersistence* (inhibitory pauses occurring during voluntary motion that account for the "milkmaid grips" seen when hand grasp is tested). Patients with Huntington's disease do not have only involuntary movements. Psychiatric features (depression, psychosis) are very common in this disease, as are cognitive problems (mild to severe) and changes in personality, with prominent disinhibition.

Diagnostic Tests

Because the disease is transmitted in an autosomal dominant manner, a family history is an important feature of the diagnosis. One should rule out other causes of chorea including hyperthyroidism, use of anticonvulsants, and Sydenham's chorea. The abnormal gene, on the short arm of chromosome 4, consists of an abnormally long CAG repeat fragment. The CT or MRI scan may show atrophy of the caudate nuclei.

Management

In many cases, the movements are not bothersome to the patient, and the psychiatric manifestations are often the focus of

treatment. However, treatment for the movements might consist of
- **Haloperidol (Haldol) 1 to 10 mg per day, divided, two to three times a day.**
- **Reserpine 0.5 to 8 mg per day, divided, three to four times a day.**

Idiopathic Torsion Dystonia (Dystonia Musculorum Deformans)

This illness is characterized by twisting dystonic movements.

Types of Movements

The illness usually begins in childhood and has a progressive course. The *dystonia* often involves the foot initially and is most apparent with certain actions but not with others (e.g., intermittent spasmodic inversion of the foot while walking but not while running or walking backward). Although the dystonia initially consists of twisting *movements* with action, sustained dystonic *postures* at rest become apparent eventually.

Diagnostic Tests

The diagnosis is based on clinical history and examination. It should be distinguished from other secondary or symptomatic causes of dystonia (e.g., Wilson's disease, Hallervorden-Spatz disease) and from adult-onset dystonia. The latter usually runs a more benign course and begins in adulthood with involvement of the neck, eyes, or hand, but it rarely involves the leg. A common gene for idiopathic torsion dystonia, the *DYT1* gene, is located on the long arm of chromosome 9 and is inherited in an autosomal dominant manner with a penetrance as low as 30%.

Management
- **Trihexyphenidyl (Artane) 1 to 100 mg per day, divided, three to four times a day.**
- **Baclofen (Lioresal) 10 to 80 mg per day, divided, three times a day.**
- **Diazepam (Valium) 2 to 10 mg per day, divided, two to three times a day.**
- **Tizanidine (Zanaflex) 8 to 24 mg per day, divided, three times a day.**
- **Carbamazepine (Tegretol) 300 to 1200 mg per day, divided, three to four times a day.**
- **Botulinum toxin (Botox) injected into selected muscles several times per year.**

Tourette's Syndrome

Tourette's syndrome was first definitively described by Gilles de la Tourette in 1885.

Types of Movements

Tics are characteristic of Tourette's syndrome. They may be *simple motor tics* (eye blinking, eyebrow raising), *complex motor tics* (head shaking, wrist shaking), *simple phonic tics* (throat clearing, grunting), or *complex phonic tics* (uttering words). *Coprolalia* (uttering obscenities) and *echolalia* (repeating sounds or words) are examples of the latter. As with most tics, these are voluntarily suppressible for brief periods and may vary in intensity over time.

Diagnostic Tests

The diagnosis is clinical. This disorder begins in childhood with both motor and phonic tics. Coprolalia is not an essential feature of the diagnosis.

Management

Clonazepam (Klonopin) 1 to 10 mg per day, divided, two to three times a day.
Pimozide (Orap) 2 to 10 mg per day, divided.
Haloperidol (Haldol) 1 to 10 mg per day, divided, two to three times a day.
Reserpine 0.5 to 8 mg, divided, three to four times a day.
Clonidine (Catapres) 0.2 to 1.0 mg per day, divided.

Wilson's Disease

Wilson's disease was first described by Samuel Alexander Kinnier Wilson in 1912.

Types of Movements

The movements are protean. Tremor, rigidity, bradykinesia, dystonia, and chorea are all seen in this disease, and one or more of these movements may be present. A *parkinsonian form* of the illness may be characterized by rest tremor, rigidity, or bradykinesia. A *pseudosclerotic* form of the illness is associated with a *wing-beating tremor* (a large-amplitude, flapping, violent tremor that is present when the shoulders are abducted, elbows are flexed, and fingers are facing each other). *Dystonia* and *chorea* may also be present. Dysarthria occurs frequently and may progress to anarthria. Psychiatric manifestations (anxiety, depression, psychosis) are a common feature of the illness.

Diagnostic Tests

The diagnosis is based on clinical history and examination and is supported by the presence of Kayser-Fleischer rings (ring-shaped copper deposits in the cornea), low serum ceruloplasmin level, abnormalities in liver function tests, or hepatitis. Lesions in the basal ganglia may be seen on an MRI scan. The gene *pWD* is located on the long arm of chromosome 13.

Management
   Penicillamine (Cuprimine) 125 to 1000 mg per day.
   Trientine (Syprine) 750 to 1250 mg per day, divided, two to
   four times a day.

Restless Leg Syndrome

The syndrome is characterized by feelings of discomfort and restlessness in the legs. These feelings are often relieved by movement.

Types of Movements

The movements involved are fidgeting, kicking, or writhing movements of the legs and pacing the floor.

The discomfort is deep seated and is often described as feelings of stretching, itching, crawling, or creeping in the bones, muscles, or tendons. These symptoms are most common when the patient first lies down in bed at night. The feelings may cause writhing movements in the legs, fidgeting, or kicking. Some patients need to pace the floor for temporary relief. Unlike akathisia, which also causes discomfort with a desire to move, restless leg syndrome occurs primarily at night.

Diagnostic Tests

Restless leg syndrome is a clinical syndrome that is diagnosed based on the clinical features described. Akathisia can resemble restless leg syndrome, but is typically constant throughout the day, has a more generalized distribution (i.e., not just localized leg discomfort), and is confined to patients taking neuroleptic medications or patients with Parkinson's disease.

Treatment
   Levodopa (Sinemet) 25/100 to 50/200 qhs.
   Pergolide (Permax) 0.1 to 1.25 mg qhs.
   Clonazepam (Klonopin) 1 to 4 mg qhs.
   Propoxyphene (Darvon) 65 mg qhs.
   Clonidine (Catapres) 0.1 to 1.0 mg qhs.

Miscellaneous Disorders

This section briefly discusses those movements from the list in **Step 4** that were not discussed under specific diseases.
   Akathisia is most commonly seen as a side effect of certain psychiatric medications.
   Asterixis, usually seen bilaterally in the arms, is most commonly a feature of toxic/metabolic states such as liver or renal failure. Patients are often encephalopathic.
   Athetosis may appear in a variety of neurologic disorders ranging from cerebral palsy to paroxysmal kinesiogenic choreo-

athetosis. Athetotic movements may merge with chorea (choreoathetosis).

Ballismus, most commonly unilateral (hemiballismus), is usually the result of a stroke in the contralateral subthalamic nucleus.

Myoclonus may occur anywhere in the body, including palatal myoclonus and ocular myoclonus. Myoclonus may be the result of anoxic ischemic injury (Lance-Adams syndrome), birth injuries, degenerative disorders (Ramsay Hunt syndrome), infections, tumors, strokes, or even medications (levodopa). Hiccups are a physiologic form of myoclonus.

Myokymia, most commonly seen in facial muscles, is often due to pontine lesions, particularly plaques in multiple sclerosis or pontine gliomas.

chapter 26 | Epilepsy and Seizure Disorders

LAWRENCE J. HIRSCH

Dramatic advances have occurred in the management of epilepsy over the past decade—diagnostically and therapeutically, medically and surgically. Seizures and epilepsy are a prominent component of any neurologist's practice and are a common problem encountered by neurology residents. This chapter covers the basics of epilepsy diagnosis and treatment. Status epilepticus is covered in Chapter 5, and further details of the antiepileptic drugs are covered in Appendix B.

Epilepsy is defined as recurrent (two or more) unprovoked seizures. It occurs in 0.5 to 1% of the population. Nearly 10% of the population will experience at least one seizure in their lifetime.

■ SEIZURE CLASSIFICATION

Seizures are divided into primary generalized seizures (seen in all parts of the cortex simultaneously) and partial-onset seizures (localization-related; starting in one region, with or without spread) (Table 26–1). These types are then subdivided into idiopathic (presumably genetic) and symptomatic/cryptogenic (with an underlying cause). The most common seizure types are described here.

Primary Generalized Seizures

Primary Generalized Tonic-Clonic Seizures (Convulsions or Grand Mal Seizures)

Primary generalized tonic-clonic (GTC) seizures are characterized by the absence of an aura, an ictal cry due to forced inhalation, and a tonic phase (lasting about 30 seconds), which gradually progresses to a clonic phase (also lasting about 30 seconds). Postictal stertorous breathing, with gradual awakening, extends over many minutes. Often incontinence or tongue biting occurs.

Primary or secondary GTCs usually result in postictal acidosis with low HCO_3, elevated creatine kinase (CK), and elevated prolactin (over three times the baseline prolactin level at similar time

Table 26-1 □ ILAE* SEIZURE CLASSIFICATION (SIMPLIFIED)

I. Localization-related seizures (i.e. focal, partial-onset)
   a. Simple partial seizures (no impairment of consciousness)
      i. With motor symptoms
      ii. With somatosensory or special sensory symptoms
      iii. With autonomic symptoms
      iv. With psychic symptoms
   b. Complex partial seizures (with impaired consciousness)
      i. Beginning as simple partial-onset
      ii. With impaired consciousness at onset
   c. Secondary generalized (secondary GTC)
II. Primary generalized seizures
   a. Absence
      i. Typical absence
      ii. Atypical absence
   b. Myoclonic
   c. Clonic
   d. Tonic
   e. Tonic-clonic (primary GTC)
   f. Atonic
III. Unclassifiable

*International League Against Epilepsy.

of day if drawn within 30 minutes of convulsion; this finding may be useful in distinguishing it from a nonepileptic event).

Absence Seizures

Absence seizures are sudden-onset brief (approximately 10 seconds) staring spells with immediate recovery. They can occur many times per day, and eye flutter is common. Electroencephalogram (EEG) shows *generalized spike and wave discharges.* Typical absence seizures show 3 Hz generalized spike and wave in a very regular pattern and usually occur in neurologically normal children (i.e., in primary generalized epilepsy). Atypical absence seizures tend to be longer, with a less clear onset and offset; show less regular slow generalized spike and wave (1 to 2.5 Hz) on EEG; and are usually associated with underlying neurologic abnormalities (i.e., in symptomatic generalized epilepsy). Longer absence seizures (20 to 30 seconds) often have associated automatisms that can mimic complex partial seizures.

Myoclonic Seizures

These seizures are characterized by brief, lightning-like muscle jerks. The movements may be symmetric, asymmetric, or multifocal, with no impairment of consciousness. EEG usually shows a *generalized polyspike and wave discharge.*

Generalized Tonic Seizures

In these seizures sudden bilateral symmetric tonic posturing is brief, with rapid recovery. Brief impairment of consciousness is typical. EEG usually shows sudden diffuse low-voltage beta waves or background attenuation. These seizures are usually seen in neurologically abnormal patients, especially children, and especially in those with Lennox-Gastaut syndrome.

Partial-Onset Seizures

These seizures are divided into *simple* partial seizures (SPS), with complete retained awareness (although patients may be aphasic), and *complex* partial seizures (CPS), with impairment of consciousness. Partial seizures may progress to *secondary generalized tonic-clonic seizures*. If there is no known aura or focal feature at the onset of a convulsion, it is not possible to distinguish primary GTC from secondary GTC without an EEG. An *aura* is a sensation experienced by the patient at the onset of a partial seizure such as a smell, déjà vu, dizziness, or nausea. Auras are actually simple partial seizures with sensory or experiential symptoms only. These are brief and either resolve (SPS) or progress. Some patients have a prolonged sensation lasting many hours prior to their seizures, referred to as a *prodrome*; these feelings are often nonspecific and difficult to describe.

Temporal Lobe Seizures

These seizures are the most common types seen in adults. They are usually accompanied by an aura, often an epigastric rising sensation. Other common auras include indescribable cephalic sensations, smells, and déjà vu. Seizures tend to last 1 to 3 minutes and consist primarily of quiet unresponsive staring. There are frequently oral automatisms (chewing, lip smacking) as well as manual automatisms (picking at clothes, rubbing, patting, etc.). There is often contralateral dystonic posturing of the arm and hand (due to basal ganglia spread). The classic semiology includes unresponsiveness, oral automatisms, contralateral dystonic posturing, and ipsilateral manual automatisms. Postictally, there is usually some confusion and lethargy lasting at least a few minutes. Patients may not even be aware of their seizures. With seizures arising from the dominant hemisphere (usually the left), there is frequently postictal aphasia for at least 1 minute. In nondominant hemisphere seizures, recovery of speech is usually rapid, though the patient may remain confused.

Frontal Lobe Seizures

These seizures usually have no aura or postictal phase and are shorter than temporal lobe seizures (often 15 to 40 seconds in duration). They tend to occur in sleep. Prominent motor manifestations are often seen, including rhythmic unilateral clonic activity if involving the primary motor cortex; this activity may march across the body as it spreads within the motor homunculus ("Jacksonian march"). There may also be frantic restless movements, bicycling of the legs, and vocalizations such as screaming. Asymmetric tonic posturing is common if the supplementary motor area is involved. Bilateral motor manifestations can occur with full retained awareness and memory. It is often difficult to distinguish a frontal lobe seizure from a nonepileptic psychogenic seizure.

Occipital Lobe Seizures

These seizures tend to begin with a visual aura, either simple (spots or lights) if from the primary visual cortex, or complex (formed visual hallucinations including detailed scenes, usually stereotyped from spell to spell) if from the temporo-occipital region. Occipital seizures can spread either to the temporal lobe, causing a typical temporal lobe CPS, or above the Sylvian fissure, causing motor manifestations that can be difficult to distinguish from a frontal lobe seizure.

Parietal Lobe Seizures

These seizures are the least common. They may begin with a sensory aura and can rarely begin with contralateral pain. They will often spread to either the temporal or frontal lobe, with corresponding symptomatology.

■ EPILEPSY SYNDROME CLASSIFICATION

Once the seizure type is determined, an effort is made to see if a patient fits a particular epilepsy syndrome, which may be useful both prognostically and therapeutically. Syndromes incorporate history, seizure type, neurologic status, and EEG findings. The ILAE (International League Against Epilepsy) classification is shown in Table 26–2. The most common syndromes are described here.

Primary Generalized Syndromes

Childhood Absence Epilepsy

In childhood absence epilepsy (CAE) typical absence seizures, often many per day (can be hundreds), begin between ages 4 and 10 (peak 6 to 7) and usually resolve by puberty; they rarely persist into adulthood. Treatment of choice is **ethosuximide** or

Table 26-2 □ ILAE* EPILEPSY SYNDROME CLASSIFICATION

I. Localization-related syndromes (focal, partial-onset)
   a. Idiopathic (with age-related onset)
      i. Benign childhood epilepsy with centrotemporal spikes (benign Rolandic epilepsy of childhood, or BREC)
      ii. Childhood epilepsy with occipital paroxysms (benign occipital epilepsy)
      iii. Primary reading epilepsy
   b. Symptomatic/cryptogenic
      i. By lobe of onset (frontal, temporal, parietal, or occipital)
      ii. Chronic progressive epilepsia partialis continua of childhood (including Rasmussen's encephalitis)
      iii. Epilepsies characterized by seizures with specific modes of precipitation
II. Generalized syndromes
   a. Idiopathic
      i. Benign neonatal familial convulsions
      ii. Benign neonatal convulsions
      iii. Benign myoclonic epilepsy in infancy
      iv. Childhood absence epilepsy (CAE; pyknolepsy)
      v. Juvenile absence epilepsy (JAE)
      vi. Juvenile myoclonic epilepsy (JME; impulsive petit mal)
      vii. Epilepsy with grand mal (GTC) seizures upon awakening
      viii. Other
      ix. Epilepsies with seizures precipitated by specific modes of activation
   b. Cryptogenic or symptomatic (in order of age)
      i. West syndrome (infantile spasms)
      ii. Lennox-Gastaut syndrome
      iii. Epilepsy with myoclonic-astatic seizures
      iv. Epilepsy with myoclonic absences
   c. Symptomatic
      i. Nonspecific etiology
          1. Early myoclonic encephalopathy
          2. Early infantile epileptic encephalopathy with suppression burst
          3. Other symptomatic generalized epilepsies (common)
      ii. Specific etiology
III. Undetermined whether focal or generalized
   a. With both generalized and focal seizures
      i. Neonatal seizures
      ii. Severe myoclonic epilepsy in infancy
      iii. Epilepsy with continuous spike-waves during slow wave sleep
      iv. Acquired epileptic aphasia (Landau-Kleffner syndrome)
      v. Other
   b. Without unequivocal focal or generalized features (e.g., nocturnal GTCs, unclear whether primary or secondary)
IV. Special syndromes
   a. Situation-related seizures
      i. Febrile convulsions
      ii. Isolated seizures or isolated status epilepticus
      iii. Seizures occurring only during acute or toxic event (alcohol/drugs, hypoglycemia, nonketotic hyperglycemia)

*International League Against Epilepsy.

valproic acid. A minority (up to 40%) develop convulsions as well (rare and easily controlled).

Juvenile Absence Epilepsy

In juvenile absence epilepsy typical absence seizures begin between ages 10 and 17 (peak at 12), with fewer seizures per day than in CAE. Most patients also have convulsions (approximately 80%) and some have occasional myoclonic seizures (15%). **Valproate** is the treatment of choice. Although a relatively benign syndrome, it is more likely to persist into adulthood than CAE.

Juvenile Myoclonic Epilepsy

In juvenile myoclonic epilepsy, onset typically occurs at ages 12 to 18 years (peak at 14 to 15). It is a common, often-missed syndrome that consists of morning myoclonic jerks and primary GTCs; some patients have preceding absence seizures (10 to 33%). It is important to ask about morning myoclonus (twitching, clumsiness, or spilling things) to make this diagnosis, as many patients with this syndrome assume that everybody has myoclonic jerks. The seizures tend to occur shortly after awakening and are often preceded by an increased frequency of myoclonic jerking. Sleep deprivation, alcohol, and photic stimulation all precipitate seizures. Family history is positive for epilepsy in 25%. Patients respond well to **valproic acid** (and probably **lamotrigine**) but usually need lifelong medication (≥90%). EEG shows primary generalized spike and wave in 95%, usually at a fast rate (approximately 4 to 5 Hz generalized spike and wave and generalized polyspike and wave; this is also known as *atypical spike and wave*, to distinguish it from the 3-Hz discharges of CAE and from the slow spike and wave of Lennox-Gastaut syndrome). *Epilepsy with grand mal seizures upon awakening* is a related syndrome, but without the myoclonic jerks.

Symptomatic Generalized Epilepsy Syndromes

Lennox-Gastaut Syndrome

This syndrome (LGS) is characterized by early onset (at ages 1 to 8 years, peak between 3 and 5 years) of multiple seizure types. Almost all patients are developmentally delayed and have multiple seizure types including tonic seizures, drop attacks (can be due to atonic, tonic, or myoclonic seizures; also called "astatic seizures" as a group), generalized convulsions, and atypical absence seizures. EEG in LGS usually shows generalized slow spike and wave (≤2.5 Hz), multifocal epileptiform discharges, and diffuse slowing. LGS is often refractory to multiple medications. About one third of these patients have a preceding diagnosis of *West syndrome* (developmental delay, infantile spasms, and hypsarrhythmia on EEG). Prognosis is poor in general.

Localization-Related Epilepsy Syndromes, Symptomatic/Cryptogenic

Temporal Lobe Epilepsy

Temporal lobe epilepsy is the most common syndrome seen in adults and is the form most amenable to surgery. It is often associated with an early life risk factor such as meningitis, head trauma, or febrile seizures. There is a particular association of prolonged febrile seizures, temporal lobe epilepsy, and hippocampal sclerosis (also known as mesial temporal sclerosis, or MTS) both pathologically and on magnetic resonance imaging (MRI). MRI in these patients shows hippocampal atrophy (best seen on oblique coronal T1 images or STIR) and increased signal (best seen on coronal FLAIR or T2 images) in these patients. Patients with an early risk factor, MTS, documented temporal lobe seizures, and interictal temporal lobe spikes on EEG are excellent candidates for temporal lobectomy, with approximately 80% of patients becoming seizure-free postoperatively.

Localization-Related Epilepsy Syndromes, Idiopathic

Benign Rolandic Epilepsy of Childhood

This is an idiopathic focal epilepsy with usual onset at 4 to 10 years old (peak at 8 to 9 years; range, 2 to 13 years). This syndrome is characterized by simple partial seizures beginning with oropharyngeal symptoms (inability to speak, unilateral facial twitching, drooling), often progressing to a hemiconvulsion and secondary GTC, often nocturnal. EEG shows stereotyped centrotemporal spikes, unilateral (60 to 70% with one EEG) or bilateral, activated by sleep (occurring in one third of these patients only in sleep). Generalized spike and wave may be present as well (in 10 to 20%). The disease remits by puberty in most patients. If seizures rarely occur, treatment may not be needed. If seizures are classic, there is no need to image. **Carbamazepine** and **gabapentin** are the most commonly used antiepileptic drugs (AEDs).

Situation-Related Epilepsies

Febrile Seizures

Febrile seizures occur in about 4% of the population, onset being between age 6 months and 6 years, peaking at 18 to 24 months. One third have recurrent febrile seizures that are more likely to recur if the first febrile seizure occurs before 1 year of age. Later epilepsy occurs in 2 to 4% overall; this risk is lowest for *simple febrile seizure* (single convulsion at onset of fever, no lateralizing features, <15 minutes in duration, neurologically normal child), and most febrile seizures fit this category. The risk is higher for *complex febrile seizure* (focal, multiple, prolonged, or neurologically impaired). There is no need to treat, image, or obtain EEG in a patient with a simple febrile seizure.

■ NEW-ONSET SEIZURES

Evaluation of New-Onset Seizures

The history should concentrate on both acute and chronic remote risk factors for seizures as listed in Table 26–3. In adults aged 20 to 60, the most common causes, listed in order of frequency, are trauma, infection, metabolic/drugs, tumor, and vascular. For adults over 60 years old, the most common causes in order are vascular (stroke is by far the most common), tumor/metastasis, trauma, metabolic, and infection.

If there is an acute symptomatic explanation for the seizure, the underlying etiology should be corrected. Although usually generalized, focal seizures may also be seen with systemic metabolic abnormalities, especially hyper- or hypoglycemia, including epilepsia partialis continua (continuous simple partial seizures consisting of focal clonic jerking; common with nonketotic hyperglycemia). These seizures are best treated by correcting the metabolic abnormality first, as they are refractory to anticonvulsants unless this has been done.

If the patient is neurologically normal and has returned to baseline, MRI and EEG should be arranged. If MRI is not available and follow-up is questionable, a head CT scan with and without contrast should be obtained before discharge. It is particularly important to image those who are older, immunosuppressed, or at risk for HIV. The only patients with new-onset seizures that do not require any imaging are those with febrile convulsions or those with clear benign Rolandic or primary generalized epilepsy diagnosed by history *and* confirmed by EEG.

Lumbar punctures are rarely helpful in patients with new-onset seizures that have returned to baseline. This excludes patients with evidence of infection or those who may be immunosuppressed.

Risk of Seizure Recurrence

In the most common group of patients with normal examination, single seizure, and normal MRI and EEG, the chance of recurrence is approximately 25 to 30% over the next 2 to 3 years. Treatment is usually not recommended in these patients, in order to avoid chronic potentially harmful medication use when the majority will not need it. If the patient is neurologically abnormal,

Table 26-3 □ EVALUATION OF NEW-ONSET SEIZURE(S)

I. **History/examination:** look/ask for evidence of the following:
   A. *Acute risk factors*
      Trauma
      Alcohol
      Illegal drugs (especially cocaine, amphetamine)
      Medications: see Table 26-5; also withdrawal from benzodiazepines or barbiturates
      Metabolic:
         Low: glucose, sodium, oxygen, calcium, magnesium
         High: glucose, osmolality, BUN
      Infections, especially CNS infections; ask about HIV status and risk factors
      Stroke
   B. *Chronic/remote risk factors*
      Cerebral palsy/mental retardation (difficult birth without CP or MR is not a risk factor for epilepsy)
      Head trauma (moderate to severe)
      CNS infections
      Family history of epilepsy
      Febrile convulsions, especially if complex
      Neurocutaneous syndromes (examine skin)
      Prior unrecognized seizures, including absence and myoclonic jerks
II. **Laboratory Tests**
      CBC w/differential blood count
      Chem-7
      Calcium
      Magnesium
      LFTs
      Urine toxicology screen
      Serum toxicology
      Ethanol level (usually 0 when seizing)
      HIV testing when appropriate
III. **Imaging**
      Head CT scan with contrast or brain MRI

or has epileptiform discharges on EEG, the risk goes up significantly (about 50% if one factor is present, higher if both are present), and use of anticonvulsants is usually recommended. In general, the use of AEDs will cut the risk of recurrence in half.

The decision to treat or not should be individualized and discussed with the patient. It is important to ask all patients about prior possible seizures including myoclonic, absence, and partial. All patients should be advised about seizure precipitants such as alcohol use and sleep deprivation. They should also be counseled about seizure safety, including not driving or swimming alone until a full evaluation has been performed. They should be educated about other possible spells that may represent seizures.

If a person has two unprovoked seizures (i.e., epilepsy), the chance of having a third is approximately 70 to 80%, and treatment is almost always recommended.

■ MEDICAL TREATMENT OF EPILEPSY

General Principles

In general, the first AED should be continued until the patient is seizure free or at risk of clinical toxicity. If this medication fails, another first-line drug should be tried in monotherapy prior to attempting combination therapy. Choice of AED should be based on the seizure type and epilepsy syndrome as well as practical factors. Medication that can be taken once daily may be necessary for patients with poor memory or noncompliance. Coexisting conditions should be taken into account. For example, valproate is also effective for migraine prophylaxis; valproate, carbamazepine, lamotrigine, and some of the other new AEDs are effective for bipolar and related disorders; gabapentin is effective for neuropathic pain. Patients with severe liver disease may want to take gabapentin because it is 100% renally cleared. In patients with porphyria, only gabapentin (and possibly a benzodiazepine) is safe.

Although no new medications for epilepsy were approved between 1978 and 1993, eight new AEDs were approved between 1993 and early 2000 (in chronologic order, felbamate, gabapentin, lamotrigine, topiramate, tiagabine, levetiracetam, oxcarbazepine, and zonisamide). These newer options certainly helped patients with epilepsy but make choosing medications more difficult.

Primary Generalized Epilepsy

The drug of choice for most primary generalized epilepsy syndromes remains valproic acid, although some epileptologists are using lamotrigine, especially in young women (to avoid the weight gain, alopecia, and hormonal effects that can occur with valproate). Some of the other newer anticonvulsants are also effective, such as topiramate, and probably zonisamide. Ethosuximide is used for absence seizures but is ineffective for other seizure types. Acetazolamide and clonazepam can be useful adjuncts as well, although tolerance to these drugs is common. Carbamazepine and phenytoin can exacerbate myoclonic and absence seizures but are effective for primary GTC seizures. Primidone and phenobarbital are effective but less well tolerated.

Localization-Related Epilepsy

The first-line treatment for localization-related (partial-onset) epilepsy is usually carbamazepine or phenytoin. However, with the advent of multiple new anticonvulsants, all of which are approved for partial epilepsy, the choices are extensive. Oxcarbazepine (Trileptal) is a reasonable alternative to carbamazepine. Lamotrigine is another reasonable alternative, as it has been shown to be equally effective in small trials and probably is better tolerated than older AEDs. Because of its safety, gabapentin is a good choice for mild epilepsies such as BREC and is also a reasonable alternative in medically ill, elderly patients owing to its safety and lack of interactions. The other newer anticonvulsants are also reasonable first-line treatment in select patients.

Newer Forms of Antiepileptic Drugs

1. **Cerebyx (fosphenytoin)** is an intravenous (IV) formulation that is rapidly dephosphorylated to phenytoin in the blood stream. It can be given three times as fast as IV phenytoin, as it is available at a normal pH rather than the highly alkaline and toxic pH of IV phenytoin. This form is much gentler on veins and safer with extravasation. Blood pressure must still be monitored closely, including for at least 10 to 15 minutes after IV load, as phenytoin continues to be formed. This drug has replaced IV phenytoin in most academic centers.
2. **Carbatrol (carbamazepine, long-acting)** is available as a capsule containing three different carbamazepine preparations: enteric release, immediate release, and delayed release. Dosing twice a day with Carbatrol is equivalent to dosing four times a day with Tegretol. It is available in 200-mg and 300-mg capsules.
3. **Tegretol XR (carbamazepine, long-acting)** is available in 100-mg, 200-mg, and 400-mg capsules. Medication is slowly released from a pinhole in the tablet via osmotic forces. The tablet itself will be excreted intact in the stool, and this should be explained to the patient (to avoid patient's misconception that the pill is not being absorbed and possibly stopping the medication).
4. **Depacon (IV valproate)** is an IV preparation of valproate that is extremely well tolerated. Although the suggested rate is ≤20 mg per minute, it appears to be safe at faster rates. It may play an important role in treating status epilepticus, especially when nonconvulsive.
5. **Diastat (rectal diazepam)** is a convenient gel preparation of rectal diazepam (Valium) that can be given via prepackaged syringes by caregivers at home. This drug is excellent for

patients with clusters ("acute repetitive seizures") or prolonged seizures.

Common Errors in Treatment

1. **Following serum levels rather than clinical response**
   A valproate level of 130 mg/L (typical therapeutic range is 50 to 100 mg/L) may be just right for a given patient as long as the drug is not clinically toxic. Similarly, a phenytoin level of 8 mg/L (therapeutic range, 10 to 20 mg/L) may be adequate for some patients. Seizure control and clinical toxicity should be used as the primary endpoint, with serum levels as an adjunct.

2. **Missing the diagnosis of primary generalized epilepsy**
   If atypical absence spells are treated as complex partial seizures, most of the selected medications (e.g., phenytoin, carbamazepine) will not work. Similarly, if the primary GTC seizures of juvenile myoclonic epilepsy are treated as secondary generalized seizures with carbamazepine, myoclonic jerks and absence seizures may be exacerbated. It is important to ask about morning myoclonus and absence spells.

3. **Missing the diagnosis of nonepileptic pseudoseizures**
   It can be very difficult to distinguish epileptic spells from pseudoseizures by history. Pseudoseizures are psychogenic spells that mimic epileptic seizures and are usually a form of conversion disorder (unconscious behavior rather than conscious malingering, which is rare). Risk factors include prior physical or sexual abuse and psychiatric disease, although these may not be present. To complicate matters, many patients have both epileptic seizures and pseudoseizures. Video/EEG monitoring is required to make this diagnosis. For this reason alone, any patient with persistent spells that have not responded to AEDs, especially if the EEG and imaging are negative, should be referred for video/EEG monitoring. Approximately 30% of patients admitted to epilepsy monitoring units have pseudoseizures.

4. **Missing the diagnosis of nonepileptic physiologic spells**
   For refractory spells, always consider other physiologic episodes such as arrhythmias/syncope (especially if "slumping" is present; syncope commonly leads to a few myoclonic jerks or brief tonic stiffening), movement disorders (e.g., paroxysmal dyskinesias), sleep disorders (e.g., REM behavior disorder, somnambulism), or panic attacks (usually lasting longer than partial seizures and with retained awareness, though differentiation can be difficult). Again, recording episodes (with EEG, ECG, and possibly EMG or sleep parameters) is the key to accurate diagnosis.

5. **Missing the diagnosis of epilepsy**
   Frontal lobe seizures are frequently misdiagnosed as psychogenic spells, a sleep disorder, or paroxysmal nocturnal dystonia, as they tend to be nocturnal with rapid recovery, and EEGs are often normal (including ictally). Temporal lobe seizures with fear and autonomic symptoms may be misdiagnosed as panic attacks.
6. **Causing toxicity with high unbound ("free") drug levels**
   The free, or unbound, portion of a drug is the active component. Free levels are most important to measure with phenytoin because of its high protein binding (90%) and saturation kinetics (small increases in dose or free fraction will lead to dramatic increase in blood level at higher levels). Free phenytoin toxicity is common in patients with chronic illness (including liver and kidney failure, due to low albumin) and in patients on other highly protein bound drugs, *especially valproate* (also tiagabine and benzodiazepines). It is not unusual for patients with refractory seizures to be given high doses of phenytoin, followed by a load of valproate, leading to very high unbound phenytoin levels. This combination can cause lethargy, myoclonus, and exacerbation of seizures.
7. **Not being aware of important drug interactions**
   Valproate (a P450 enzyme inhibitor) dramatically slows the metabolism of lamotrigine, leading to higher risk of severe rash if not dosed properly (starting at 25 mg every other day). Erythromycin and calcium-channel blockers are also P450 inhibitors that frequently lead to AED toxicity (erythromycin causing carbamazepine toxicity is the most notorious combination). Table 26–4 gives further examples of medications that can influence AED levels. Antacids and

Table 26–4 ▫ IMPORTANT P450 ENZYME INHIBITORS AND INDUCERS

Enzyme inducers *can cause decreased effectiveness of Coumadin, oral contraceptives, theophylline, haloperidol, steroids, cyclosporine, chemotherapeutics, and many AEDs*

carbamazepine	rifampin
phenytoin	theophylline
phenobarbital	ethanol (chronic use)
primidone	topiramate

Enzyme inhibitors *can cause toxicity or elevated levels of Coumadin, oral contraceptives, theophylline, haloperidol, steroids, cyclosporine, chemotherapeutics, and many AEDs*

valproate	cimetidine	Ca^{2+}-channel blockers	erythromycin
felbamate	antifungals	propoxyphene	clarithromycin
fluoxetine	ethanol	isoniazid	azithromycin

Table 26-5 □ COMMONLY USED DRUGS THAT CAN LOWER THE SEIZURE THRESHOLD

Antibiotics, especially in the elderly or those with renal impairment
  Imipenem
  Penicillins
  Cephalosporins
  Isoniazid
  Metronidazole
Antihistamines, including over-the-counter diphenhydramine (Benadryl)
Antipsychotics, especially clozapine and low potency phenothiazines (e.g., chlorpromazine)
Antidepressants:
  Maprotiline (Ludiomil)
  Bupropion (Wellbutrin)
  Tricyclics, especially clomipramine; possibly least with desipramine
Baclofen
Fentanyl
Flumazenil (benzodiazepine antagonist)
Ketamine
Lidocaine
Lithium (especially in overdosage)
Meperidine (Demerol)
Propoxyphene (Darvon)
Theophylline

sucralfate can block the absorption of AEDs, especially phenytoin. Finally, remember to check for medications that can lower the seizure threshold (Table 26–5).

■ EPILEPSY SURGERY

Focal Resections

There have been dramatic improvements in epilepsy surgery in the past decade, especially in patients with temporal lobe epilepsy. Carefully selected patients with temporal lobe epilepsy (discussed previously) have an 80% cure rate. All patients with lesions associated with epilepsy are also good candidates for surgery, with a postoperative seizure-free rate of about 90%. Patients with normal MRIs are a more difficult group, although surgery remains a possibility.

Other Neurosurgical Options

When resection of a single seizure focus is not possible, there are multiple other surgical options. *Corpus callosotomy* can be useful in preventing drop attacks and associated injuries. *Hemispherectomy* is highly effective and often beneficial in patients with hemimegalencephaly, Rasmussen's encephalitis, or other severe unilateral epilepsies. *Subpial transections* are a technique used in eloquent regions of the brain where resection cannot be done. In this procedure, horizontal fibers are transected to prevent lateral spread of seizures, whereas vertical pathways are maintained to allow continued functioning of vertically oriented cortical columns.

■ OTHER TREATMENT OPTIONS

Ketogenic Diet

This treatment is most useful in children with severe epilepsies. This high-fat, low-carbohydrate diet causes the brain to rely on ketones for energy. This diet is effective for multiple seizure types, with approximately 30% of patients becoming seizure-free and another 30% showing marked improvement.

Vagal Nerve Stimulator

This option requires a minor surgery that is similar to having a pacemaker implant, though the wires are placed around the left vagal nerve. The mechanism is unclear, but vagal nerve stimulation decreases seizures by an average of 30% in multiple seizure types. Approximately 30% will have a significant reduction in seizures; it is extremely rare for patients to become seizure-free. Patients may activate stimulation themselves with a hand-held magnet when they feel an aura. Side effects are usually minimal but include change in voice and cough during stimulation. Stimulation parameters are adjustable using a magnet–computer interface.

■ PREGNANCY AND SEIZURES

Virtually all fertile women with epilepsy should be taking folate (1 mg per day; 4 mg per day if planning pregnancy) in order to decrease the risk of neural tube defects in the fetus. All older anticonvulsants are known to be teratogenic. Infants of mothers with epilepsy have a malformation rate of 4 to 6% (versus 2% in the general population). Thus, about 95% of mothers with epilepsy will have normal babies.

Teratogenicity is minimized by using a *single drug at the lowest effective dose*. Drug of choice should be based on the patient's seizure syndrome and drug response, independent of the pregnancy. Drugs should not be changed after conception, as this leads to multiple drug exposure. The greatest risk to the fetus from AEDs is clearly in the first trimester. Seizures during pregnancy can also be harmful, especially later in pregnancy.

Although animal studies suggest that some of the newer anticonvulsants will be significantly safer than the older ones, experience in humans is limited at this point. Pregnant women with epilepsy are encouraged to register with the national AED pregnancy registry during their first trimester (1–888–233–2334).

Screening for neural tube defects and other anatomic abnormalities is usually recommended at 16 to 18 weeks with serum triple screen and anatomic fetal ultrasound. It is also recommended that patients be placed on oral vitamin K (10 mg/day from 36 weeks through delivery) to prevent neonatal peripartum hemorrhage due to vitamin K deficiency. This regimen is most important in women taking enzyme-inducing drugs.

■ SEIZURES IN SPECIAL SITUATIONS

Perioperative Seizures. Approximately 3 to 6% of patients undergoing supratentorial craniotomy will develop seizures perioperatively, and 8 to 17% will have new-onset seizures within the first year. Patients at highest risk for perioperative seizures include those with large meningiomas, ruptured aneurysms with parenchymal blood, large arteriovenous malformations, and traumatic ICH.

Patients usually recommended for prophylactic perioperative AEDs (usually phenytoin or fosphenytoin) are listed in Table 26–6. **Phenytoin/fosphenytoin dosing: Load 18 to 20 mg/kg; maintenance is 5 to 6 mg/kg per day; keep levels between 10 and 25 mg/L.**

If no seizures have occurred, AEDs should be discontinued after the patient has recovered from surgery, usually within 2 weeks.

Head Trauma. Patients with significant head trauma who are at increased risk for seizures include those with intracranial bleeding, depressed skull fracture, penetrating wound, Glasgow Coma Scale score <10, and early seizures. These patients should receive phenytoin for 1 week prophylactically. Phenytoin does not appear to be effective in preventing the first seizure after this and may impair rehabilitation.

Stroke. About 5% of patients with acute infarcts will have early seizures, most within 48 hours; 9 to 15% with supratentorial hemorrhage have seizures. Late epilepsy after ischemic stroke is seen in 5 to 10% overall and up to 32% with early seizures. Prophylactic AEDs are not recommended in general, although

Table 26–6 □ NEUROSURGICAL CONDITIONS FOR WHICH SHORT-TERM* PERIOPERATIVE AED PROPHYLAXIS IS REASONABLE

Aneurysms:
  Subarachnoid hemorrhage and unclipped aneurysm
  Unruptured aneurysm only if significant cortical retraction is required
Arteriovenous malformations
Neoplasms:
  Supratentorial: all
  Sellar region: only if significant cortical retraction is required (not posterior fossa tumors)
Infections:
  Abscess
  Subdural empyema
Intracerebral hematoma, spontaneous, supratentorial, requiring evacuation
Subdural hematoma, chronic, requiring craniotomy
Trauma
  Any brain injury that requires neurosurgical intervention

*"Short term" refers to less than 2 weeks unless there is persistently raised ICP or an unstable vascular lesion such as an unclipped aneurysm.

short-term use should be considered with large supratentorial strokes with elevated ICP, especially if hemorrhagic, when a seizure could precipitate herniation.

Alcohol. Alcohol-related seizures usually occur about 24 hours after the last drink, although they can occur at any time in chronic alcoholics. Alcohol-related seizures should be treated by abstinence; AEDs tend to be ineffective, and patients who continue to drink are usually noncompliant. Prescribing AEDs to alcoholics is usually counterproductive because frequent withdrawal from the medications can exacerbate seizures, and the combination of AEDs and alcohol can be particularly toxic to the liver. If seizures persist unrelated to alcohol use, chronic AEDs are usually indicated; many of these cases are posttraumatic epilepsy.

Renal Failure. Daily doses of medications should be given after dialysis (on dialysis days); checking free and total levels before and after dialysis can be helpful. Most medications do not need dramatic adjustment in dose; the exceptions are the renally cleared medications (gabapentin, topiramate, levetiracetam, zonisamide).

Hepatic Failure. Because most AEDs are metabolized by the liver, they must be given "low and slow." Free phenytoin levels should be as used. Avoid valproate. Seizures are not often a major problem in patients with liver failure. Consider renally cleared medications (see previous paragraph).

Postanoxic Myoclonus. Continuous myoclonic jerks after cardiac arrest are associated with a poor prognosis. If there is any question of seizures, AEDs should be administered. Valproate and clonazepam are the most effective medications; phenytoin is ineffective. Treatment of postanotic myoclonus will not improve outcome.

chapter 27

Pediatric Neurologic Emergencies

JUAN M. PASCUAL

A developmental, social, and family history should be obtained for every pediatric patient seen as an emergency. The guardians' understanding of any underlying diseases and of the cause of the current events should also be investigated. At a first glance, determine the degree of neurologic compromise by estimating the level of alertness of the child and the need for rapid intervention. Then, the interview is directed toward obtaining the child's baseline values and how the current event departs from it. Infants become more cooperative when they are spoken to in a pleasant voice, and children are less intimidated when the examiner appears to ignore them at first. When possible, children should be examined while seated on a caretaker's lap and should be engaged in conversation and play. Careful observation and holding of normal-appearing children may reveal unsuspected tone anomalies (Fig. 27–1), but should be reserved for the end of the examination. Developmental milestones should be documented in the history (Table 27–1).

■ BIRTH TRAUMA

Large (over 4500 g) infants, instrumentation during delivery, uncommon presentations, augmented delivery, and first vaginal delivery are associated with neurologic birth trauma. **Clavicular fracture** is the most common form of trauma and is diagnosed by palpation and radiographs. The prognosis for spontaneous recovery is good. **Brachial plexus injuries** are common also in babies with low Apgar scores. Erb's (proximal) palsy involves cervical roots C5, C6, and sometimes C7 and results in "waiter's tip" appearance, with the limb in adduction, internal rotation, elbow extension, pronation, and finger flexion (Fig. 27–2). Total plexus lesion is commonly misnamed as Klumpke's (distal) paralysis and is much less frequent. All plexus roots are affected, with occasional Horner syndrome from T1 root lesion and diaphragmatic paralysis from C4 injury. Electromyography (EMG) shows a diminished number of motor units and fibrillations after 2 to 3 weeks. Magnetic resonance imaging (MRI) is informative in suspected root avulsion, which carries a poor prognosis. The

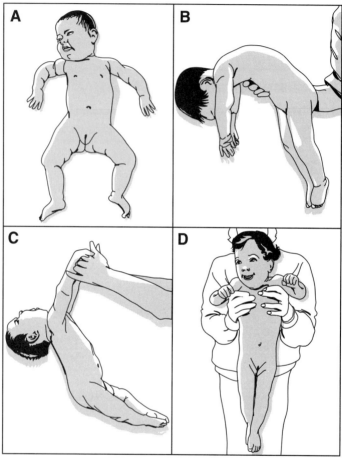

Figure 27-1 □ Examination of tone. *A* to *C*, Severe hypotonia in an infant with spinal muscular atrophy. *A*, Hypotonic frog-legged posture with arms adducted, legs in external rotation and knee flexion. All limbs make contact with the examination table. *B*, Ventral suspension revealing limp arms and legs and poor neck extension. *C*, Pulling maneuver demonstrating significant head lag and extended legs. *D*, Hypertonicity after periventricular leukomalacia. The thumbs are in a "cortical" position, and the legs display "scissoring."

Table 27-1 □ NORMAL DEVELOPMENTAL MILESTONES

Age (Months)	Milestones
1 to 1½	Smiling; attempts at lifting up the head briefly
4	Head control; identification of familiar persons and objects
6	Reaching for objects; rolling from prone to supine
8	Transfer between hands; sitting with support; combination of syllables
10	Standing holding; fine grasp
12	Walking supported; two or three word vocabulary
15	Walking unsupported
18	Command following
24	Phrases
36	Handedness develops

outcome of brachial plexus injuries is good, with near complete recovery in 88% and 92% of cases by 4 and 12 months, respectively. Physical therapy measures are started in the second week, and surgical exploration may be considered in infants who do not improve by the third month.

Spinal cord injury, associated with rotation of the head during forceps extraction, may be difficult to appreciate in low-Apgar-score infants. Long-term sequelae include hydromyelia and myelomalacia. Benign C1–C2 subluxation, however, is more common

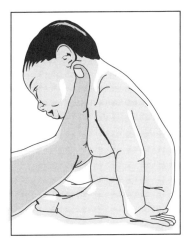

Figure 27-2 □ Erb's palsy in a newborn. The limb is adducted and internally rotated.

and has a good prognosis. Cord ultrasounds may be obtained until the sixth month. Thereafter, MRI is preferred for diagnosis.

Tentorial subdural hematoma that resolves within the first week of life is very common in neonates who are extracted with vacuum. **Subgaleal hemorrhage** is palpable as a soft collection that crosses skull sutures and may cause progressive anemia and consumption coagulopathy. Cephalohematoma is confined to the subperiosteum and therefore respects suture lines. It is firm to palpation and self-limited. Both should be differentiated from **caput succedaneum** due to subcutaneous edema, which involves the presenting part.

■ CEREBROVASCULAR COMPLICATIONS OF PREMATURITY

Premature infants are susceptible to intraventricular hemorrhage, periventricular hemorrhagic infarction, and periventricular leukomalacia. All are diagnosed by ultrasonography. **Intraventricular hemorrhage** is associated with extreme prematurity (less than 1500 g) and occurs within the first few days of life. It is divided into grades I (germinal matrix), II (intraventricular blood that does not distort the ventricular system), III (blood that causes ventricular enlargement), and IV (parenchymal extension). Higher grade hemorrhages cause hydrocephalus, manifested as enlargement of the head and a bulging fontanelle. Decreased tone or spontaneous movements, loss of pupillary reactivity, respiratory arrest, hypotension, and anemia may be associated features. Serial lumbar punctures relieve the hydrocephalus in some cases; the remaining necessitate ventriculoperitoneal or ventriculosubgaleal shunt. Long-term outcome correlates with the degree of parenchymal damage.

Periventricular hemorrhagic infarction must be distinguished from intraventricular hemorrhage type IV and is a venous infarct probably caused by compression of terminal veins that run under the germinal matrix of the lateral ventricles. The infarct involves the dorsal and lateral aspect of the lateral ventricle and is usually asymmetric and evolves into a single cavity that communicates with the ventricle. It is associated with a significant mortality rate and with spastic hemiparesis in survivors.

Periventricular leukomalacia affects the white matter of the centrum semiovale. It is probably caused by perfusion failure at the border zone between the long penetrator vessels branching off the middle cerebral artery that enter the brain from its surface and the basal lenticulostriate arteries (short penetrators). It causes a spastic quadriparesis with predominant leg involvement or paraplegia (see Fig. 27–1). The lesions tend to cavitate, causing a Swiss-cheese appearance of the white matter.

■ NEONATAL SEIZURES

Newborns do not display generalized seizures, possibly owing to insufficient myelination; they may, however, exhibit multiple focality when the epileptogenic process affects the brain diffusely. Important etiologic clues are provided by the time of onset of neonatal seizures (see Table 27–2). Newborns and infants who are younger than 3 months of age with new onset seizures should be evaluated and treated for infection until blood, urine, and cerebrospinal fluid (CSF) cultures are negative for at least 2 days even in the absence of fever. Treatment includes emergency evaluation of electrolytes and indicators of infection and **phenobarbital**, given as a **20 mg/kg IV** load, followed by **5 mg/kg** daily orally or IV. Two repeat loading doses of **10 mg/kg** may be administered for refractory seizures. To avoid respiratory depres-

Table 27–2 □ ETIOLOGIC CLASSIFICATION OF NEONATAL SEIZURES BY TIME OF ONSET

Less than 24 hours
  Sepsis and meningitis
  Drug effect
  Hypoxic-ischemic encephalopathy
  Intracranial hemorrhage
  Pyridoxine dependency

24 to 72 hours
  Sepsis and meningitis
  Drug withdrawal
  Intracranial hemorrhage
  Glycine encephalopathy
  Cerebral dysgenesis
  Glycogen synthase deficiency
  Hypoparathyroidism-hypocalcemia
  Cerebral venous thrombosis
  Intraventricular hemorrhage of prematurity
  Pyridoxine dependency
  Tuberous sclerosis
  Incontinentia pigmenti
  Urea cycle errors

72 hours to 1 week
  Familial neonatal seizures
  Cerebral dysgenesis
  Cerebral infarction
  Hypoparathyroidism
  Cerebral venous thrombosis
  Intracerebral hemorrhage
  Kernicterus
  Methylmalonic acidemia
  Hypocalcemia
  Propionic acidemia
  Tuberous sclerosis
  Urea cycle errors

1 to 4 weeks
  Neonatal adrenoleukodystrophy
  Cerebral dysgenesis
  Fructose dysmetabolism
  Gaucher disease type 2
  GM_1 gangliosidosis
  Herpes simplex encephalitis
  Cerebrovenous thrombosis
  Ketotic hyperglycinemia
  Neonatal maple syrup urine disease
  Tuberous sclerosis
  Urea cycle errors

Source: Adapted from Fenichel G: Clinical Pediatric Neurology. Philadelphia, WB Saunders, 1997.

sion, care must be taken not to add a benzodiazepine while loading with phenobarbital.

■ FEBRILE SEIZURES

Febrile seizures occur in children between 6 months and 5 years of age in association with fever and without nervous system infection. Although they may be of any type, they usually are generalized tonic-clonic or tonic. They recur in one third of children, and of those, one half have a second recurrence or more. Early age at onset of seizures, pre-existing neurologic anomalies, persistence for more than 15 minutes, or focal features may increase the likelihood of subsequent epilepsy. The main management decisions are whether to perform a spinal tap at presentation to evaluate infection or whether to treat them with prophylactic antiepileptics. Recurrent febrile seizures do not necessitate the use of prophylactic anticonvulsants but may be treated with **5 mg rectal diazepam gel.** EEG is recommended in children who exhibit focal features or deficits at baseline.

■ INFECTIONS OF THE CENTRAL NERVOUS SYSTEM

Meningitis, encephalitis, and cerebral abscess are most common central nervous system (CNS) infections in children. The signs of meningitis may be absent in children who are younger than 3 years of age and in neutropenic children (absolute neutrophil count below 1000 per mm^3). In the newborn, the most common organisms are group B *Streptococcus, Escherichia coli,* and *Listeria monocytogenes. Citrobacter* spp. cause cerebral abscesses owing to hemorrhagic necrosis; in general, these abscesses should not be drained. During infancy and preschool, responsible agents are *Haemophilus influenzae, Neisseria meningitidis,* and *Streptococcus pneumoniae* and in school age, *N. meningitidis* and *S. pneumoniae.* Treatment of meningitis in infants and children should include **dexamethasone 0.15 mg/kg every 6 hours** for 4 days. For empiric antibiotic coverage, see Table 22–2. Sequelae of meningitis include hydrocephalus, mental retardation, seizures, and hearing loss. Except for *Citrobacter* infection, meningitis does not cause abscess, and therefore, predisposing cardiopulmonary conditions should be investigated in every case of cerebral abscess.

■ DISORDERS THAT RESEMBLE CNS INFECTION

Several disorders may first manifest with fever, depressed consciousness, seizures, meningeal signs, and CSF pleocytosis without ever identifying a responsible infectious agent or its antigens. **Acute disseminated encephalomyelitis** preferentially affects children over 2 years and follows trivial infections, immunizations, or the administration of certain drugs by 4 to 21 days. The lesions are widespread, with gray and white matter and peripheral nerve involvement. However, computed tomographic (CT) abnormalities may be undetectable until the second week after onset. MRI is abnormal from the beginning of the neurologic illness, and 60% of the lesions may enhance with contrast material. A polymorphonuclear pleocytosis is commonly found in CSF, which later becomes mononuclear. The CSF glucose level is normal, and the protein is elevated. The course may be polyphasic, particularly in patients treated with steroids. **Acute toxic encephalopathy** is more common in children who are younger than 2 years and may also be preceded by banal infections. It causes cerebral edema without inflammation. The CSF is under high pressure but its composition is normal. **Acute hemorrhagic leukoencephalitis** is the least common postinfectious and postvaccinal disorder. The pathologic process consists of a small-vessel necrotizing vasculitis in the white matter with circulating atypical lymphocytes and albuminuria. The CSF pleocyosis is at the expense of polymorphonuclear cells. **Serum sickness** occurs as a drug reaction, accompanied by CSF polymorphonuclear, lymphocytic, or eosinophilic pleocytosis, elevated protein, and peripheral eosinophilia. CT is usually normal. **Systemic lupus erythematosus** occasionally first presents as aseptic meningitis, seizure disorder, or psychosis. **Behçet disease** may also present as meningitis or seizures caused by vasculitis and associates with orogenital ulcers and uveitis.

■ VENTRICULOPERITONEAL SHUNT MALFUNCTION

Permanent drainage of CSF is accomplished by ventriculojugular or, more commonly, by ventriculoperitoneal shunt. Proximal shunt malfunction is caused by either disconnection or obstruction of the intracranial portion of the shunt by hemorrhage or debris. Intermediate (valve) malfunction is due to disconnection, blood clot, or dense CSF with a high protein content. Distal shunt fracture or tip occlusion may also occur. Complete malfunction in the infant manifests as irritability, feeding difficulty, enlarged head, and tense fontanelle. In an older child, it first manifests as headache, vomiting, and progressively depressed consciousness. Seizures may also occur. An infected shunt additionally causes fever but rarely local signs of infection. Partial malfunction is insidious, develops over weeks or months, and causes poor cognition (first manifested as school difficulties), papilledema, sixth nerve and upgaze palsies, hyperreflexia, and lower extremity hypertonicity. Shunt evaluation involves a radiographic shunt series to assess continuity of the system, head CT to determine ventricular size (most helpful when prior scans are available for comparison), and tapping of the shunt reservoir with measurement of the pressure if distal malfunction is suspected. CSF should be analyzed and cultured.

Management. If malfunction cannot be excluded, admission for observation is warranted. When it is suspected or confirmed, urgent neurosurgical consultation is required. Infected shunts should generally be removed as soon as infection is found. *Overshunting* refers to low CSF pressure due to excess drainage. It may cause subdural hematoma and postural headaches that are alleviated when the patient is in a supine position.

■ TUMORS

The mode of presentation of brain tumors depends on local mass effect, infiltration, or hydrocephalus. In infancy, they may cause irritability, failure to thrive, developmental arrest and regression, poor feeding, vomiting, and macrocephaly. In childhood, they may not produce localizing neurologic signs and instead cause progressive and recurrent episodes of headache and vomiting. **Supratentorial hemispheric** tumors, most commonly low-grade astrocytomas and malignant gliomas, may produce focal neurologic deficits and seizures. **Supratentorial midline** tumors such as low-grade gliomas, craniopharyngiomas, and pineal tumors may compress the optic chiasm producing visual disturbance; may affect the hypothalamus altering endocrine function, appetite, and behavior; and may cause Parinaud syndrome or obstructive hydrocephalus. **Infratentorial** tumors cause a variety of symptoms: diffuse brain stem glioma causes cranial neuropathies and long tract signs; cerebellar astrocytomas and medulloblastomas produce ataxia and hydrocephalus; and ependymomas cause vomiting from compression of the floor of the fourth ventricle and obstructive hydrocephalus. **Neuroblastomas** are extraneural tumors (most commonly abdominal) that in two thirds of cases are associated with neurologic complications such as metastasis, carcinomatous meningitis, and paraneoplastic opsoclonus-myoclonus. The latter causes erratic, conjugate eye movements ("dancing eyes"). Emergency **management** of brain tumors includes CT followed by staging MRI including the spinal cord for tumors that are suspected to expand multifocally. **Dexamethasone administered at 0.1 mg/kg four times a day** relieves symptoms caused by peritumoral edema. Neurosurgical consultation for biopsy, resection, or relief of hydrocephalus must be obtained.

■ HEAD INJURY

Initial management of minor accidental head trauma requires establishing the likelihood of cerebral injury and the need for CT scanning of the head. In general, children with normal findings on examination who have fallen out of bed onto a hard surface, who wore protective equipment such as a helmet, or who sustained the injury more than 6 hours prior to the examination have not sustained cerebral damage. Similarly, brief amnesia, headache, vomiting up to three times, and scalp laceration (alone or in combination) do not suggest brain injury. On the other hand, in the presence of seizure, depression of consciousness, skull fracture (including raccoon eyes or Battle signs), or localizing neurologic deficit, cerebral injury must be suspected. **Diagnosis** of suspected brain injury relies on CT. Skull radiographs are not sufficient. **Management** of suspected brain injury with negative CT includes admission to the hospital for a 24- to 48-hour observation period. The neurologic status should be assessed periodically. Any CT showing signs of hemorrhage or significant contusion must be repeated in 6 to 12 hours, along with prompt evaluation of coagulation. Seizure prophylaxis must be initiated in those with an abnormal CT, and neurosurgical consultation must be considered.

■ CHILD ABUSE

In infants and young children, most accidental head injuries are due to falls that impose weak impact forces on the head; these rarely cause the findings of the shaken-baby syndrome. Conversely, the rotation imposed by shaking the head accounts for the intracranial injury of battered children. Compounding forces include deceleration against a hard or soft force while shaking and compression of the neck with the hands. **Shaken-baby syndrome** typically affects infants and children who are younger than 3 years of age. The history is usually vague, and trivial head trauma that is disproportionate to the degree of injury is usually caused by caretakers. Often, the aggressor is not the father of the child and maintains a sporadic relationship with the mother. Poverty and lack of education are common, but it happens in every socioeconomic level. Abused children may fail to thrive and are sometimes admitted to the hospital solely for that reason. While hospitalized, the children quickly gain weight and display catchup growth.

Extracranial lesions include finger marks over the chest and limbs, bruising, burns, lacerations, and skeletal fractures, particularly those involving the lateral ribs and metaphyses of long bones. A characteristic pattern of burns involves the buttocks and both feet and is caused by submersion in hot water with the child flexing feet, knees, and hips while being submersed. Lesions may be of different ages, showing a yellowish discoloration. **Intracranial injuries** are subdural hematoma, subarachoid hemorrhage with a preference for the interhemispheric fissure, loss of gray-white matter differentiation due to axonal shearing, cerebral contusion, skull fracture, and retinal hemorrhages. Layering of subdural blood is indicative of trauma of different ages after a coagulopathy has been excluded. **Clinical presentation** includes lethargy, irritability, seizures, meningeal signs, vomiting, poor feeding, apnea, a bulging fontanelle, and coma.

The **differential diagnosis** includes the retinal hemorrhages seen in up to 40% of vaginally delivered newborns that resolve within a month, coagulopathy, sepsis, osteogenesis imperfecta (with blue sclerae, dental anomalies, short stature, and angulation of healed fractures), glutaric aciduria type I (with developmental delay, hypotonia, cortical atrophy, and chronic subdural collections), benign subdural fluid collections of infancy (usually bifrontal), and accidental trauma.

The **diagnosis** requires head CT scanning including bone windows, a radiographic skeletal survey, fundoscopy after midriasis, and coagulation profile (platelet count, prothrombin time [PT], partial thromboplastin time [PTT]). Photographs of all visible injuries should be taken. Cerebral gradient ECHO MRI aids with the identification of hemorrhage of different ages. Lumbar puncture performed to evaluate cases confounded with sepsis reveals a bloody fluid. Ophthalmologic consultation should be obtained to assess and document retinal findings.

The **management** of suspected abuse requires admission, attention to fluid balance, and immediate report to the appropriate child protection agency according to hospital policy. Seizure prophylaxis with phenytoin is started in every case with intracranial injury, skull fracture, and coma or if seizures have occurred. A mild, self-resolving coagulopathy can be found in severe cases of head injury. Caretakers should be informed of the diagnostic investigations ahead of time in a nonaccusatory manner. All findings and progress must be documented with extreme care.

■ BRAIN DEATH

Determination of brain death in a child who is younger than 1 year of age represents a special challenge, as the developing brain has a greater potential for recovery from reversible conditions than the adult brain does. **Requisites** for the diagnosis of brain death include knowing the cause of coma, normothermia, normotension, and a normal metabolic and toxicologic profile, including prescribed agents that depress the nervous system. **Examination**

must reveal coma, apnea, midposition or dilated unreactive pupils, absence of oculocephalic and caloric reflexes, absent corneal reflexes, absent gag reflex, flaccidity, and absence of spontaneous movements. In preterm infants before the 32nd gestational week, most brain stem reflexes remain undeveloped and therefore may not be assessed. The respiratory drive in response to apnea may also develop as late as the 33rd week. Structural lesions in the posterior fossa that may resemble brain death include tumors, subdural hematoma, Dandy-Walker deformity, and Chiari malformations. **Adjunctive** diagnostic methods include radioisotope cerebral blood flow determination and EEG. In neonates, however, cerebral flow may persist after brain death, and it is only of value for the early diagnosis of brain death when absent. Age-appropriate brain death **criteria** are as follows:
1. For patients over 1 year
   - Two examinations spaced 12 to 24 hours
   - EEG and cerebral blood flow determinations are optional
2. For patients 2 months to 1 year
   - Two examinations and EEGs 24 hours apart *or*
   - One examination with an EEG and a cerebral blood flow study
3. For patients 7 days to 2 months
   - Two examinations and EEGs 48 hours apart.

The latter criteria may be extended to term newborns who are younger than 7 days of age, but consensus has not been reached. In anencephaly, adjunctive techniques such as EEG and cerebral blood flow studies are not needed, and they may be impractical for anatomic reasons; the diagnosis is therefore clinical.

APPENDIX A-1
Muscles of the Neck and Brachial Plexus

Appendix A

Muscle	Action to Test	Roots*	Nerve
Deep neck	Flexion, extension, rotation of neck	C1, C2, C3, C4	Cervical
Sternocleidomastoideus	Rotation of head to contralateral shoulder	XI, C2, C3	Spinal accessory
Trapezius	Elevation of the shoulders	XI, C3, C4	Spinal accessory
Diaphragm	Inspiration	C3, C4, C5	Phrenic
Serratus anterior	Forward shoulder thrust	C5, C6, C7	Long thoracic
Rhomboideus minor	Adduction and elevation of scapula	C4, C5	Dorsal scapular
Levator scapulae	Elevation of scapula	C4, C5	Dorsal scapular
Supraspinatus	Abduction of arm (0 to 90 degrees)	**C5**, C6	Suprascapular
Infraspinatus	Lateral arm rotation	**C5**, C6	Suprascapular
Deltoideus	Abduction of arm (>30 degrees)	**C5**, C6	Axillary
Teres minor	Medial arm rotation	C4, C5	Axillary
Biceps brachii	Flexion of supinated forearm	**C5**, C6	Musculocutaneous
Brachialis	Flexion of pronated forearm	C5, C6	Musculocutaneous
Teres major	Medial rotation and adduction of arm	C5–C7	Subscapular
Latissimus dorsi	Adduction of arm	C6, **C7**, C8	Thoracodorsal
Flexor carpi ulnaris	Ulnar flexion of hand	C7, **C8**, T1	Ulnar
Flexor digitorum profundus (ulnar part)	Flexion of distal phalanx of fingers 4 and 5	**C8**, T1	Ulnar
Adductor pollicis	Adduction of thumb	C8, T1	Ulnar
Abductor digiti minimi manus	Abduction of little finger	C8, T1	Ulnar
Flexor digiti minimi brevis manus	Flexion of little finger	C8, **T1**	Ulnar
Interossei	Abduction (dorsal) or adduction (palmar) of fingers	C8, T1	Ulnar
Lumbricales 3 and 4	Flexion of proximal phalanges and extension of two distal phalanges (fingers 4 and 5)	C8	Ulnar
Flexor digitorum superficialis	Flexion of middle phalanx fingers 2 to 5, flexion of hand	C7, **C8**, T1	Median

Muscle	Action	Roots	Nerve
Pronator teres	Pronation of forearm	C6, C7	Median
Flexor carpi radialis	Radial flexion of hand	C6, C7	Median
Palmaris longus	Wrist flexion	C7, C8, T1	Median
Abductor pollicis brevis	Abduction of thumb metacarpal	C8, **T1**	Median
Flexor pollicis brevis	Flexion of proximal phalanx of thumb	C8, **T1**	Median
Opponens pollicis	Opposition of thumb	C8, **T1**	Median
Lumbricales 1 and 2	Flexion of proximal phalanx and extension of distal phalanges (fingers 2 and 3)	C8, **T1**	Median
Flexor digitorum profundus (radial part)	Flexion of distal phalanx of fingers 2 and 3; flexion of hand	C7, **C8**	Median (anterior interosseous nerve)
Flexor pollicis longus	Flexion of distal phalanx of thumb	C7, **C8**	Median (anterior interosseous nerve)
Triceps brachii	Forearm extension	C6, **C7**, C8	Radial
Brachioradialis	Forearm flexion (with thumb pointing upwards)	**C6**, C7	Radial
Extensor carpi radialis	Radial hand extension	**C6**, C7	Radial
Supinator	Forearm supination	**C6**, C7	Radial
Extensor digitorum	Extension of hand and phalanges of fingers 2 to 5	C7, C8	Radial (posterior interosseous nerve)
Extensor carpi ulnaris	Ulnar hand extension	C7, C8	Radial (posterior interosseous nerve)
Abductor pollicis longus	Abduction of thumb metacarpal	C7, C8	Radial (posterior interosseous nerve)
Extensor pollicis brevis and extensor pollicis longus	Thumb extension and radial wrist extension	C7, C8	Radial (posterior interosseous nerve)
Extensor indicis	Index finger extension and hand extension	C7, C8	Radial (posterior interosseous nerve)

* **Boldface** letters indicate primary innervation.

APPENDIX A-2
Muscles of the Perineum and Lumbosacral Plexus

Muscle	Action to Test	Roots	Nerve
Iliopsoas	Hip flexion	L1, **L2**, * **L3**	Femoral and L1, L2 and L3
Sartorius	Hip flexion and lateral thigh rotation	L2, L3	Femoral
Quadriceps femoris	Leg extension	L2, **L3**, **L4**	Femoral
Adductor longus	Thigh adduction	L2, **L3**, L4	Obturator
Adductor brevis	Thigh adduction	L2, L3, L4	Obturator
Adductor magnus	Thigh adduction	L2, L3, L4	Obturator
Gracilis	Thigh adduction	L2, L3, L4	Obturator
Obturator externus	Thigh adduction and lateral rotation	L3, L4	Obturator
Gluteus medius and gluteus minimus	Thigh abduction and medial rotation	L4, **L5**, S1	Superior gluteal
Tensor fasciae latae	Thigh abduction	L4, L5	Superior gluteal
Gluteus maximus	Hip extension	**L5**, **S1**, S2	Inferior gluteal
Biceps femoris	Knee flexion (and assistance with thigh extension)	L5, S1, S2	Sciatic (trunk)
Semitendinosus	Knee flexion (and assistance with thigh extension)	L5, S1, S2	Sciatic (trunk)
Semimembranosus	Knee flexion (and assistance with thigh extension)	L5, S1, S2	Sciatic (trunk)
Tibialis anterior	Foot dorsiflexion and inversion	L4, **L5**	Deep peroneal
Extensor digitorum longus	Extension of toes 2 to 5 and foot dorsiflexion	**L5**, S1	Deep peroneal
Extensor hallucis longus	Great toe extension and foot dorsiflexion	**L5**, S1	Deep peroneal
Extensor digitorum brevis	Extension of toes	L5, S1	Deep peroneal
Peroneus longus and peroneus brevis	Foot eversion (and assistance with plantar flexion)	**L5**, S1	Superficial peroneal
Tibialis posterior	Foot plantar flexion and inversion	L5, S1	Tibial
Flexor digitorum longus	Foot plantar flexion and flexion of toes 2 to 4	S2, S3	Tibial
Flexor hallucis longus	Foot plantar flexion and flexion of terminal phalanx of great toe	S1, S2	Tibial
Gastrocnemius	Knee flexion and ankle plantar flexion	**S1** (S2)	Tibial
Soleus	Ankle plantar flexion	**S1** (S2)	Tibial
Perineal muscles and sphincters	Voluntary contraction of the pelvic floor	S2, S3, S4	Pudendal

***Boldface** letters indicate primary innervation.

APPENDIX A-3
Brachial Plexus

Appendix A 387

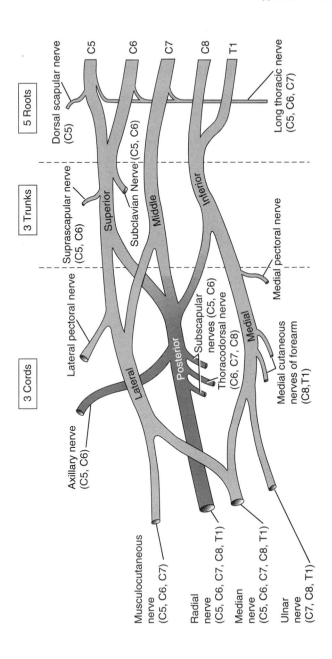

APPENDIX A-4
Lumbar Plexus

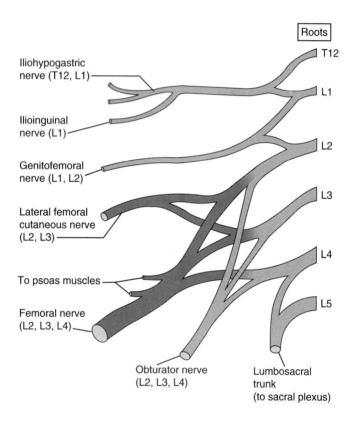

APPENDIX A-5
Sensory Dermatome Map

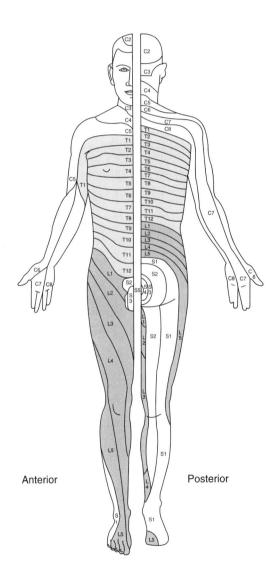

APPENDIX A-6
Mini-Mental State Examination

Patient: _____

Date __/__/__

Examiner: _____

	Normal Score*
Younger Patients	28–30
Older Patients	24–30
(*Score = number correct)	

Instructions: Say to the person "I would like to ask you some questions to check your memory and concentration. Some questions may be easy and some may be difficult." Record the patient's response, where applicable, and darken one circle to indicate correctness of each response.

	Patient's Response	Incorrect	Correct
1. What is today's date?	_____	⓪	①
2. What is the year?	_____	⓪	①
3. What is the month?	_____	⓪	①
4. What is the day of the week?	_____	⓪	①
5. What season is it?	_____	⓪	①
6. What is the name of this place?	_____	⓪	①
7. What floor are we on?	_____	⓪	①
8. What town or city are we in?	_____	⓪	①
9. What county (district, borough, area) are we in?	_____	⓪	①
10. What state are we in?	_____	⓪	①

Appendix A 391

	Patient's Response	Incorrect	Correct

11. Say, "I am going to name three objects. After I have said them, I want you to repeat them. Remember what they are because I am going to ask you to name them again in a few minutes. Then say "apple," "table," "penny" clearly and slowly, about one second for each. Score the first try. Repeat the objects until the patient can repeat all three, for up to three trials.

	"Apple"	⓪	①
	"Table"	⓪	①
	"Penny"	⓪	①

12. Say, "I am going to say a word and ask you to spell it forward and backward. The word is WORLD. First can you spell it forward? Now spell it backward." Repeat if necessary, and help the patient to spell WORLD forward. Indicate and score the first five letters of the backward spelling.

1st _____		⓪	①
2nd _____		⓪	①
3rd _____		⓪	①
4th _____		⓪	①
5th _____		⓪	①

13. Show the patient a wristwatch and ask "What is this called?"   "Watch"   ⓪   ①

14. Show the patient a pencil and ask "What is this called?"   "Pencil"   ⓪   ①

15. Say, "I would like you to repeat a phrase after me. The phrase is 'No ifs ands or buts.'" Allow only one trial.   ⓪   ①

16. Say "I'm going to give you a piece of paper. When I do, take the paper in your right hand, fold the paper in half, and then put the paper on your lap." Read the full statement, then give him or her the paper. Do not repeat or coach.

Takes paper in right hand	⓪	①
Folds paper in half	⓪	①
Puts paper on lap	⓪	①

	Patient's Response	Incorrect	Correct
17. Hold the piece of paper that reads "Close your eyes," so the patient can see it clearly. Say "Read the words on this page, then do what they say." Score correct only if the patient actually closes his or her eyes.		0	1
18. Ask "What were the three objects I asked you to remember?"	"Apple" "Table" "Penny"	0 0 0	1 1 1
19. Give the patient a blank piece of paper and say "Write a complete sentence on this piece of paper." It is to be written spontaneously and must contain a subject and a verb to be correct. Correct grammar and punctuation are not necessary.		0	1
20. Show the intersecting pentagons and say "Here is a drawing. Draw this same drawing on this same page." Two five-sided figures must intersect and all angles must be preserved. Tremor and rotation are ignored.		0	1

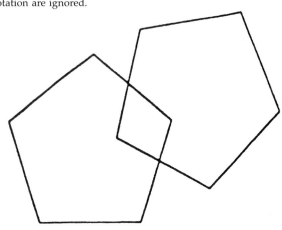

APPENDIX A-7
Surface Map of the Brain

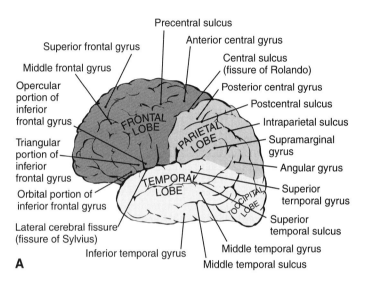

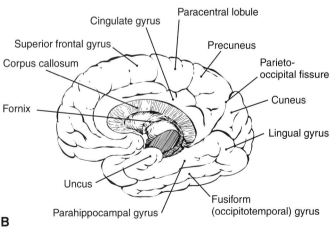

A, Lateral view of left cerebral hemisphere. *B*, Medial view of right cerebral hemisphere.

APPENDIX A-8
Nuclei of the Brainstem

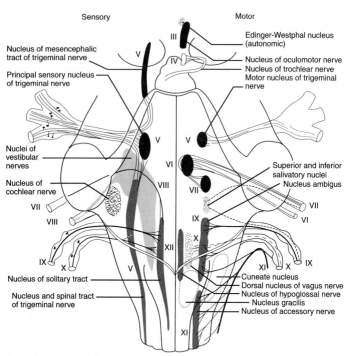

Cranial nerve nuclei.

APPENDIX A-9
Surface Anatomy of the Brainstem

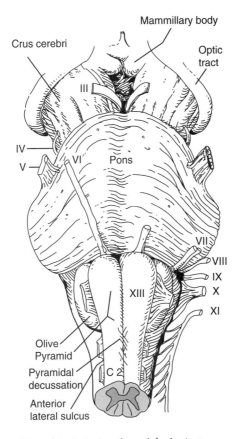

Ventral (anterior) surface of the brainstem.

APPENDIX B
On-Call Formulary: Commonly Prescribed Medications in Neurology

Acetazolamide [Diamox] (Chapters 11 and 14)

Indications	Pseudotumor cerebri, seizures
Actions	Diuretic that is thought to reduce cerebrospinal fluid (CSF) volume, and intracranial pressure
Side effects	Paresthesias, tinnitus or hearing dysfunction, anorexia, nausea, vomiting, diarrhea, polyuria
Dose	500 mg two times a day

Amantadine [Symmetrel] (Chapter 25)

Indications	Parkinson's disease
Actions	Antiviral agent that also increases dopamine release, blocks dopamine reuptake, and stimulates dopamine receptors
Side effects	Livedo reticularis, ankle edema, confusion, hallucinations, insomnia
Comments	More effective for akinesia and rigidity, less effective for tremor; best used for 6 months to a year as monotherapy in patients with mild to moderate Parkinson's disease; may delay need for initiation of levodopa
Dose	100 to 300 mg two times a day

Amitriptyline [Elavil] (Chapters 14 and 17)

Indications	Neuropathic pain, migraine prophylaxis, depression
Actions	Inhibitor of membrane pump responsible for uptake of norepinephrine and serotonin, anticholinergic effects; unknown mechanism for action on neuropathy and migraine
Side effects	Drowsiness, paresthesias, urinary retention, dry mouth, constipation, blurred vision, confusion, cardiac conduction block, arrhythmias
Comments	Sedative effect may limit use for migraine and neuropathy to evening doses
Dose	25 to 75 mg every day at night time for migraine and

peripheral neuropathy; up to 150 mg daily in divided doses may be required for antidepressant effect

Aspirin (Ecotrin, Ascriptin, Bayer) (Chapter 24)

Indications	Secondary stroke prevention
Actions	Platelet aggregation inhibitor
Side effects	Dyspepsia, gastrointestinal bleeding
Comments	Reduces risk of recurrent stroke by 10 to 20% compared with placebo
Dose	81 or 325 mg once a day

Aspirin/extended release dipyridamole (Aggrenox) (Chapter 24)

Indications	Secondary stroke prevention
Actions	Platelet aggregation inhibitor
Side effects	Headache, dizziness, nausea, abdominal pain, dyspepsia
Comments	Reduces risk of recurrent stroke by 10% compared with either agent alone, or 24% compared with placebo
Dose	25 to 200 mg twice a day

Azathioprine (Imuran) (Chapter 15)

Indications	Myasthenia gravis (long-term management)
Actions	Immunosuppressant
Side effects	Leukopenia, thrombocytopenia, nausea, vomiting, increased secondary infection risk
Comments	Adequate immunosuppression is reflected by mild decrease in white blood cell count and increase in mean corpuscular volume
Dose	100 to 250 mg per day

Baclofen (Lioresal) (Chapters 21 and 25)

Indications	Dystonia, spasticity of multiple sclerosis
Actions	γ-Aminobutyric acid agonist, antispasmodic
Side effects	Confusion, sedation, increased muscle weakness
Comments	Can be given via intrathecal pump for severe cases
Dose	10 to 20 mg three times a day

Benztropine (Cogentin) (Chapter 25)

Indications	Parkinsonism, extrapyramidal reactions
Actions	Anticholinergic

Side effects	Dry mouth, constipation, urinary retention, tachycardia, psychosis
Comments	Effective for Parkinsonian tremor
Dose	Start 0.5 mg once or twice daily, increase 0.5 mg a day every 5 days to max 6 mg a day

Bethanechol (Urecholine) (Chapter 21)

Indications	Urinary retention due to neurogenic atonic bladder
Actions	Cholinergic agonist that stimulates parasympathetic muscarinic receptors
Side effects	Cramps, nausea, diarrhea, lacrimation, hypotension, sweating
Comments	Antidote for overdose is atropine 0.6 mg IV
Dose	10 to 50 mg PO three to four times a day

Biperiden (Akineton) (Chapter 25)

Indications	Parkinsonism, extrapyramidal reactions
Actions	Anticholinergic
Side effects	Dry mouth constipation, urinary retention, tachycardia, psychosis
Comments	Helpful for extrapyramidal reactions caused by neuroleptic agents
Dose	2 mg one to three times a day

Botulinum Toxin (Botox) (Chapter 25)

Indications	Focal dystonia, blepharospasm
Actions	Neuromuscular blocking agent
Side effects	Increased muscle weakness
Comments	Antibody-mediated tolerance may develop over time
Dose	1.25 to 2.50 units per injection site

Bromocriptine (Parlodel) (Chapters 20 and 25)

Indications	Parkinson's disease, neuroleptic malignant syndrome
Actions	Dopamine agonist
Side effects	Nausea, headache, dizziness, fatigue, vomiting
Comments	May delay the need for levodopa
Dose	2.5 mg to 10 mg three times a day

Capsaicin (Zostrix) (Chapter 18)

| Indications | Painful peripheral neuropathy |

Actions	Topical analgesic; probable substance P mediator in sensory neurons
Side effects	None significant
Comments	Now available without prescription
Dose	0.025% or 0.075% cream, apply topically three to four times a day

Carbamazepine (Tegretol) (Chapters 24 and 26)

Indications	Partial and generalized seizures, trigeminal neuralgia, neuropathic pain
Actions	Reduces polysynaptic responses and blocks post-tetanic potentiation
Side effects	Double or blurred vision, dizziness, vertigo, gastrointestinal upset, diarrhea, rare agranulocytosis, syndrome of inappropriate antidiuretic hormone, rash
Comments	Half-life of 10 to 35 hours; drug levels needed for anticonvulsant use are 4 to 12 $\mu g/ml$; raises levels of phenytoin, lowers levels of valproate
Dose	300 to 1600 mg daily in divided doses three to four times a day; usual starting dose is 200 mg three times a day; Tegretol XR (100, 200, 400 mg caps) can be given twice a day

Clonazepam (Klonopin) (Chapter 25)

Indications	Tourette's syndrome, tics, anxiety, seizures
Actions	Benzodiazepine sedative-hypnotic drug
Side effects	Sedation
Comments	May be habit forming
Dose	1 to 10 mg per day, divided, two to three times a day

Clopidogrel (Plavix) (Chapter 24)

Indications	Secondary stroke prevention
Actions	Platelet aggregation inhibitor
Side effects	Dyspepsia, thrombotic thrombocytopenic purpura (rare)
Comments	Also reduces risk of fatal and nonfatal vascular events in patients with MI or peripheral vascular disease
Dose	75 mg once a day

Cyproheptadine (Periactin) (Chapter 14)

Indications	Migraine prophylaxis
Actions	Serotonin and histamine antagonist
Side effects	Dizziness, drowsiness, decreased coordination

Appendix B **401**

Comments	Second line of therapy; contraindicated with monoamine oxidase inhibitors, closed-angle glaucoma, pyloric or bladder obstruction
Dose	4 to 8 mg PO three times a day

Dantrolene (Dantrium) (Chapter 20)

Indications	Neuroleptic malignant syndrome
Actions	Direct-acting skeletal muscle relaxant
Side effects	Pulmonary edema, thrombophlebitis
Comments	Approved by Food and Drug Administration for use in malignant hyperthermia; use in neuroleptic malignant syndrome described in medical literature
Dose	1 to 10 mg/kg IV every 4 to 6 hours

Dexamethasone (Decadron) (Chapters 5, 7, and 23)

Indications	Spinal cord compression, neoplasm or abscess of the brain or spinal cord, acute bacterial meningitis
Actions	Anti-inflammatory agent
Side effects	Peptic ulcer disease, sodium and fluid retention, hypertension, hyperglycemia, myopathy, impaired wound healing, avascular necrosis of femoral or humeral heads, endocrine abnormalities
Comments	Reduces vasogenic edema but not cytotoxic edema
Dose	For spinal neoplasm: 100 mg IV bolus; for intracranial mass: 4 to 10 mg IV every 6 hours

Diazepam (Valium) (Chapters 4 and 8)

Indications	Seizures, anxiety, alcohol withdrawal
Actions	Benzodiazepine
Side effects	Sedation, hypotension, respiratory depression, paradoxical agitation
Comments	May be administered IV, PO, or rectally as a gel; patients with history of benzodiazepine use or ethanol abuse may have cross-tolerance, requiring higher doses; habit forming with chronic use
Dose	For ongoing seizure or status epilepticus: 5 mg IV push, repeat every 5 minutes up to 20 mg; for ongoing seizures at home, rectal gel 2.5, 5, 10, or 20 mg via syringe for agitation, anxiety, or ethanol withdrawal: 2 to 10 mg PO or IV every 4 hours.

Diphenhydramine (Benadryl) (Chapter 18)

Indications	Acute drug-induced dystonic reaction, insomnia
Actions	Antihistamine and anticholinergic

Side effects	Drowsiness, dizziness, dry mouth, urinary retention
Comments	Avoid use in elderly, confused patients: may have CNS side effects
Dose	For dystonic reaction: 50 mg IV or IM, may repeat after several minutes; for insomnia: 25 to 50 mg PO per day at night

Donepezil Hydrochloride (Aricept) (Chapter 18)

Indications	Alzheimer's disease
Actions	Cholinesterase inhibitor
Side effects	Nausea, diarrhea
Comments	May promote GI bleeding in patients with peptic ulcer disease
Dose	5 mg to 10 mg PO per day

Edrophonium (Tensilon) (Chapter 15)

Indications	Evaluation for myasthenia gravis
Actions	Short-acting anticholinesterase (cholinergic action)
Side effects	Nausea, bradycardia, arrhythmias
Comments	Atropine 0.4 mg should be kept at the bedside to reverse adverse cholinergic side effects
Dose	2 mg IV test dose, then 8 mg IV after 45 seconds

Ergotamine (Dihydroergotamine or D.H.E. 45 IV or IM injection; with caffeine: Cafergot, Wigraine) (Chapter 14)

Indications	Migraine (abortive therapy)
Actions	Alpha-adrenergic/serotonin antagonist; cranial vasoconstrictor
Side effects	Precordial tightness, myalgias, paresthesias, nausea
Comments	D.H.E. 45 may require pretreatment with metoclopramide 10 mg IV or IM and promethazine 50 mg IV as antiemetic; contraindicated in complicated migraine or patients with coronary artery disease
Dose	1 tablet PO at onset, then repeat every 30 minutes up to 6 tabs; alternatively, 1 suppository PR, may repeat one time; D.H.E. 45: 1 mg IV or IM, repeat in 1 hour if needed

Ethosuximide (Zarontin) (Chapter 26)

Indications	Absence seizures
Actions	Anticonvulsant
Side effects	Drowsiness, gastrointestinal (GI) upset, anorexia, headache, dizziness, hiccups

Comments	Pediatric population
Dose	250 mg PO per day (ages 3 to 6), 500 mg PO per day if over 6 years of age

Felbamate (Felbatol) (Chapter 26)

Indications	Adjunctive therapy for Lennox-Gastaut syndrome
Actions	Anticonvulsant
Side effects	Aplastic anemia (can be fatal), hepatotoxicity, anorexia, headache, insomnia, somnolence
Comments	Use only with written informed consent due to risk of potentially fatal hepatotoxicty
Dose	400 mg PO three times a day, taper up to 3600 mg per day; in pediatric patients: begin 15 mg/kg per day

Fludrocortisone (Florinef) (Chapter 16)

Indications	Orthostatic hypotension
Action	Potent mineralocorticoid
Side effects	Volume overload, congestive heart failure, hypertension, edema
Comments	The lowest possible effective dose should be used
Dose	0.1 mg PO one to three times per day

Fosphenytoin (Chapter 4)

Indications	Status epilepticus
Actions	Anticonvulsant
Side effects	Nystagmus, ataxia, cardiac arrhythmias, hypotension
Comments	Phenytoin pro-drug that is rapidly converted to phenytoin within minutes; causes less hypertension than IV phenytoin; can also be given IM
Dose	15 to 20 mg/kg IV load infused at 50 mg per minute

Gabapentin (Neurontin) (Chapter 4)

Indications	Adjunctive therapy in adult epilepsy, neuropathic pain
Actions	Anticonvulsant
Side effects	Somnolence, dizziness, ataxia, fatigue, nystagmus
Comments	Useful for partial-onset seizures; renally cleared with no drug interactions, and very safe; FDA approved for painful diabetic peripheral neuropathy
Dose	Taper from 100 to 300 mg PO three times a day over a few days; average dose is 300 to 900 mg three times a day to a maximum of 1600 mg three times a day

Glatiramer (Copaxone) (Chapter 21)

Indications	Relapsing-remitting multiple sclerosis
Actions	Immune modulator
Side effects	Injection-site pain, vasodilation, chest pain, weakness
Comments	Reduces frequency and severity of MS episodes; in 10% of patients, transient weakness, flushing, and palpitations may occur after injection
Dose	20 mg injected SC every day

Glycopyrrolate (Robinul) (Chapter 15)

Indications	Control of secretions in myasthenia gravis or bulbar amyotrophic lateral sclerosis
Actions	Anticholinergic (antimuscarinic) agent
Side effects	Anticholinergic: decreased sweating, urinary retention, tachycardia, blurred vision
Dose	1 to 2 mg PO three times a day

Haloperidol (Haldol) (Chapters 8 and 25)

Indications	Psychosis, acute agitation, Tourette's syndrome, Huntington's disease
Actions	Antipsychotic neuroleptic butyrophenone
Side effects	Sedation, extrapyramidal effects (acute or with chronic use), galactorrhea, jaundice, neuroleptic malignant syndrome
Comments	Extrapyramidal effects may occur acutely or with chronic use
Dose	For agitation or acute psychosis: 2 to 10 mg IM, may repeat every hour; for chronic agitation or psychosis: 0.5 to 2 mg PO two to three times a day

Heparin (Chapters 6, 11, and 24)

Indications	Acute embolic or progressing stroke, transient ischemic attack
Actions	Antithrombin effect; acts in conjunction with antithrombin III
Side effects	Hemorrhage, thrombocytopenia
Comments	Monitor aPTT, usually to a target of 1.5 to 2 times control
Dose	20,000 units in 500 ml D5W at 20 ml per hour (800 units per hour maintenance, no bolus)

Immune Globulin (IVIG) (Chapters 17 and 20)

Indications	Guillain-Barré syndrome (GBS), chronic inflammatory demyelinating polyneuropathy (CIDP), myasthenia gravis
Actions	Immunosuppressive
Side effects	Renal failure, aseptic meningitis, anaphylaxis, hyperviscosity syndrome, leukopenia
Comments	Hydrate patient well to avoid renal toxicity
Dose	For GBS: 0.4 g/kg IV per day for 5 days; for CIPD 0.4 g/kg IV weekly

Interferon Beta-1a (Avonex) (Chapter 21)

Indications	Relapsing-remitting multiple sclerosis
Actions	Cytokine, immune modulator
Side effcts	Flu-like symptoms, muscle ache, fevers, chills, weakness
Comments	Reduces frequency and severity of MS episodes; use with caution in patients with depression or seizures
Dose	30 μg injected IM once a week

Interferon Beta-1b (Betaseron) (Chapter 21)

Indications	Relapsing-remitting multiple sclerosis (MS)
Actions	Antiviral, immunoregulatory agent
Side effects	Injection site pain and inflammation, influenza-like symptoms, headache
Comments	Reduces frequency and severity of MS episodes
Dose	0.3 mg (9.6 million IU [one vial]) SC every other day

Lamotrigine (Lamictal) (Chapter 26)

Indications	Partial-onset or generalized epilepsy
Actions	Anticonvulsant
Side effects	Rash (including Stevens-Johnson syndrome), dizziness, ataxia, nausea, vomiting, somnolence, headache, insomnia
Comments	Dose must be reduced with concurrent phenytoin, carbamazepine, or phenobarbital; risk of rash is especially high when given with valproic acid, or in children
Dose	Start 50 mg PO per day for 14 days, then 50 mg two times a day for 14 days, up to 150 mg to 250 mg two times a day

Levetiracetam (Keppra) (Chapter 26)

Indications	Add-on for partial-onset seizures in adults
Actions	Antiepileptic
Side effects	Sedation, dizziness, behavioral, infection (mostly mild URIs)
Comment	Primarily renal excretion. No drug interactions. May help for primary generalized seizures also.
Dose	1000 to 3000 mg daily divided twice a day; start at 500 mg twice a day

Levodopa-Carbidopa (Sinemet, Sinemet CR) (Chapter 25)

Indications	Parkinson's disease
Actions	Levodopa is converted to dopamine in the basal ganglia; carbidopa inhibits dopamine production (dopa decarboxylation) in the periphery
Side effects	Dyskinesias: dystonia, chorea; confusion, paranoia
Comments	Dosing highly dependent on clinical response; top number denotes milligrams of carbidopa, bottom number denotes milligrams of levodopa; controlled-release preparation (CR) may mediate on/off changes; available in 10/100, 25/100, 25/250, and 50/200 (CR)
Dose	Start with 25/100 tablets three times a day, taper up as clinically indicated

Lidocaine Patch 5% (Lidoderm transdermal patch) (Chapter 17)

Indications	Postherpetic neuralgia
Action	Local anesthetic, inhibits sodium channels
Side effects	Local skin irritation
Comment	Apply only to intact skin
Dose	Apply to cover painful areas, may use up to three patches at a time, for up to 12 hours daily

Lorazepam (Ativan) (Chapters 4 and 8)

Indications	Ongoing seizure or status epilepticus, anxiety
Actions	Benzodiazepine sedative, anxiolytic; anticonvulsant
Side effects	Drowsiness, respiratory depression
Comments	Habit forming
Dose	For status epilepticus: 0.1 mg/kg IV given versus repeated 2-µg boluses; for anxiety 0.5 to 2 mg PO two times a day

Mannitol (Osmitrol) (Chapter 12)

Indications	Increased intracranial pressure
Actions	Osmotic diuretic
Side effects	Hypotension, dehydration, hyponatremia, hyperosmolar renal tubular damage, CHF exacerbation
Comments	Rebound intracranial hypertension with prolonged administration; monitor serum osmolality, electrolytes, and fluid balance
Dose	0.25 to 1.5 g/kg of 20% solution (20 g per 100 ml), repeat every 1 to 6 hours

Meclizine (Antivert) (Chapter 13)

Indications	Benign positional vertigo, labyrinthitis
Actions	Antihistamine
Side effects	Drowsiness, dry mouth, blurred vision
Comments	Efficacy in about 50% of patients
Dose	12.5 to 25 mg PO three times a day

Methylprednisolone (Solu-Medrol) (Chapters 11, 14, and 20)

Indications	Traumatic spinal cord injury, multiple sclerosis exacerbation, inflammatory optic neuritis, pseudotumor cerebri
Actions	Anti-inflammatory/immunosuppressive agent
Side effects	Peptic ulcer disease, sodium and fluid retention, hypertension, hyperglycemia, myopathy, impaired wound healing, avascular necrosis of femoral or humeral heads, endocrine abnormalities
Comments	Stronger mineralocorticoid effect than dexamethasone or prednisone
Dose	For multiple sclerosis and inflammatory optic neuritis: 1 g IVSS per day for 5 to 10 days, followed by prednisone taper; for traumatic cord injury: 30 mg/kg IV bolus over 15 minutes, then 45-minute pause, and then 5.4 mg/kg per hour continuous IV infusion over next 23 hours; for pseudotumor cerebri: 250 mg IVSS four times a day

Methysergide (Sansert) (Chapter 14)

Indications	Migraine prophylaxis
Actions	Serotonin antagonist
Side effects	Retroperitoneal and pleuropulmonary fibrosis, nausea, vomiting, drowsiness, insomnia, hallucinations

Comments	Should not be used for 2 to 6 months after 6 months of use
Dose	2 mg PO one to three times a day

Midazolam (Versed) (Chapters 4 and 15)

Indications	Agitation while on ventilator, refractory status epilepticus
Actions	Short-action benzodiazepine sedative-hypnotic
Side effects	Drowsiness, respiratory depression, hypotension
Comments	Rapid acting, with very short half-life
Dose	For sedation: 1 to 2 mg IV/IM every 30 to 60 minutes; for status epilepticus: 0.1 to 0.3 mg/kg IV push load, then maintenance of 0.05 to 0.4 mg/kg per hour

Midodrine (ProAmatine) (Chapter 16)

Indications	Orthostatic hypotension
Actions	Alpha receptor agonist
Side effects	Supine hypertension, paresthesias, pruritus
Comments	Last dose should be given no later than 6 PM to avoid nocturnal supine hypertension
Dose	10 mg PO three times per day

Modafinil (Provigil) (Chapter 21)

Indications	Narcolepsy, fatigue in MS, abulia
Actions	Stimulant
Side effects	Headache, nausea, diarrhea, dry mouth, anorexia
Comments	May impair thinking or motor skills
Dose	100 to 200 mg PO once a day

Naloxone (Narcan) (Chapter 5)

Indications	Suspected narcotic coma
Actions	Narcotic antagonist
Side effects	Nausea, vomiting, may precipitate withdrawal in narcotic addicts
Comments	Reversal of narcotic coma may wear off after 1 to 2 hours
Dose	0.4 to 2.0 mg IV, IM, or SC every 5 minutes to a maximum dose of 10 mg

Naratriptan (Amerge) (Chapter 14)

Indications	Migraine (abortive therapy)
Actions	Selective serotonin agonist
Side effects	Paresthesias, dizziness, drowsiness, fatigue, throat tightness
Comments	Longer duration of action than other riptans, but slower onset and lower efficacy rate; contraindicated in patients with coronary artery disease
Dose	1 or 2.5 mg, may repeat after 4 hours, maximum 5 mg daily

Neostigmine (Prostigmin) (Chapter 15)

Indications	Myasthenia gravis
Actions	Acetylcholinesterase inhibitor
Side effects	Abdominal cramps, diarrhea, salivation, fasciculations
Comments	Has longer duration of action than does pyridostigmine
Dose	15 mg to 90 mg PO four times a day; 0.5 to 1.0 mg IV or IM every 2 to 3 hours

Nimodipine (Nimotop) (Chapter 24)

Indications	Subarachnoid hemorrhage
Actions	Calcium-channel blocker with CNS penetration
Side effects	Hypotension
Comments	Reduces the frequency of delayed ischemia from vasospasm by 30%
Dose	60 mg every 4 hours for 21 days

Oxcarbazepine (Trileptal) (Chapter 26)

Indications	Monotherapy or add-on for partial-onset seizures in adults; add-on for kids ages 4 years or older
Actions	Antiepileptic; sodium-channel blocker
Side effects	Dizziness, sedation, nausea, vomiting, diplopia, rash, hyponatremia
Comment	Similar to carbamazepine but fewer side effects and fewer drug interactions; active ingredient is the 10-monohydroxy metabolite
Dose	300 to 3600 mg a day divided in two doses (usually need 150% of carbamazepine dose)

Oxybutynin (Ditropan) (Chapter 21)

Indications	Bladder spasticity (detrusor dysynergia), e.g., in multiple sclerosis

Actions	Smooth muscle antispasmodic, antimuscarinic
Side effects	Palpitations, decreased sweating, dry mouth, dizziness, urinary retention, constipation
Comments	Contraindicated in patients with obstructive uropathy
Dose	5 mg PO two to three times a day

Pramipexole (Mirepex) (Chapter 25)

Indications	Parkinson's disease
Actions	Dopamine agonist
Side effects	Hallucinations, dizziness, somnolence, nausea
Comments	Can be used alone or in combination with levodopa
Dose	0.125 mg three times daily, increase weekly to a maximum of 1.5 mg three times a day

Pemoline (Cylert) (Chapter 21)

Indications	Narcolepsy, abulia after brain injury, attention deficit disorder
Actions	CNS stimulant
Side effects	Insomnia, anorexia, weight loss, seizure, dyskinesias, hallucinations, rare aplastic anemia
Comments	Contraindicated in patients with impaired hepatic function
Dose	18.75 mg PO every day, taper weekly as indicated up to maximum of 75 mg per day

Penicillamine (Cuprimine) (Chapter 25)

Indications	Wilson's disease
Actions	Copper chelator
Side effects	Lupus-like rash, polyarteritis, leukopenia, thrombocytopenia, epigastric pain, nausea, diarrhea, nephrotic syndrome, tinnitus, neuropathy
Comments	May precipitate myasthenia gravis
Dose	125 to 1000 mg per day, divided, two to four times a day

Pentobarbital (Chapter 4)

Indications	Status epilepticus, increased intracranial pressure
Actions	Anticonvulsant, sedative
Side effects	Respiratory suppression, sedation, hypotension
Comments	EEG monitoring indicated; hypotension may require pressors. Levels of 25 to 35 mg/L are generally suffi-

	cient to control intracranial pressure; levels of <5 mg/L are compatible with a clinical diagnosis of brain death
Dose	5 to 20 mg/kg IV load, 1 to 4 mg/kg per hour maintenance

Pergolide (Permax) (Chapter 25)

Indications	Parkinson's disease
Actions	Dopamine agonist
Side effects	Nausea, headache, dizziness, fatigue, vomiting
Comments	May delay onset or reduce required dose of levodopa
Dose	0.75 to 3.0 mg per day, divided, three to four times a day

Phenobarbital (Chapter 4)

Indications	Epilepsy, status epilepticus
Actions	Anticonvulsant
Side effects	Sedation, respiratory suppression, hypotension, behavioral changes, hyperactivity
Comments	For chronic therapy, therapeutic range is 20 to 40 µg/ml; lowers levels of phenytoin, carbamazepine, and valproate
Dose	For status epilepticus: 10 to 20 mg/kg IV load infused at 100 mg/min; for epilepsy 60 mg PO two to three times a day; for pediatric patients: 3 to 6 mg/kg per day

Phenytoin (Chapter 4)

Indications	Epilepsy, status epilepticus
Actions	Anticonvulsant
Side effects	Nystagmus, ataxia, gingival hyperplasia, hirsutism, rash, adenopathy, liver function test abnormalities
Comments	For chronic therapy, therapeutic range is 10 to 20 µg/ml; lowers levels of carbamazepine and valproate and increases or decreases phenobarbital level
Dose	Typical maintenance dose is 300 mg every day at night

Pimozide (Orap) (Chapter 25)

Indications	Tourette's syndrome
Actions	Piperidine antipsychotic
Side effects	Dry mouth, sedation, dyskinesias, akinesia, behavioral effects, prolongation of QT interval

Comments	None
Dose	Start with 1 mg PO two times a day, up to 2 to 10 mg per day in divided doses

Prednisone (Chapter 11)

Indications	Temporal arteritis, Bell's palsy
Actions	Anti-inflammatory agent
Side effects	Peptic ulcer disease, sodium and fluid retention, hypertension, hyperglycemia, myopathy, impaired wound healing, avascular necrosis of femoral or humeral heads, endocrine abnormalities, increased susceptibility to infection
Comments	Initiate therapy as soon as diagnosis is suspected to avoid irreversible visual loss
Dose	100 mg PO per day, tapered slowly to alternate-day therapy over several weeks

Primidone (Mysoline) (Chapters 4 and 25)

Indications	Generalized tonic-clonic epilepsy, essential tremor
Actions	Anticonvulsant
Side effects	Ataxia, vertigo, nausea, anorexia, vomiting, irritability, sedation
Comments	Second line of therapy; metabolized to phenobarbital
Dose	Start with 100 to 125 mg PO once a day, taper up to 250 mg three to four times a day

Propantheline Bromide (Pro-Banthine) (Chapter 15)

Indications	Control of secretions in myasthenia gravis
Actions	Antimuscarinic agent
Side effects	Anticholinergic: decreased sweating, urinary retention, tachycardia, blurred vision
Comments	None
Dose	15 mg PO four times a day

Propranolol (Inderal) (Chapters 14 and 25)

Indications	Benign essential tremor, migraine prophylaxis
Actions	Nonspecific beta-adrenergic blocker
Side effects	Hypotension, bradycardia, bronchospasm, may mask symptoms of hypoglycemia, impotence
Comments	Avoid use in asthmatics and diabetics
Dose	For tremor: 40 to 240 mg PO per day, divided, three to four times a day; for migraine 20 to 40 mg per day

Pyridostigmine (Mestinon) (Chapter 15)

Indications	Myasthenia gravis
Actions	Acetylcholinesterase inhibitor
Side effects	Excess salivation, pulmonary secretions, diarrhea
Comments	Muscarinic side effects controlled by glycopyrrolate or propantheline bromide
Dose	Start at 30 mg PO three times a day, up to 120 mg every 3 to 6 hours

Riluzole (Rilutek) (Chapter 20)

Indications	Amyotrophic lateral sclerosis
Actions	Glutamate antagonist
Side effects	Malaise, abdominal pain, nausea, dizziness, circumoral numbness, liver function abnormalities
Comments	May extend survival 60 to 90 days and delay time to intubation; avoid use in patients with liver dysfunction
Dose	50 mg PO two times a day

Rizatriptan (Maxalt) (Chapter 14)

Indications	Migraine (abortive therapy)
Actions	Selective serotonin agonist
Side effects	Weakness, fatigue, chest or throat pressure, dizziness, somnolence
Comments	Faster acting and slightly more effective than other triptans, but more likely to cause side effects. Contraindicated in patients with coronary artery disease.
Dose	5 to 10 mg, may repeat in 2 hours, maximum 30 mg daily

Ropinirole (Requip) (Chapter 25)

Indications	Parkinson's disease
Actions	Dopamine agonist
Side effects	Syncope, hallucinations, dyskinesias, nausea, dizziness, somnolence, headache
Comments	May be used alone or in combination with levodopa
Dose	0.25 mg three times daily

Selegiline (Eldepryl) (Chapter 25)

Indications	Parkinson's disease
Actions	Monoamine oxidase B inhibitor: antioxidant
Side effects	Nausea, dizziness, confusion, hallucinations
Comments	Thought to slow progression of disease

| Dose | Taper up to 5 mg PO two times a day |

Sumatriptan (Imitrex) (Chapter 14)

Indications	Migraine (abortive therapy)
Actions	Selective serotonin agonist
Side effects	Coronary vasospasm, tingling, flushing, tightness in jaw, neck, and chest, dizziness, injection site reaction
Comments	Contraindicated in patients with coronary artery disease
Dose	6 mg SC, may repeat in 1 hour, maximum 12 mg per day, 6 doses per month; 25 mg PO, may repeat up to 100 mg in 2 hours

Tacrine (Cognex) (Chapter 18)

Indications	Alzheimer's disease
Actions	Reversible cholinesterase inhibitor
Side effects	Nausea, vomiting, diarrhea, abdominal pain, fatigue, agitation, confusion
Comments	May improve cognitive scores in some patients
Dose	Start 10 mg PO three times a day, tapering up to 30 mg three times a day

Thiamine (Chapters 4 and 8)

Indications	Coma, thiamine deficiency neuropathy
Actions	Enzymatic cofactor in oxidative metabolism (thiamine pyrophosphate)
Side effects	None
Comments	Give with glucose in setting of coma to prevent Wernicke's encephalopathy
Dose	For coma: 100 mg IV push; 100 mg PO or IM for 3 days

Tiagabine (Gabitril) (Chapter 26)

Indications	Add-on for partial-onset seizures in adults
Actions	Antiepileptic; GABA-reuptake inhibitor
Side effects	Sedation, cognitive dysfunction, dizziness, nausea, vomiting, tremor, anxiety
Comment	Highly protein-bound
Dose	4 to 56 mg daily, divided two to four times a day

Ticlopidine (Ticlid) (Chapter 24)

Indications	Secondary stroke prevention
Actions	Platelet aggregation inhibitor

Side effects	Neutropenia, diarrhea, rash, nausea, vomiting, thrombotic thrombocytopenic purpura
Comments	Check CBC every 2 weeks during the first 3 months of treatment
Dose	250 mg twice a day

Tissue Plasminogen Activator (t-PA) (Chapters 6 and 24)

Indications	Hyperacute ischemic stroke
Actions	Thrombolytic
Side effects	Intracerebral hemorrhage
Comments	Must be given within 3 hours of stroke onset; increases chance of full recovery or minimal residual deficit at 3 months by 33%; patients with acute hemorrhage, uncontrolled hypertension ($>180/105$ mm Hg), or those on anticoagulant therapy should be excluded
Dose	0.9 mg/kg IV (10% IV push, then infuse the remaining 90% over 1 hour), maximum dose 90 mg

Tolcapone (Tasmar) (Chapter 25)

Indications	Parkinson's disease
Actions	Catechol-O-methyltransferase (COMT) inhibitor
Side effects	Fulminant hepatic failure (may be fatal), dyskinesias, nausea, sleep disorders, anorexia, somnolence
Comments	Should be reserved for patients with symptom fluctuations on levodopa who do not respond to other adjunctive agents; withdraw if no substantial benefit is seen after 3 weeks
Dose	100 to 200 mg three times daily

Topiramate (Topamax) (Chapter 26)

Indications	Add-on for partial-onset or primary generalized seizures
Actions	Antiepileptic, weak carbonic-anhydrase inhibitor
Side effects	Sedation, cognitive dysfunction, anorexia, dizziness, paresthesias, ataxia, renal stones
Comment	Probably effective for all seizure types; mostly renal excretion
Dose	Start 25 to 50 mg per day; maintenance 100 to 600 mg per day divided in two doses; 1 to 10 mg/kg per day in children; also available in sprinkles

Trihexyphenidyl HCl (Artane) (Chapter 25)

Indications	Parkinson's disease, idiopathic torsion dystonia
Actions	Anticholinergic
Side effects	Visual blurring, dry mouth, urinary retention
Comments	May be effective in treating parkinsonian tremor; botu-

	linum toxin has largely replaced anticholinergics for the treatment of focal dystonias
Dose	1 to 15 mg PO per day, divided, three to four times a day

Valproic Acid (Depakote, Depakene [syrup], Depacon [IV]) (Chapter 4)

Indications	Partial or generalized seizures, migraine prophylaxis
Actions	Anticonvulsant
Side effects	Nausea, weight gain, hair loss, tremor, hepatitis, agranulocytosis, thrombocytopenia, Stevens-Johnson syndrome
Comments	Therapeutic range is 50 to 100 µg/ml; increases levels of carbamazepine, phenytoin, and lamotrigine
Dose	250 to 2000 mg PO four times a day; 5 to 15 mg/kg IV every 6 hours

Warfarin (Coumadin) (Chapters 6 and 24)

Indications	Stroke prophylaxis
Actions	Inhibits vitamin K–dependent clotting factors
Side effects	Hemorrhage, rash
Comments	Used for secondary stroke prevention in cardioembolic stroke and in large vessel atherosclerosis when antiplatelet therapy has failed; used for primary stroke prevention in atrial fibrillation; close monitoring of prothrombin times (PT or International Normalized Ratios [INRs]) required
Dose	Begin with 4 mg PO per day, with dose adjusted according to target PT/INR

Zolmitriptan (Zomig) (Chapter 14)

Indications	Migraine (abortive therapy)
Actions	Selective serotonin agonist
Side effects	Paresthesias, nausea, neck or chest tightness, dry mouth, somnolence
Comments	May be useful for keeping headaches away in patients with early recurrence after sumatriptan; contraindicated in patients with coronary artery disease
Dose	2.5 mg may repeat after 2 hours, maximum 10 mg daily

Zolpidem (Ambien) (Chapter 18)

Indication	Insomnia
Action	Sedative
Side effects	Confusion in the elderly
Comments	Do not use for benzodiazepine or ethanol withdrawal

Dose	5 to 10 mg at night

Zonisamide (Zonegran) (Chapter 26)

Indications	Add-on for partial-onset seizures in adults
Actions	Antiepileptic, weak carbonic anhydrase inhibitor
Side effects	Sedation, dizziness, anorexia, irritability, rash, kidney stones
Comments	Sulfa drug; mostly renal excretion; may help for absence seizures and for other generalized seizures
Dose	100 to 600 mg daily, divided twice a day

INDEX

Note: Page numbers in *italics* refer to illustrations. Page numbers followed by the letter b refer to boxed material; those followed by t refer to tables.

A

Abdomen, in amnesia/dementia evaluation, 230
  in ataxia/gait failure evaluation, 130
  in dizziness/vertigo evaluation, 164
  in head injury evaluation, 120
  in pain syndrome evaluation, 218
Abdominal reflexes, in neurologic examination, 26
Abducens (VI) nerve, in neurologic examination, 19
Abduction nystagmus, 165t
Abductor digiti minimi manus muscle, 390t
Abductor pollicis brevis muscle, 391t
Abductor pollicis longus muscle, 391t
Abscess, brain, 293
  spinal epidural, 295
Absence epilepsy, childhood, 353, 355
  juvenile, 355
Absence seizures, 351
Abstract reasoning, in mental status examination, 14t
Acetaminophen, for headache, 170
  for migraine headache, 178t
  in increased intracranial pressure management, 157
  with codeine, for brachial neuritis, 227
  for root compression, 224
Acetazolamide, for epilepsy, 360t
  for pseudotumor cerebri, 149
  information summary on, 404
Acetylcholine receptor antibodies, in myasthenia gravis diagnosis, 196
Acetylsalicylic acid (ASA), for migraine headache, 178t
  for transient global amnesia, 238
  for transient ischemic attacks, 330b
  for transient monocular blindness, 148
Acidosis, metabolic, in stupor/coma, 65
Acoustic neuromas, 312–313
  evoked potentials in, 43
Acquired immunodeficiency syndrome (AIDS). See also *HIV* entries.
  neurologic complications of, 299–301
Activity, in stroke management, 91
Acyclovir, for Bell's palsy, 256
  for herpes simplex encephalitis, 297
  for herpes zoster in AIDS, 300
  for herpetic neuralgia, 222
Adductor brevis muscle, 393t
Adductor longus muscle, 393t
Adductor magnus muscle, 393t
Adductor pollicis muscle, 390t
Adenomas, pituitary, 313–314
  binocular visual loss from, 139
Adventitial movements, in amnesia/dementia evaluation, 232–233
  in neurologic examination, 22
Advil, for migraine headache, 178t
Affect, in mental status examination, 14t
Afferent pupillary defect, in neurologic examination, 19–20
  in vision disturbance evaluation, 143
Age, in acute visual disturbance evaluation, 137–138

420 Index

Age *(Continued)*
  in neurologic history, 4–5
Aggrenox, information summary on, 405
Agitation, treatment of, 107–108, 108t
AIDS (acquired immunodeficiency syndrome). See also *HIV* entries.
  neurologic complications of, 299–301
AIDS dementia complex, 300–301
  treatment of, 238
Airway, in head injury evaluation, 119
  in headache evaluation, 172
  in neuromuscular respiratory failure evaluation, 187–188
  management of, 191–193
  in stroke evaluation, 79
  in syncope evaluation, 205
  protection of, for comatose patient, 72
  reassessment of, in severe head injury management, 123
Akathisia, causes of, 349
  description of, 343
Akinetic mutism, 71–72
Akinetic seizures, syncope from, 210
Akineton, information summary on, 406
Albendazole, for cysticercosis, 296
Alcohol. See *Ethanol*.
Alertness, in amnesia/dementia evaluation, 231
Alkalosis, respiratory, in stupor/coma, 65
Alprazolam, for agitation and delirium, 108t
ALS. See *Amyotrophic lateral sclerosis (ALS)*.
Alzheimer's disease, treatment of, 237
Amantadine, for fatigue in multiple sclerosis, 279
  for movement disorders, dosage of, 341t
  for Parkinson's disease, 345
  information summary on, 404
Amerge, for migraine, 179t
  information summary on, 409
Amitriptyline, for neuropathic pain, 264

Amitriptyline *(Continued)*
  for postherpetic neuralgia, 222
  in migraine prevention, 180t
  information summary on, 404–405
Amnesia, anterograde, 228
  bedside evaluation of, 230–233
  chart review in, 235–236
  definition of, 228
  differential diagnosis of, 229–230
  elevator thoughts on, 229–230
  from head injury, 121
  history of, selective, 235–236
  major threat to life in, 230
  management of, 234–239, 234–239
  neurologic examination in, 231–233
  phone call on, 228–229
  physical examination in, 230–233
  retrograde, 228
  transient global, treatment of, 238–239
Amphetamine, for pain syndromes, 219
Amphotericin B, for brain abscess, 294
  for fungal meningitis, 292
Ampicillin, for bacterial meningitis, 109, 175, 286, 288t
Amyloid angiopathy, cerebral, 338b
Amyotrophic lateral sclerosis (ALS), 251–252
Amyotrophy, diabetic, 262
  neuralgic, 227
Anal wink, in neurologic examination, 26
Anaplastic astrocytoma, 305
Anaprox, for migraine headache, 178t
Anatomic localization, 6–11
  in brain stem, 8–10, *9*
  in lower motor neuron system, 7–8
  in spinal cord, 10–11
  in upper motor neuron system, 7
Aneurysms, common sites of, *328*
  management of, 327–330, 329b, 330t

Angiography, cerebral, in subarachnoid hemorrhage evaluation, 327
 in brain death confirmation, 243
 magnetic resonance, 35
  in ataxia/gait failure evaluation, 135
  in stroke evaluation, 90
Angiopathy, cerebral amyloid, 338b
Angioplasty, carotid, for central retinal artery occlusion, 147–148
Angiitis, granulomatous, of brain, 334b
Anisocoria, in neurologic examination, 19
Anomic aphasia, 17t
Anterior cord syndrome, 99t
Anterograde amnesia, 228
 from head injury, 121
Antibiotics, in severe head injury management, 124
Anticholinesterase drugs, for myasthenia gravis, 199t
Anticoagulants, oral, in ischemic stroke management, 334, 336
Anticonvulsants, 359, 360t–366t
 in severe head injury management, 124
 overdose of, ataxia from, treatment of, 136
 prophylactic, 376
  for migraine, 180t
Antidepressants, tricyclic, for pain syndromes, 219
 in migraine prevention, 180t
Antiemetics, for migraine headache, 176
Antineoplastic drugs, toxicity of, 323, 323t
Antipsychotics, for agitation and delirium, 108t
Anti-serotonin drugs, in migraine prevention, 180t
Antivert, information summary on, 414
Anton's syndrome, 141t
Anxiety disorder, syncope in, 212
Aortic arch atherosclerosis, emboli from, 333
Aphasia(s), Broca's, 16, 17t
 classification of, 17t
 in amnesia/dementia evaluation, 231–232

Aphasia(s) *(Continued)*
 in seizure evaluation, 55
 Wernicke's, 16, 17t
Apnea, testing for, protocol in, 314b
Apneustic breathing, in stupor/coma, 65
Apoplexy, pituitary, 313
Apraxia, in amnesia/dementia evaluation, 232
Apraxic gait, 29t
Ara-C, for leptomeningeal metastases, 319
Arbovirus encephalitis, 298
Argyll Robertson pupils, in neurosyphilis, 290
Aricept, information summary on, 409
Arm(s), pain syndromes involving, 215
Arm drift, in head injury evaluation, 121
Arm-rolling test, for hemiparesis, 24
Arnold-Chiari malformation, spinal cord compression from, 94
Arrhythmia(s), during syncope, 204
 syncope from, 202
Artane, for idiopathic torsion dystonia, 347
 for movement disorders, dosage of, 341t
 for Parkinson's disease, 345
 information summary on, 415–416
Arteritic ischemic optic neuropathy, management of, 148
Arteritis, temporal, management of, 182–183
Artery(ies), retinal, central, occlusion of, management of, 147–148
 occlusion of, fundoscopic appearance of, 144t
 temporal, biopsy of, in temporal arteritis evaluation, 182–183
Arthritis, rheumatoid, spinal cord compression from, 95
ASA. See *Acetylsalicylic acid (ASA)*.
Ascriptin, information summary on, 405

Aspiration, during syncope, 204
Aspirin. See also *Acetylsalicylic acid (ASA)*.
 in ischemic stroke management, 337
 information summary on, 405
Asterixis, causes of, 349
 description of, 343
Astrocytoma(s), 302–306
 anaplastic, 305
 grade I to II, 305–306
 grade III, 305
 grade IV, 303–305
 low-grade, 305–306
Asymmetric horizontal nystagmus, 165t
Asymmetry, reflex, in seizure evaluation, 55
Ataxia, 126–136
 chart review in, 129–130
 diagnostic testing in, 135
 differential diagnosis of, 129t
 history in, selective, 129–130
 management of, 133–134, 135–136
 medications causing, 130t
 phone call on, 126–127
 physical examination in, 130–133, 134
 reversible causes of, treatment of, 136
 sensory, gait failure features in, 128t
Ataxic breathing, in stupor/coma, 65
Ataxic gait, 29t
Ataxic hemiparesis, 332
Atenolol, in migraine prevention, 180t
Atherosclerosis, aortic arch, emboli from, 333
 large-vessel, ischemic stroke from, 331–332
Athetosis, causes of, 349–350
 description of, 343
 gait failure features in, 128t
Ativan. See also *Lorazepam*.
 for agitation/delirium, 108t
 information summary on, 413
Atonic seizures, syncope from, 210
Atrophy, in motor neuron disease, 251
Atropine, in myasthenia gravis diagnosis, 196

Attention, in head injury evaluation, 121
 in mental status examination, 13–15
Attentiveness, in amnesia/dementia evaluation, 231
Audiography, in acoustic neuroma diagnosis, 312
Autoimmune disorders, delirium from, 103
Autonomic dysfunction, syncope from, 211
Autonomic neuropathy, 264
 from antineoplastic drugs, 323, 323t
Autoregulation, cerebral, 154, 155
Avonex, in multiple sclerosis management, 276, 278
 information summary on, 412
Axillary nerve, 395
Axonal shearing injury, from head trauma, 119
Azathioprine, for chronic inflammatory demyelinating polyneuropathy, 263
 for paraprotein-associated neuropathy, 263
 for polymyositis, 266
 information summary on, 405
AZT, for AIDS dementia complex, 238

B

Babinski's sign, 25–26
Back, in head injury evaluation, 120
 low, pain syndromes involving, 215
Baclofen, for idiopathic torsion dystonia, 347
 for movement disorders, dosage of, 341t
 for spasticity/pain in multiple sclerosis, 278
 for trigeminal neuralgia, 183
 information summary on, 405
Bacterial meningitis, 286
 antibiotic therapy for, 288t
 as threat to life, 171
 cerebrospinal fluid findings in, 287t
 delirium in, 104

Bacterial meningitis *(Continued)*
  diagnostic testing for, 174–175
  treatment of, 109
Balint's syndrome, 141t
"Ball-bearing eyes," in stupor/
  coma evaluation, 67–68
Ballismus, causes of, 350
  description of, 343
Bárány maneuver, 164, 166, *167*
Batson's vertebral venous plexus,
  metastatic spread via, 320
Bayer, information summary on,
  405
Becker muscular dystrophy, 268
Behavior, in mental status
  examination, 14t
Behavioral dysfunction, treatment
  of, 237
Behçet's disease, 284
  in pediatric patient, 384
Bell's palsy, 255–256
Benadryl, information summary
  on, 408–409
Benzathine penicillin, for
  neurosyphilis, 291
Benzodiazepines, for agitation and
  delirium, 108t
Benztropine, information
  summary on, 405–406
Berry aneurysm, diplopia from,
  141
Beta blockers, for vasovagal
  syncope, 209
  in migraine prevention, 180t
Betaseron, for multiple sclerosis,
  276
  information summary on, 412
Bethanechol chloride, for bladder
  dysfunction in multiple
  sclerosis, 279
  information summary on, 406
Biceps brachii muscle, testing,
  roots, and innervation of, 390t
Biceps femoris muscle, testing,
  roots, and innervation of, 393t
Biopsy, brain, 43
  muscle, 43
  nerve, 43, 262t
  temporal artery, 182–183
Biot's breathing, in stupor/coma,
  65
Biperiden, information summary
  on, 406
Birth trauma, 378, 380–381

Bladder care, for neuromuscular
  respiratory failure, 193
  in stroke management, 91
  in stupor/coma, 73
Bladder dysfunction, in multiple
  sclerosis, 278–279
Blindness, monocular, transient,
  148
Blood pressure, in headache
  evaluation, 172
  in neuromuscular respiratory
    failure evaluation, 188
  in stroke evaluation, 79–80
  in syncope evaluation, 205
  monitoring of, in severe head in-
    jury management, 123
Blood tests, in amnesia/dementia
  diagnosis, 236
  in spinal cord compression eval-
    uation, 97
Blood vessels, disorders of. See
  Vascular disorders.
  large, stenosis of, ischemic
    stroke from, 331–332
  small, disease of, ischemic
    stroke from, 332
Bone marrow transplantation,
  toxic effects of, 323–324
Bonnet's syndrome, 141t
Border-zone infarction, 86, *87*
Botox, for idiopathic torsion
  dystonia, 347
  information summary on, 406
Botulinum toxin, for idiopathic
  torsion dystonia, 347
  information summary on, 406
Botulism, respiratory failure in,
  198, 200
Bowel care, for neuromuscular
  respiratory failure, 193
  in stupor/coma, 73
Brachial plexopathy, 253–254
Brachial neuralgia, 227
Brachial neuritis, 227
Brachial plexus, *395*
  injuries to, as birth trauma, 378
  muscles of, 390t–391t
Brachialis muscle, 390t
Brachioradialis muscle, 391t
Bradykinesia, description of, 343
Brain, abscess of, 293
  biopsy of, 43
  granulomatous angiitis of, 334b
  herniation of, stupor/coma
    from, 61

Brain *(Continued)*
  injury to. See also *Head, injury to.*
    focal, gait failure features in, 128t
  metastases to, 316, 318
  surface map of, *401*
  tumors of, glial, 302–308
    nonglial, 308–316
Brain death, 240–245
  clinical diagnosis of, criteria for, 240–242
  clinical significance of, 240
  confirmatory testing for, 243
  EEG in, 42
  in pediatric patient, 387–388
  potential organ donor management and, 244–245
  psychosocial issues in, 243–244
Brain stem, compression of, stupor/coma from, 61
  encephalitis of, 317t
  lesions of, evoked potentials in, 43
  tumors of, diplopia from, 141
  ventral surface of, *403*
Brain stem auditory evoked potentials, 312
Brain stem auditory evoked responses, 42
Branch retinal artery, occlusion of, 144t
Breath, in stupor/coma evaluation, 62
Breathing patterns, in stupor/coma evaluation, 65
Broca's aphasia, 16, 17t
Bromocriptine, for movement disorders, dosage of, 341t
  for neuroleptic malignant syndrome, 268
  for Parkinson's disease, 344
  for pituitary adenoma, 314
  information summary on, 406
Bronchoscopy, in neuromuscular respiratory failure management, 191
Brown-Séquard's paralysis, 99t
Brudzinski's sign, 173, *174*
Bulbocavernosus reflex, 26
Butterfly glioma, 304

C

Cafergot, information summary on, 409

Calan, for migraine prevention, 180t
Calcium gluconate, for hypocalcemia, 111
Calcium-channel blockers, in migraine prevention, 180t
Calculations, in amnesia/dementia evaluation, 232
  in mental status examination, 14t
California encephalitis virus, 298
Capsaicin, for painful peripheral neuropathy, 323
  information summary on, 406–407
Caput succedaneum, from birth trauma, 381
Carbamazepine, for epilepsy, 361
  for idiopathic torsion dystonia, 347
  for movement disorders, dosage of, 341t
  for neuropathic pain, 264
    in multiple sclerosis, 279
  for postherpetic neuralgia, 222
  for trigeminal neuralgia, 183, 221
  information summary on, 407
Carbatrol. See also *Carbamazepine.*
  for epilepsy, 360t, 368
Carbidopa, for movement disorders, dosage of, 341t
  for Parkinson's disease, 344
Carcinoma-associated retinopathy, 317t
Carcinomatosis, meningeal, 318–319
Carcinomatous meningitis, 318–319
Cardioembolic stroke, 331–332
Cardiopulmonary system, in amnesia/dementia evaluation, 230
Carotid angioplasty, for central retinal artery occlusion, 147–148
Carotid artery dissection, 333
Carotid cavernous fistulae, 125
Carotid Doppler ultrasonography, duplex, 35–36
  in stroke evaluation, 89
Carotid endarterectomy, for central retinal artery occlusion, 147–148

Carotid sinus syncope, 206, 210
Carotid stenosis/occlusion, syncope from, 210
Carpal tunnel syndrome, 254–255
Catapres, for movement disorders, dosage of, 341t
  for Tourette's syndrome, 348
Catheter, ventricular, in intracranial pressure monitoring, 152–153
Cauda equina, lesion localization to, signs and symptoms of, 11
Caudal neglect, 29
Causalgia, 219–220
Cavernous sinus region, tumor in, diplopia from, 141
Cefotaxime, for bacterial meningitis, 288t
Ceftazidime, for bacterial meningitis, 288t
Ceftriaxone, for bacterial meningitis, 109, 175, 286, 288t
  for brain abscess, 294
  for epidural CNS infection, 295
  for Lyme disease, 291
Celebrex, for migraine headache, 178t
Celecoxib, for migraine headache, 178t
Central cord syndrome, 99t
Central deafferentation, gait failure features in, 128t
Central nervous system (CNS), demyelinating disorders of, 270–282. See also *Demyelinating disorder(s).*
  infection(s) of, 285–301
    cysticercosis as, 296
    disorders resembling, 383–384
    epidural, 295
    in AIDS, 299–301
    in children, 383
    leptospirosis as, 292–293
    Lyme disease as, 291–292
    meningitis as, 286, 288t, 289–293. See also *Meningitis.*
    neurosyphilis as, 290–291
    subdural empyema as, 294–295
    suspected, approach to patient with, 285–286
    toxoplasmosis as, 295–296
    viral encephalitis as, 297–299
  inflammatory disorder(s) of, 280–281, 283–284

Central nervous system (CNS) *(Continued)*
    Behçet's disease as, 284
    optic neuritis as, 280–281
    sarcoidosis as, 283–284
  lymphoma of, primary, 309–310
    complicating AIDS, 301
  neoplasm(s) of, gliomas as, 302–308
    nonglial, 308–316
    solitary, *303*
Central neurogenic hyperventilation, in stupor/coma, 65
Central pontine myelinolysis, 282
Central retinal artery, occlusion of, 144t
  management of, 147–148
Cerebellar degeneration, 317t
Cerebellar syndrome, from antineoplastic drugs, 323, 323t
Cerebellopontine angle meningioma, 311
Cerebellum, disease of, gait failure features in, 128t
  hemorrhage in, gait failure/ataxia from, 127
  infarction in, gait failure/ataxia from, 127
  testing of, in ataxia/gait failure evaluation, 131–132, *132*
Cerebral amyloid angiopathy, 338b
Cerebral autoregulation, 154, *155*
Cerebral infarction, border-zone, 86, *87*
  lacunar, 86, *87*
  stroke from, management of, 85–90
    radiographic assessment of, *85*, 85–86
  territorial, 85–86, *87*
Cerebral palsy, gait failure features in, 128t
Cerebral perfusion pressure, 154
Cerebral vasculitis, 334b
Cerebrospinal fluid (CSF), examination of, 32
  leaks of, complicating severe head injury, 124–125
Cerebrospinal fluid otorrhea/rhinorrhea, in stupor/coma evaluation, 62
Cerebrovascular disease, 325–339. See also *Stroke.*

Cerebrovascular disease *(Continued)*
  intracerebral hemorrhage as, 336–339
  subarachnoid hemorrhage as, 325–329
Cerebyx. See also *Fosphenytoin*.
  for epilepsy, 368
Cervical root compression, 223–227, 226t
Cervical spine, radiographs of, 114
Charcot-Marie-Tooth disease, 263
Chemotherapy, for brain metastases, 318
  for glioblastoma multiforme, 304
  for leptomeningeal metastases, 319
  for oligodendrogliomas, 307
  for pineal region tumors, 315
  for primary central nervous system lymphoma, 310
  toxicity of, 323, 323t
Chest, in head injury evaluation, 120
  radiograph of, in ataxia/gait failure evaluation, 135
Chest physical therapy, for neuromuscular respiratory failure, 193
Cheyne-Stokes respiration, in stupor/coma, 64
Child. See *Pediatric* entries.
Child abuse, 386–387
Childhood absence epilepsy, 354, 356
Chlordiazepoxide, for delirium tremens, 110
Chorea, 343
  gait failure features in, 128t
  in Wilson's disease, 348
Ciprofloxacin, for tubercular meningitis, 289
Clavicular fracture, 378
Clindamycin, for toxoplasmosis, 296
Clinoril, for migraine headache, 178t
Clivus meningioma, 311
Clonazepam, for epilepsy, 360t
  for movement disorders, dosage of, 341t
  for restless leg syndrome, 349
  for Tourette's syndrome, 348

Clonazepam *(Continued)*
  information summary on, 407
Clonidine, for movement disorders, dosage of, 341t
  for reflex sympathetic dystrophy, 220
  for restless leg syndrome, 349
  for Tourette's syndrome, 348
Clopidogrel, in ischemic stroke management, 337
  information summary on, 407
Clozapine, for agitation and delirium, 108t
  for benign essential tremor, 346
Clozaril, for agitation and delirium, 108t
  for benign essential tremor, 346
Clumsy hand dysarthria, 332
Cluster breathing, in stupor/coma, 65
Cluster headache, 177, 181. See also *Headache*.
Cogentin, information summary on, 405–406
Cognex, information summary on, 414
Cognitive functions, radiation toxicity and, 322
  testing for, 16, 18
Cogwheel rigidity, in neurologic examination, 23
Colace, in neuromuscular respiratory failure management, 193
Cold caloric reflex, in stupor/coma evaluation, 68
Color vision, in neurologic examination, 18–19
Colorado tick fever virus, 298
Coma, airway protection in, 72
  causes of, 59–60, 60t
  diagnostic testing in, 69, 71–72
  elevator thoughts on, 59–60
  emergency treatment for, 72
  from head injury, 117–118
  history of, selective, 61–62
  hypoxic-ischemic, evoked potentials in, 43
  intravenous hydration for, 72
  major threat to life from, 60–61
  management of, 72–73
  nutrition in, 72
  phone call on, 58–59
  prognosis in, 42, 73–75

Coma *(Continued)*
  psychogenic, 71
Compliance, intracranial, 154
Comprehension, in delirium evaluation, 106
  in mental status examination, 16
Computed tomography (CT), 33
  follow-up, in severe head injury management, 124
  in amnesia/dementia diagnosis, 236
  in dizziness/vertigo evaluation, 166, 169
  in head injury, *85,* 85–86
  in headache evaluation, 174
  in intracerebral hemorrhage diagnosis, 337–338
  in multiple sclerosis diagnosis, 275
  in retrobulbar mass lesion evaluation, 148
  in seizure evaluation, 56
  in stroke management, *39, 40,* 82
  in subarachnoid hemorrhage diagnosis, 326
Comtan, for Parkinson's disease, 345
Concentration, in head injury evaluation, 121
  in mental status examination, 15
Concussion, 113
  from head injury, 118
  headache after, management of, 181
Conduction aphasia, 17t
Conduction deafness, in neurologic examination, 21
Confabulatory responses, 16
Congenital disorders, gait failure features in, 128t
  spinal cord compression from, 94–95
Congenital myopathies, 269
Consciousness, level of, in head injury evaluation, 119, 121
  in mental status examination, 13
  in seizure examination, 55
  in stroke evaluation, 78–79
  in stupor/coma evaluation, 63–64
  loss of, 201–212. See also *Syncope.*

Contusion, parenchymal, from head injury, 118–119
Conus medullaris, lesion localization to, signs and symptoms of, 11
Convergence-retraction nystagmus, 165t
Conversion disorder, syncope from, 211
Convulsions, 350–351. See also *Seizure(s).*
Coordination, in amnesia/dementia evaluation, 233
  in neurologic examination, 24–25
  in neuromuscular respiratory failure evaluation, 190
  in stroke evaluation, 82
  in vision disturbance evaluation, 147
Copaxone, in multiple sclerosis management, 276, 278
  information summary on, 411
Coprolalia, in Tourette's syndrome, 348
Corgard, for migraine prevention, 180t
Corneal reflex, in neurologic examination, 21
  in stupor/coma evaluation, 68
Corpus callosotomy, for epilepsy, 372
Cortical sensory modalities, in neurologic examination, 28–29
Coumadin, information summary on, 416
Cranial epidural abscess, 295
Cranial nerves, in ataxia/gait failure evaluation, 97
  in delirium evaluation, 106
  in dizziness/vertigo evaluation, 164, 166, *167*
  in head injury evaluation, 121
  in neurologic examination, 18–22
  in spinal cord compression evaluation, 100
  in stroke evaluation, 81
  in vision disturbance evaluation, 143–145, *146*
  nuclei of, *402*
Cranial neuropathy, from antineoplastic drugs, 323t
Craniopharyngioma, 314–315

Craniospinal radiation, for leptomeningeal metastases, 319
Cremasteric reflex, in neurologic examination, 26
Critical illness myopathy, 267
Critical illness polyneuropathy, 263
Cryptococcal meningitis, cerebrospinal fluid findings in, 287t
Cryptococcus, complicating AIDS, 299
CSF. See *Cerebrospinal fluid (CSF)*.
CT. See *Computed tomography (CT)*.
Cuprimine, for movement disorders, dosage of, 341t
for Wilson's disease, 349
information summary on, 410
Cutaneous reflexes, in neurologic examination, 26
Cyclosporine, neurotoxicity of, 324
Cylert, information summary on, 410
Cyproheptadine, in cluster headache prevention, 181
in migraine prevention, 180t
information summary on, 407–408
Cysticercosis, 296
Cytomegalovirus (CMV) encephalitis, 299
Cytomegalovirus (CMV) infection, complicating AIDS, 300

D

Dantrium, information summary on, 408
Dantrolene, for malignant hyperthermia, 268
for spasticity/pain in multiple sclerosis, 278
information summary on, 408
Deafness, conduction, in neurologic examination, 21
Death, brain, 240–245. See also *Brain death*.
Decadron, information summary on, 408
Decorticate posturing, in stupor/coma evaluation, 69, *70*
Deep neck muscle, testing, roots, and innervation of, 390t
Deep tendon reflexes, in neurologic examination, 25, 26t
in stupor/coma evaluation, 69
Deep vein thrombosis (DVT), prophylaxis for, for neuromuscular respiratory failure, 193
in severe head injury management, 124
in stroke management, 91
in stupor/coma, 73
Degenerative disease, spinal cord compression from, 94
Delirium, 102–112
bedside evaluation of, 105–107
causes of, 103–104
chart review in, 107, 110
control of, 107–109
drugs for, 108t
elevator thoughts on, 103–104
history of, selective, 107, 110
major threat to life in, 104
management of, 108–112
delirium control in, 108–109
life-threatening disorder treatment in, 109–110
treatment of other disorders in, 110–112
medications causing, 107t
neurologic examination in, 106–107
phone call on, 102–103
physical examination in, 105–106
Delirium tremens, 104, *105*
treatment of, 109
Deltoideus muscle, 390t
Dementia, bedside evaluation of, 230–233
chart review in, 235–236
definition of, 228
differential diagnosis of, 229–230
elevator thoughts on, 229–230
history of, selective, 235–236
HIV-associated, 300–301
major threat to life in, 230
management of, 234–239
neurologic examination in, 231–233
phone call on, 228–229
physical examination in, 230–233

Demyelinating disorder(s), 270–282
acute disseminated encephalomyelitis as, 281
acute necrotizing hemorrhagic encephalomyelitis as, 281–282
central pontine myelinolysis as, 282
Devic's disease as, 281
multiple sclerosis as, 270–280. See also *Multiple sclerosis.*
optic neuritis as, 280–281
Depacon, for epilepsy, 366
information summary on, 416
Depakene, for epilepsy, 366
in migraine prevention, 180t
information summary on, 416
Depakote, for epilepsy, 366
in migraine prevention, 180t
information summary on, 416
Dermatomes, sensory, 397
Dermatomyositis, 266, 317t
Developmental milestones, 380t
Devic's disease, 271, 281
Dexamethasone, for bacterial meningitis, 286
for brain abscess, 294
for brain tumors, 302
for CNS infections in children, 383
for cysticercosis, 296
for epidural CNS infection, 295
for fungal meningitis, 292
for painful peripheral neuropathy, 223
for primary central nervous system lymphoma, 310
for spinal neoplasm, 97
for toxoplasmosis, 296
for tubercular meningitis, 289
for tumors, in pediatric patient, 385
information summary on, 408
Dextroamphetamine, for AIDS dementia complex, 238
Dextrose, for coma, 59
Diabetes insipidus, complicating severe head injury, 125
Diabetes mellitus, diplopia in, 141
neuropathy in, 262
Diabetic amyotrophy, 262
Diagnostic study(ies), 31–43
angiography as, 36–38, 37

Diagnostic study(ies) *(Continued)*
brain biopsy as, 43
computed tomography as, 33
Doppler ultrasonography as, 35–36
electroencephalography as, 39–42
electromyography as, 38–39
evoked potentials as, 42–43
lumbar puncture as, 31–33
magnetic resonance imaging as, 33–35
muscle biopsy as, 43
myelography as, 35
nerve biopsy as, 43
nerve conduction, 39
Diamox, for epilepsy, 360t
information summary on, 404
Diaphragm, in neuromuscular respiratory failure evaluation, 190
testing, roots, and innervation of, 390t
Diastat, for epilepsy, 368
Diazepam, for agitation and delirium, 108t
for idiopathic torsion dystonia, 347
for movement disorders, dosage of, 341t
for root compression, 224
for seizures, 52
for spasticity/pain in multiple sclerosis, 278
information summary on, 408
rectal, for epilepsy, 361–362
for febrile seizures in children, 383
Diclofenac, for migraine headache, 178t
Diet, ketogenic, for epilepsy, 372
Diffuse encephalopathy, EEG in, 40–42
Diffusion-weighted imaging, 34
Dihydroergotamine, for cluster headache, 177
for migraine, 179t
information summary on, 409
Dilantin. See also *Phenytoin.*
for epilepsy, 364
Diphenhydramine, for agitation, 108
information summary on, 408–409

Diplopia, 139, 141
Dislocations, spinal, surgical intervention for, 101
Disseminated encephalomyelitis, acute, 281
 in pediatric patient, 384
Dissociated nystagmus, 165t
Ditropan, for bladder dysfunction, 279
 information summary on, 409–410
Dizziness, 161–169
 bedside evaluation of, 162–166
 chart review in, 162–163
 differential diagnosis of, 161–162
 elevator thoughts on, 161–162
 history in, selective, 162–163
 major threat to life in, 162
 management of, 166, *168*, 169
 neurologic examination in, 164, 166
 phone call on, 161
 physical examination in, 163–166
Docusate sodium, in neuromuscular respiratory failure management, 193
Doll's eye reflex, in stupor/coma evaluation, 66–68
Donepezil hydrochloride, for Alzheimer's disease, 237
 information summary on, 409
Dopamine, in increased intracranial pressure management, 158–159
 in organ donor management, 244
Doppler ultrasonography, 35–36
 duplex, in central retinal artery occlusion, 147
 in ataxia/gait failure evaluation, 135
 in stroke evaluation, 89
 transcranial, in brain death confirmation, 243
Double simultaneous stimulation, in neurologic examination, 29
Doxycycline, for leptospirosis, 293
Drawing, in amnesia/dementia evaluation, 232
Drop metastases, from ependymomas, 307
Drug(s). See also specific drug or drug group.

Drug(s) *(Continued)*
 antiepileptic, 360t–366t
  in pregnancy, 373–374
  newer forms of, 368
 causing ataxia, 130t
 causing delirium, 104t
 causing memory impairment, 235t
 causing myopathies, 267, 267t
 causing pain or paresthesia, 217t
 causing peripheral polyneuropathy, 258t–259t
 causing seizures, 49t
 causing syncope, 203t
 causing vertigo/dizziness, 163t
 exacerbating weakness in myasthenia gravis, 198t
 for migraine headache, 178t–179t
  preventive, 180
 lowering seizure threshold, 373t
Duchenne muscular dystrophy, 268
Duplex Doppler ultrasonography, in central retinal artery occlusion, 147
DVT. See *Deep vein thrombosis (DVT)*.
Dysarthria, 16
 clumsy hand, 332
Dyschromatopsia, 141t
Dyskinesia, description of, 343
Dysmetria, ocular, 165t
Dysphagia, in neurologic examination, 22
Dystonia, description of, 343
 gait failure features in, 128t
 in Wilson's disease, 348
 torsion, idiopathic, 347
Dystonia musculorum deformans, 347

E

Ear, in head injury evaluation, 120
 in stupor/coma evaluation, 62
Echocardiography, in stroke evaluation, 89
Echolalia, in Tourette's syndrome, 348
Ecotrin, information summary on, 405
Edrophonium, information summary on, 409

Edrophonium testing, in myasthenia gravis diagnosis, 196
Elavil. See also *Amitriptyline*.
 in migraine prevention, 180
 information summary on, 404–405
Eldepryl, for movement disorders, dosage of, 341t
 for Parkinson's disease, 345
 information summary on, 413
Electrocardiography, in syncope diagnosis, 207
Electrodes, intracranial, in epilepsy surgery evaluation, 371–372
Electroencephalography, 39–42
 in amnesia/dementia diagnosis, 236
 in brain death confirmation, 243
 in epilepsy, 376–377
 in seizure evaluation, 57
 in stupor/coma evaluation, 71
Electrolytes, for neuromuscular respiratory failure, 193
Electromyography, in ataxia/gait failure evaluation, 135
 in painful peripheral neuropathy diagnosis, 223
 single-fiber, in myasthenia gravis diagnosis, 196
Electronystagmogram, 169
Embolization, endovascular, for subarachnoid hemorrhage, 328–329
Embolus, artery-to-artery, ischemic stroke from, 333
Emotional functions, testing for, in mental status examination, 16, 18
Empyema, subdural, 294–295
Encephalitis, brain stem, 317t
 coma from, 72
 delirium in, 104
 limbic, 317t
 stupor/coma from, 61
 viral, 297–299
Encephalomyelitis, acute disseminated, 281
 in pediatric patient, 384
 acute necrotizing hemorrhagic, 281–282
 necrotizing, 317t
 postinfectious, 281

Encephalomyelitis *(Continued)*
 postvaccinal, 281
Encephalopathy, acute toxic, in pediatric patient, 384
 diffuse, EEG in, 40–42
 from antineoplastic drugs, 323t
 hepatic, 111b
Endarterectomy, carotid, for central retinal artery occlusion, 147–148
 in ischemic stroke management, 337
Endocrine diseases/dysfunction, causing peripheral polyneuropathies, 258t
 radiation-induced, 322
Endocrine myopathies, 266
Endocrinologic investigation, in pituitary adenoma diagnosis, 314
Endovascular embolization, for subarachnoid hemorrhage, 328
Entacapone, for Parkinson's disease, 345
Enterovirus encephalitis, 298
Ependymoblastomas, 307
Ependymomas, 307–308
Epidural hematoma, complicating lumbar puncture, 33
 from head injury, 118
Epidural transducer, in intracranial pressure monitoring, 153
Epilepsy, 350–377. See also *Seizure(s); Status epilepticus*.
 benign Rolandic, of childhood, 357
 childhood absence, 354, 356
 definition of, 47
 drugs, 361–362
 electroencephalography in, 376–377
 focal resection for, 370–372
 generalized, primary, 367
 juvenile absence, 356
 juvenile myoclonic, 356
 ketogenic diet for, 365
 localization-related, 367
 medical treatment of, 360–364, 363t, 364t, 364–365
 missing diagnosis of, 369
 surgery for, 364
 temporal lobe, 357

Epilepsy *(Continued)*
  treatment of, errors in, common, 362–364
  vagal nerve stimulator for, 365
Epilepsy syndrome(s),
  classification of, 354, 355t, 356–358
  generalized, primary, 354, 356
  symptomatic, 356
  localization-related, 357
  situation-related, 357–358
Epley maneuver, modified, for benign positional vertigo, 168, 169
Epstein-Barr virus encephalitis, 299
Equine encephalomyelitis virus encephalisitis, 298
Erb's palsy, in newborn, *380*
Ergomar, for migraine, 179t
Ergot medications, for migraine headache, 176, 179t
Ergotamine, for cluster headache, 177
  for migraine, 179t
  in cluster headache prevention, 181
  information summary on, 409
Esthesioneuroblastoma, 309
Ethambutol, for tubercular meningitis, 289
Ethanol, neuropathy from, 262
  seizures from, 367
Ethosuximide, for epilepsy, 361t
  information summary on, 409–410
Evoked potentials, 42–43
  brain stem auditory, in acoustic neuroma diagnosis, 312
Extensor carpi radialis muscle, 391t
Extensor carpi ulnaris muscle, 391t
Extensor digitorum brevis muscle, 393t
Extensor digitorum longus muscle, 393t
Extensor digitorum muscle, 391t
Extensor hallucis longus muscle, 393t
Extensor indicis muscle, 391t
Extensor pollicis brevis muscle, 391t
Extensor pollicis longus muscle, 391t

Extensor posturing, in stupor/coma evaluation, 69, *70*
Extraocular movements, in ataxia/gait failure evaluation, 131
  in head injury evaluation, 121
  in neurologic examination, 20
Extraocular muscles, in neuromuscular respiratory failure evaluation, 190
Extremity(ies), in amnesia/dementia evaluation, 231
  in head injury evaluation, 120
  in syncope evaluation, 207
Extubation, weaning to, 192–193
Eye(s), care of, in stupor/coma, 73
  motility of, in vision disturbance evaluation, 145, *146*
  movements of, in stupor/coma evaluation, 66–68
  primary central nervous system lymphoma involving, 310
Eyelids, in neurologic examination, 19

F

Face, asymmetry of, in delirium evaluation, 106
  pain syndromes involving, 215
Face-hand test, in neurologic examination, 29
Facial palsy, 255–256
Facial (VII) nerve, in ataxia/gait failure evaluation, 131
  in head injury evaluation, 121
  in neurologic examination, 21
Fainting, 201–212. See also *Syncope.*
Famciclovir, for herpetic neuralgia, 222
Fasciculations, in motor neuron disease, 251
  in neurologic examination, 22
  in neuromuscular respiratory failure evaluation, 190
Fatigue, in multiple sclerosis, therapy for, 279
Febrile seizures, 357–358, 383
Feet, pain syndromes involving, 215
Felbamate, for epilepsy, 361t
  information summary on, 410
Felbatol, for epilepsy, 361t

Index **433**

Felbatol *(Continued)*
  information summary on, 410
Feldene, for migraine headache, 178t
Femoral cutaneous nerve, lateral, *396*
Femoral nerve, *396*
Fentanyl, in increased intracranial pressure management, 158
Fever, in stroke patient, management of, 90
  in syncope evaluation, 205
  treatment of, in increased intracranial pressure management, 157
Finger taps, rapid, in screening for hemiparesis, 23
Finger-to-nose test, in neurologic examination, 24
Fistula, carotid cavernous, complicating severe head injury, 125
FLAIR images, 34
Flexor carpi radialis muscle, 391t
Flexor carpi ulnaris muscle, 390t
Flexor digiti minimi brevis manus muscle, 390t
Flexor digitorum longus muscle, 393t
Flexor digitorum profundus muscle, 390t, 391t
Flexor digitorum superficialis muscle, 390t
Flexor hallucis longus muscle, 393t
Flexor pollicis brevis muscle, 391t
Flexor pollicis longus muscle, 391t
Flexor posturing, in stupor/coma evaluation, 69, *70*
Florinef, information summary on, 410
Flow voids, 35
Fluconazole, for fungal meningitis, 292
Flucytosine, for fungal meningitis, 292
Fludrocortisone, for autonomic dysfunction, 211
  for autonomic neuropathy, 264
  information summary on, 410
Fluency, in mental status examination, 16
Fluid(s), for neuromuscular respiratory failure, 193
Fluid management, in severe head injury management, 123
  of subarachnoid hemorrhage, 329, 330t
Flumazenil, for ataxia, 136
  for coma, 59
Fluoxetine, for psychiatric complications of multiple sclerosis, 279
Focal brain stem signs, in stupor/coma evaluation, 71
Focal hemispheric signs, in stupor/coma evaluation, 71
Folinic acid, for toxoplasmosis, 296
Foramen magnum, lesion localization to, signs and symptoms of, 10–11
  meningioma of, 311
Foscarnet, for CMV infection in AIDS, 300
Fosphenytoin, for epilepsy, 361
  for perioperative seizures, 374–375
  for seizures, 52, 56
  for status epilepticus, 54t
  in increased intracranial pressure management, 157
  in severe head injury management, 124
  information summary on, 410
Foster-Kennedy syndrome, fundoscopic appearance of, 144t
Fracture(s), clavicular, 378
  skull, 119
  spinal, 101
Freezing, description of, 343
Frontal lobe seizures, 353–354
Frontal release signs, in amnesia/dementia evaluation, 233, *234*
  in neurologic examination, 27
Fundoscopy, in stupor/coma evaluation, 65
  in vision disturbance evaluation, 144, 144t
Fundus, in neurologic examination, 18
Fungal meningitis, 292

G

Gabapentin, for benign essential tremor, 346

Gabapentin *(Continued)*
for epilepsy, 361t
for neuropathic pain, 264
for neuropathic pain in multiple sclerosis, 279
for painful peripheral neuropathy, 223
for trigeminal neuralgia, 183
information summary on, 410
Gabitril, for epilepsy, 365t
information summary on, 414
Gag reflex, 68
Gait, abnormalities of, 29t
failure of, 126–136
bedside evaluation of, 127, 129–133
chart review in, 129–130
clinical features of, 127, 128t
diagnostic testing in, 135
elevator thoughts on, 127
history in, selective, 129–130
major threat to life in, 127
management of, 133–134, 135–136
phone call on, 126–127
physical examination in, 130–133, 134
in amnesia/dementia evaluation, 233
in delirium evaluation, 107
in head injury evaluation, 121–122
in neurologic examination, 30
in vision disturbance evaluation, 147
magnetic, 233
Gancyclovir, for CMV infection, 300
Ganglioneuritis, 317t
Gastrocnemius muscle, testing, roots, and innervation of, 393t
Gegenhalten, in neurologic examination, 23
Gender, in neurologic history, 5
Genetic diseases, causing peripheral polyneuropathies, 259t
Genetic neuropathies, 263
Genitofemoral nerve, *396*
Genitourinary tract, in syncope evaluation, 207
Germ cell tumors, 315
Germinomas, 315
Giant cell arteritis, management of, 182–183

Glabellar reflex, in neurologic examination, 27
Glasgow Coma Scale, 63, 63t
Glatiramer, in multiple sclerosis management, 276, 278
information summary on, 411
Glioblastoma multiforme, 303–305
Glioma(s), 302–308
butterfly, 304
Global aphasia, 17t
Globellar sign, 233, *234*
Glossopharyngeal (IX) nerve, in ataxia/gait failure evaluation, 131
in neurologic examination, 22
Glossopharyngeal neuralgia, 183
Glucose, for seizures, 51
in stroke management, 91
Glutethimide, for tremor in multiple sclerosis, 279
Gluteus maximus muscle, 393t
Gluteus medius muscle, 393t
Gluteus minimus muscle, 393t
Glycopyrrolate, for myasthenia gravis, 197
information summary on, 411
Gracilis muscle, 393t
Graft-versus-host disease, 323–324
Grand mal seizures, 350–351
Granulomatous angiitis, of brain, 334b
Graphesthesia, 29
Grasp reflex, 27
Guanidine hydrochloride, for botulism, 200
Guillain-Barré syndrome, clinical features of, 194
laboratory data on, 194
Miller-Fisher variant of, 131
ataxia from, treatment of, 136
neuromuscular respiratory failure in, 185, 193–194
onset of, 194
prognosis in, 196
treatment of, 194–195, 195b

H

Hair, in ataxia/gait failure evaluation, 134
Haldol, for agitation, 108t, 235
for delirium, 108t
for Huntington's disease, 347

Haldol *(Continued)*
  for movement disorders, dosage of, 341t
  for Tourette's syndrome, 348
  information summary on, 411
Haloperidol, for agitation, 108t, 235
  for delirium, 108t
  for Huntington's disease, 347
  for movement disorders, dosage of, 341t
  for psychiatric causes of delirium, 112
  for Tourette's syndrome, 348
  information summary on, 411
Hands, pain syndromes involving, differential diagnosis of, 215
Head, elevation of, for neuromuscular respiratory failure, 193
  in increased intracranial pressure management, 156–157
  in stupor/coma evaluation, 62
  injury to, 113–125
    bedside evaluation of, 119–122
    elevator thoughts on, 118–119
    ER diagnostic and treatment algorithm for, *115*
    hospital admission following, criteria for, 122b
    in pediatric patient, 386
    major threat to life in, 119
    management of, 122–125
    mild, management of, 122
    moderate, management of, 122
    neurologic examination in, 120–122
    phone call on, 113–118
      orders in, 114, 116–118
      questions in, 113–114
    physical examination in, 120–122
    prognosis for, 125
    seizures from, 366
    sequelae of, 118–119
    severe, complications of, 124–125
      management of, 122–125
    severity of, determining, 113–114
  scan of, in stupor/coma evaluation, 71

Headache, 170–184
  bedside evaluation of, 172–173
  causes of, 171
  chart review in, 172–173
  cluster, management of, 177, 181
  diagnostic testing in, 173–175
  elevator thoughts on, 171
  from pseudotumor cerebri, management of, 181–182
  history of, selective, 172–173
  in subarachnoid hemorrhage, 325
  major threat to life in, 171
  management of, 175–184
  migraine, binocular visual loss from, 139
    management of, 175–176
    emergency room protocol for, 181t
  neurologic examination in, 173
  phone call on, 170
  physical examination in, 173, *174*
  postconcussion, management of, 181
  spinal, complicating lumbar puncture, 32–33
  tension, management of, 177
Heart, disorders of, syncope from, 202–203
  in ataxia/gait failure evaluation, 134
  in syncope evaluation, 207
Heart rate, in neuromuscular respiratory failure evaluation, 188
  in stroke evaluation, 80
  in syncope evaluation, 205
Heel-to-shin test, in neurologic examination, 25
Heel-to-toe gait, in head injury evaluation, 121–122
HEENT, in amnesia/dementia evaluation, 230
  in ataxia/gait failure evaluation, 130, 134
  in dizziness/vertigo evaluation, 163
  in headache evaluation, 173
  in neuromuscular respiratory failure evaluation, 189–190
  in spinal cord compression evaluation, 97–98
  in syncope evaluation, 207

Hematoma, epidural, complicating
lumbar puncture, 33
from head injury, 118
parenchymal, from head injury,
118–119
subdural, from head injury, 118
tentorial, as birth trauma, 381
Hemicord syndrome, 99t
Hemineglect, in amnesia/
dementia evaluation, 232
spatial, 14–15
Hemiparesis, ataxic, 332
in seizure evaluation, 55
pure motor, 332
screening tests for, 23–24
Hemiparetic gait, 29t
Hemisensory loss, pure, 332
Hemispherectomy, for epilepsy,
372
Hemorrhage, appearance of, on
MRI, 34t
cerebellar, gait failure/ataxia
from, 127
intracerebral, 337–339. See also
Intracerebral hemorrhage.
intraventricular, complicating
prematurity, 381
radiographic assessment of,
82, *83*
subarachnoid, 325–330. See also
Subarachnoid hemorrhage.
subgaleal, from birth trauma,
381
Hemorrhagic infarction,
periventricular, complicating
prematurity, 381
Hemorrhagic leukoencephalitis,
acute, in pediatric patient, 384
Hemotympanum, in stupor/coma
evaluation, 62
Heparin, for central retinal artery
occlusion, 147
for transient monocular blindness, 148
in ischemic stroke management,
333
information summary on, 411
Hepatic encephalopathy, 111b
Hepatic failure, seizures in,
367–368
Hereditary diseases, causing
peripheral polyneuropathies,
259t
Hereditary myopathies, 268–269

Hereditary neuropathies, 263
Herniation, brain, stupor/coma
from, 61, *61*
from intracranial mass lesions,
as threat to life, 171
tentorial, complicating lumbar
puncture, 33
Herpes simplex encephalitis, 297
Herpes zoster, complicating AIDS,
300
Herpetic neuralgia, 221–222
History taking, 4–6
HIV myelopathy, 301
HIV sensory neuropathy,
complicating AIDS, 300
Hollenhorst plaques, 144
Hormonal manipulation, for
meningiomas, 312
Horner's syndrome, in neurologic
examination, 19
Huntington's disease, 346–347
treatment of, 238
Hydration, intravenous, for
comatose patient, 72
in stroke management, 90–91
Hydrocephalus, normal-pressure,
gait failure features in, 128t
magnetic gait in, 233
treatment of, 237–238
Hydroxyzine, for pain syndromes,
219
Hyperacute ischemia, diffusion-
weighted imaging of, 34
Hypercoagulable states, ischemic
stroke from, 333
Hyperglycemia, treatment of,
110–111
Hyperkalemic periodic paralysis,
268
Hyperkinesias, characteristics of,
340
Hypernatremia, treatment of, 111
Hyperreflexia, 25
Hypertension, idiopathic
intracranial, management of,
181–182
in acute stroke, ER treatment
guidelines for, 79b
in stupor/coma evaluation, 62
in syncope evaluation, 205
Hyperthermia, malignant, 267
Hyperthyroidism, diplopia in, 141
Hypertonia, in neurologic
examination, 22–23

Hyperventilation, for comatose patient, 117
in increased intracranial pressure management, 159–160
in stupor/coma, 65
syncope from, 211–212
Hypocalcemia, treatment of, 112
Hypoglossal (XII) nerve, in ataxia/gait failure evaluation, 131
in neurologic examination, 22
Hypoglycemia, treatment of, 110
Hypokalemic periodic paralysis, 268
Hypokinesias, characteristics of, 340
Hyponatremia, formula for correcting, 282t
treatment of, 111
Hyporeflexia, 25
Hypotension, in syncope evaluation, 205
intracranial, spontaneous, management of, 183–184
orthostatic, syncope from, 203
Hypothyroidism, ataxia from, treatment of, 136
Hypotonia, in neurologic examination, 22
Hypoxic-ischemic coma, evoked potentials in, 43
Hysterical faints, 211
Hysterical gait, 29t

I

Ibuprofen, for brachial neuritis, 227
for migraine headache, 176, 178t
for painful peripheral neuropathy, 223
for root compression, 224
ICP. See *Intracranial pressure.*
Iliohypogastric nerve, *396*
Ilioinguinal nerve, *396*
Iliopsoas muscle, testing, roots, and innervation of, 393t
Imitrex, for migraine headache, 179t
information summary on, 414
Immune globulin, information summary on, 412
intravenous, for Guillain-Barré syndrome, 195–196

Immune globulin *(Continued)*
for relapsing-remitting multiple sclerosis, 278
tetanus, 200
Immunologic diseases, causing peripheral polyneuropathies, 259t
Immunosuppression, for bone marrow transplantation, drugs for, 324
for myasthenia gravis, 197–198
Imuran, information summary on, 405
Inclusion body myositis, 266
Inderal. See also *Propranolol.*
for benign essential tremor, 346
for movement disorders, dosage of, 341t
in migraine prevention, 180t
information summary on, 412
Indocin, for migraine headache, 178t
Indomethacin, for migraine headache, 178t
in increased intracranial pressure management, 157
Infant. See *Pediatric* entries.
Infarction, cerebellar, gait failure/ataxia from, 127
cerebral. See *Cerebral infarction.*
hemorrhagic, periventricular, complicating prematurity, 381
stroke from, 77–78
Infection(s), causing peripheral polyneuropathies, 259t
central nervous system, 285–301. See also *Central nervous system (CNS), infection(s) of.*
delirium from, 103
spinal cord compression from, 94
Infectious myopathies, 269
Inflammatory disorder(s), 280–281, 282–284
Behçet's disease as, 284
optic neuritis as, 280–281
sarcoidosis as, 282–284
spinal cord compression from, 95
Inflammatory myopathies, 266
Inflammatory optic neuritis, management of, 148–149
Infraspinatus muscle, 390t

Infratentorial tumors, in pediatric patient, 385
Insight, in mental status examination, 14t
Insulin, in organ donor management, 245
Interferon beta-1a, in multiple sclerosis management, 276, 278
  information summary on, 412
Interferon beta-1b, in multiple sclerosis management, 276
  information summary on, 412
Internuclear ophthalmoplegia, 145
Interossei muscle, 390t
Intoxication, acute, gait failure/ataxia from, 127
  sedative, ataxia from, treatment of, 136
Intracerebral hemorrhage, 337–339
  acute management of, 84–85
  clinical presentation of, 337–338
  diagnosis of, 338–339
  management of, 339
  radiographic assessment of, 82, 83
  stroke from, 78
Intracranial anatomy, 153–154
Intracranial compliance, 154
Intracranial hypotension, spontaneous, management of, 183–184
Intracranial mass lesions, syncope from, 211
Intracranial metastases, leptomeningeal, 318–319
  skull base, 319–320
Intracranial pressure, increased, 150–160
  conditions associated with, 150t
  diplopia from, 141
  elevator thoughts on, 153–156
  emergency treatment of, 152b
  management of, 156–160
    emergency, 151–153
    general measures in, 156–157
    steps in, 157b, 157–160
  pathologic, 156, 156
  stupor/coma from, 61
  monitor for, placement of, 152–153, 153
  normal, 150

Intracranial pressure *(Continued)*
  phone call on, 151
  physiologic principles of, 153–156
  reduction of, emergency measures for, 151–152
  waveforms of, 154, 155, 156
Intracranial pressure–volume curve, 154, 155
Intraparenchymal probe, in intracranial pressure monitoring, 153
Intravenous hydration, in stroke management, 90–91
Intraventricular hemorrhage, complicating prematurity, 381
  radiographic assessment of, 82, 83
Intubation, for neuromuscular respiratory failure, indications for, 191
Ischemia, hyperacute, diffusion-weighted imaging of, 34
  optic nerve head, monocular visual loss from, 139
  retinal, monocular visual loss from, 138–139
Ischemic stroke, 330–337. See also *Stroke, ischemic.*
Isoniazid, for tremor in multiple sclerosis, 279

J

Japanese encephalitis virus, 298
Joint(s), mobility of, in stupor/coma, 73
  position of, in sensory examination, 28
Judgment, in mental status examination, 14t
Jugular foramen syndrome, from skull base metastases, 320
Juvenile absence epilepsy, 355
Juvenile myoclonic epilepsy, 355

K

Kayser-Fleischer rings, in Wilson's disease, 348
Keppra, for epilepsy, 362t
  information summary on, 413

Kernig's sign, in headache evaluation, 173, *174*
Ketogenic diet, for epilepsy, 365
Ketorolac, for migraine headache, 178t
Kidney failure, seizures in, 367
uremia with, treatment of, 112
Klonopin, for epilepsy, 360t
for movement disorders, dosage of, 341t
for Tourette's syndrome, 348
information summary on, 407

L

Labetalol, in increased intracranial pressure management, 158
Lacunar infarction, 86, *87*
Lacunar stroke, 333
Lambert-Eaton myasthenic syndrome, 317t
Lamictal, for epilepsy, 362t
information summary on, 412
Laminectomy, neurosurgical decompressive, 101
Lamotrigine, for epilepsy, 362t
information summary on, 412
Language testing, in mental status examination, 15–16
Lateral femoral cutaneous nerve, *396*
Latissimus dorsi muscle, 390t
Lennox-Gastaut syndrome, 356
Leptomeningeal metastases, 318–319
Leptospirosis, 292–293
Lethargy, in stupor/coma evaluation, 63
Leukoencephalitis, acute hemorrhagic, in pediatric patient, 384
Leukoencephalopathy, from antineoplastic drugs, 323
progressive multifocal, complicating AIDS, 299
Leukomalacia, periventricular, complicating prematurity, 381
Levator scapulae muscle, 390t
Levetiracetam, for epilepsy, 362t
information summary on, 413
Levodopa, for movement disorders, dosage of, 341t
for Parkinson's disease, 344

Levodopa *(Continued)*
for restless leg syndrome, 349
Levodopa-carbidopa, information summary on, 413
Lewy body disease, treatment of, 237
Lidocaine, for cluster headache, 177
Lidocaine patch, information summary on, 413
Lidoderm, for painful peripheral neuropathy, 223
Lightheadedness, vertigo differentiated from, 162
Limb tone, in head injury evaluation, 121
in stupor/coma evaluation, 68
Limbic encephalitis, 317t
Lioresal, for idiopathic torsion dystonia, 347
for movement disorders, dosage of, 341t
information summary on, 405
Lithium, in cluster headache prevention, 181
toxicity of, ataxia from, treatment of, 136
Locked-in syndrome, 71
Lorazepam, for agitation, 108, 235
and delirium, 108t
for seizures, 51, 52
for status epilepticus, 54t
information summary on, 413
Lou Gehrig's disease, 251–252
Lower motor neuron disease, gait failure features in, 128t
Lower motor neuron system, lesion localization in, 7–8
Lumbar plexus, *396*
Lumbar puncture, 31–33
complications of, 32–33
in amnesia/dementia diagnosis, 236
in ataxia/gait failure evaluation, 135
in headache evaluation, 174–175
in leptomeningeal metastases diagnosis, 317
in multiple sclerosis diagnosis, 273–274
in neurosyphilis diagnosis, 290
in seizure evaluation, 57
in stupor/coma evaluation, 71
in suspected CNS infection, 285–286

Lumbar puncture *(Continued)*
positioning for, *31*, 31–32
Lumbosacral plexopathy, 254
Lumbosacral plexus, muscles of, 393t
Lumbosacral root compression, 223–227, 226t
Lumbosacral trunk, *396*
Lumbricales 1 and 2 muscles, 391t
Lumbricales 3 and 4 muscles, 390t
Luminal. See also *Phenobarbital.*
for epilepsy, 363t
Lundberg A and B waves, 156, *156*
Lungs, in neuromuscular respiratory failure evaluation, 190
Lyme disease, 291–292
neurologic manifestations of, 291t
Lymphocytic choriomeningitis virus, 299
Lymphoma, CNS, primary, complicating AIDS, 301
primary central nervous system, 309–310

M

Maddox rod, in vision disturbance evaluation, 145, *146*
Magnetic gait, 233
Magnetic resonance angiography, 35
in ataxia/gait failure evaluation, 135
in stroke evaluation, 90
Magnetic resonance imaging (MRI), 33–35
cervical or lumbosacral spinal, 224
gadolinium-enhanced, in acoustic neuroma diagnosis, 312
in dizziness/vertigo evaluation, 169
in epilepsy surgery evaluation, 371
in intracerebral hemorrhage diagnosis, 337–338, *338*
in leptomeningeal metastases diagnosis, 317
in multiple sclerosis diagnosis, 275–276

Magnetic resonance imaging (MRI) *(Continued)*
in pituitary adenoma diagnosis, 313–314
in primary central nervous system lymphoma diagnosis, 310
in retrobulbar mass lesion evaluation, 148
in seizure evaluation, 56
in spinal cord compression evaluation, 97
in spinal metastases diagnosis, 321
in subarachnoid hemorrhage diagnosis, 326
Magnetic resonance venography, 35
Malignant hyperthermia, 268
Malignant thymoma, in myasthenia gravis, 196
Mannitol, for comatose patient, 117–118
in increased intracranial pressure management, 159
information summary on, 414
Marburg variant, of multiple sclerosis, 271
Marcus Gunn pupil, in neurologic examination, 19–20
in vision disturbance evaluation, 143
Massage, ocular, for central retinal artery occlusion, 147
Maxalt, information summary on, 413
McArdle's disease, 269
Measles virus encephalitis, 298
Mechanical ventilation, for neuromuscular respiratory failure, 191–193
Meclizine, for benign positional vertigo, 169
information summary on, 414
Medial cutaneous nerves of forearm, *395*
Median nerve, *395*
Medications. See *Drug(s);* specific drug or drug group.
Medulla, lesion localization in, 9–10
Medulloblastoma, 308–309
Memory, impairment of, medications associated with, 235t

Memory *(Continued)*
  in amnesia/dementia evaluation, 228, 232
  in head injury evaluation, 121
  testing of, in mental status examination, 16
Meningeal carcinomatosis, 318–319
Meningiomas, 311–312
  radiation-induced, 322–323
Meningitis, 286, 288t, 289–293
  acute, 286, 389
  bacterial, 286
    antibiotic therapy for, 288t
    as threat to life, 171
    cerebrospinal fluid findings in, 287t
    delirium in, 104
    diagnostic testing for, 174–175
    treatment of, 109
  carcinomatous, 318–319
  coma from, 72
  complicating lumbar puncture, 33
  cryptococcal, cerebrospinal fluid findings in, 287t
  diplopia from, 141
  fungal, 292
  in HIV, 301
  in leptospirosis, 292
  stupor/coma from, 61
  tubercular, 289
    cerebrospinal fluid findings in, 287t
  viral, 286, 289
Meningovascular syphilis, 290
Mental status, emotional and higher cognitive functions in, 14t
  in amnesia/dementia evaluation, 231–232
  in ataxia/gait failure evaluation, 130
  in delirium evaluation, 106
  in dizziness/vertigo evaluation, 164
  in head injury evaluation, 121
  in neurologic examination, 12–18
  in spinal cord compression evaluation, 100
  in stroke evaluation, 81
  in vision disturbance evaluation, 143
Mestinon, for myasthenia gravis, 197, 199t

Mestinon *(Continued)*
  information summary on, 413
Metabolic acidosis, in stupor/coma, 65
Metabolic disorders, causing peripheral polyneuropathies, 258t
  delirium from, 103
Metabolic myopathies, 268–269
Metastasis(es), 316–321
  brain, 316, 318
  drop, from ependymomas, 307
  leptomeningeal, 318–319
  skull, 319–320
  spinal, 320–321
Methazolamide, for benign essential tremor, 346
  for movement disorders, dosage of, 341t
Methotrexate, for leptomeningeal metastases, 319
  for polymyositis, 266
Methylphenidate, for AIDS dementia complex, 238
Methylprednisolone, for arteritic ischemic optic neuropathy, 148
  for inflammatory optic neuritis, 148–149
  for multiple sclerosis relapses, 278
  for optic neuritis, 280
  for pseudotumor cerebri, 149
  for traumatic spinal cord injury, 96–97
  information summary on, 414
Methysergide, in cluster headache prevention, 181
  in migraine prevention, 180t
  information summary on, 414–415
Metoclopramide, for autonomic neuropathy, 264
  for migraine headache, 176
Metronidazole, for brain abscess, 293–294
Midazolam, for status epilepticus, 54t
  information summary on, 408
Midbrain, lesion localization in, 8
Middle cranial fossa syndrome, 320
Midodrine, for autonomic dysfunction, 211

Midodrine *(Continued)*
  for autonomic neuropathy, 264
  information summary on, 408
Migraine headache. See also
    Headache.
  binocular visual loss from, 139
  management of, 175–176
    emergency room protocol for, 181t
    medications used for, 178t–179t
    preventive, 180t
Milk of magnesia, in
    neuromuscular respiratory
    failure management, 193
Mini Mental State Examination, 398–400
Miosis, 19
Mirapex, for Parkinson's disease, 345
  information summary on, 410
Mitochondrial myopathy, 269
Mitoxantrone, for progressive
    multiple sclerosis, 278
Modafenil, information summary on, 408
Monoamine oxidase inhibitors, in
    migraine prevention, 180t
Monocular blindness, transient, 148
Mononeuropathy(ies), 254–256
  in diabetes, 262
  motor and sensory deficit pattern in, 250t
Mononeuropathy multiplex, 256–257
  in diabetes, 262
  motor and sensory deficit pattern in, 250t
Monoradiculopathy, 253
  motor and sensory deficit pattern in, 250t
Mood, in mental status
    examination, 14t
Morphine, in increased
    intracranial pressure
    management, 158
Motion myoclonus, 317t
Motor function(s), in amnesia/
    dementia evaluation, 232–233
  in ataxia/gait failure evaluation, 133
  in delirium evaluation, 106
  in head injury evaluation, 121
  in neurologic examination, 22–24

Motor function(s) *(Continued)*
  in spinal cord compression evaluation, 98
  in stroke evaluation, 82
Motor neuron disease, 251–252, 317t
  motor and sensory deficit pattern in, 250t
Motor neuron lesion, respiratory
    weakness from, 186
Motor responses, in stupor/coma
    evaluation, 68
Motrin, for migraine headache, 178t
Movement disorders, 340–350
  basic principles for, 340–342
  classification of, 342
  description of, 342
  diagnosis of, 344–349
  gait failure features in, 128t
  medications for, 341t
  naming of, 342–344
  observation of, 342
MRI. See *Magnetic resonance
    imaging (MRI)*.
Multifocal motor neuropathy, 252
Multiple sclerosis, acute relapses
    of, therapy for, 277t, 278
  ataxia from, treatment of, 136
  clinical features of, 205–208, 270–272
  clinical patterns of, *207*
  diagnosis of, 208–211, 273–276
    clinical and laboratory, criteria for, 274t
  differential diagnosis of, 275b
  diplopia from, 141
  evoked potentials in, 42–43
  laboratory investigations of, 273–276
  management of, 276–279, 277t
    treatment of disease progression in, 276, 278
  Marburg variant, 271
  neurologic signs in, characteristic, 271b
  pain in, therapy for, 278–279
  pathogenesis of, 208, 272–273
  primary progressive, 271, *272*
    therapy for, 277t
  prognosis of, 279
  progressive-relapsing, 271, *272*, 273
  relapsing-remitting, 271, *272*

Index **443**

Multiple sclerosis *(Continued)*
  therapy for, 277t
  secondary progressive, 271, *272*
   therapy for, 277t
  spasticity in, therapy for, 278–279
  symptomatic therapy for, 278–279
Mumps virus encephalitis, 297–298
Muscle(s), biopsy of, 43
  diseases of, 249–269. See also *Myopathy(ies); Neuromuscular diseases.*
  extraocular, in neuromuscular respiratory failure evaluation, 190
  fatigability of, in myasthenia gravis, 195
  of brachial plexus, 390t–391t
  of lumbosacral plexus, 393t
  of neck, 390t–391t
  of perineum, 393t
  power of, 24
  rhythmic twitching of, in stupor/coma evaluation, 63
  tone of, 22–23
  wasting of, 22
Muscular dystrophy, 268
Musculocutaneous nerve, *395*
Musculoskeletal system, in ataxia/gait failure evaluation, 134–135
  in pain syndrome evaluation, 217–218
  in spinal cord compression evaluation, 98
Mutism, akinetic, 71–72
Myasthenia gravis,
  anticholinesterase drugs used for, 199t
  clinical features of, 195–196
  diplopia from, 141
  drugs exacerbating weakness in, 198t
  laboratory data on, 196
  neuromuscular respiratory failure in, 185, 195–198
  treatment of, 197–198
Myasthenic crisis, 196
  management of, checklist for, 197b
Mydriasis, in neurologic examination, 19

Myelinolysis, central pontine, 282
Myelography, 35
  in leptomeningeal metastases diagnosis, 319
Myelopathy, acute, from antineoplastic drugs, 323t
  HIV, 301
  radiation, 322
Myerson's sign, 233, *234*
Myoclonic epilepsy, juvenile, 355
Myoclonic seizures, 351
Myoclonus, causes of, 350
  description of, 343
  in stupor/coma evaluation, 63
  motion, 317t
  postanoxic, seizures and, 368
Myoglobinuria, in metabolic myopathies, 269
Myokymia, causes of, 350
  description of, 343
Myopathy(ies), 264–269
  causes of, 265–269
  congenital, 269
  critical illness, 267
  endocrine, 266–267
  examination in, 264–265
  gait failure features in, 128t
  hereditary, 268–269
  infectious, 269
  inflammatory, 266
  management of, 265–269
  medications causing, 267, 267t
  metabolic, 268–269
  mitochondrial, 269
  motor and sensory deficit pattern in, 250t
  suspected, questions for patient with, 264
  toxic, 267–268
Myositis, inclusion body, 266
Myotonic dystrophy, 268
Mysoline, for benign essential tremor, 346
  for epilepsy, 365t
  for movement disorders, dosage of, 341t
  information summary on, 412
Myxopapillary ependymomas, 307

N

Nadolol, in migraine prevention, 180t

Nailbed pressure, in stupor/coma evaluation, 69
Naloxone, for agitation, 108
 for ataxia from sedative intoxication, 136
 for coma, 59
 information summary on, 408
Naprosyn, for migraine headache, 178t
Naproxen, for migraine headache, 176, 178t
Naratriptan, for migraine, 179t
 information summary on, 409
Narcan, for agitation, 108
 for ataxia from sedative intoxication, 136
 for coma, 59
 information summary on, 408
Narcotic equivalence doses, 220t
Nardil, in migraine prevention, 180t
Neck, immobilization of, in spinal cord compression, 92
 in head injury evaluation, 120
 in headache evaluation, 173, *174*
 in stupor/coma evaluation, 62
 in syncope evaluation, 207
 muscles of, 390t–391t
 pain syndromes involving, 215
 x-rays of, in spinal cord compression evaluation, 93
Necrotizing encephalomyelitis, 317t
 hemorrhagic, 281–282
Neonatal seizures, 382t, 382–383
Neoplasms, brain stem, diplopia from, 141
 central nervous system, 302–379. See also *Central nervous system (CNS), neoplasm(s) of.*
 delirium from, 104
 in pediatric patient, 385
 radiation-induced, 322–323
 spinal cord compression from, 94, *95*
  surgical intervention for, 101
 spinal cord injury from, management of, 97
Neostigmine, for myasthenia gravis, 199t
 information summary on, 409
Neptazane, for benign essential tremor, 346
 for movement disorders, dosage of, 341t

Nerve(s), biopsy of, 43
 causes of peripheral neuropathy diagnosed by, 262t
 cranial. See *Cranial nerves;* specific nerve.
 diseases of, 249–269. See also *Neuromuscular diseases; Neuropathy(ies).*
 of brachial plexus, *395*
 of lumbar plexus, *396*
 peripheral. See also *Peripheral nerve(s).*
 stimulation of, repetitive, in myasthenia gravis diagnosis, 196
Nerve conduction studies, in ataxia/gait failure evaluation, 135
 in painful peripheral neuropathy diagnosis, 223
Nerve entrapment syndromes, 254–256
Neuralgia, brachial, 227
 glossopharyngeal, 183
 herpetic, 221–222
 postherpetic, 221–222
 trigeminal, 220–221
  management of, 183
Neuralgic amyotrophy, 227
Neuritis, brachial, 227
 optic, 280–281
Neuroblastomas, 309
 in pediatric patient, 385
Neurocardiogenic syncope, 209
Neuroectodermal tumors, primitive, 308–309
Neuroimaging, in multiple sclerosis diagnosis, 274–275
Neuroleptic malignant syndrome, 267–268
Neurologic complications, of AIDS, 299–301
 of bone marrow transplantation, 324
Neurologic disorders, syncope from, 203–204
Neurologic emergencies, pediatric, 378–388. See also *Pediatric neurologic emergency(ies).*
Neurologic examination, 12–30
 coordination in, 24–25
 cranial nerves in, 18–22
 gait in, 30
 in acute stroke, 81–82

Neurologic examination
  (Continued)
  in acute visual disturbances,
    143–147
  in amnesia, 231–233
  in ataxia, 130–133
  in delirium, 106–107
  in dementia, 231–233
  in dizziness/vertigo, 164, 166
  in gait failure, 130–133
  in head injury, 120–122
  in neuromuscular respiratory
    failure, 190
  in pain syndromes, 218–219
  in spinal cord compression, 98,
    100
  in stupor/coma evaluation,
    62–69
  in syncope, 207
  mental status in, 12–18
  motor function in, 22–24
  reflexes in, 25–27
  sensory function in, 27–29
  station in, 30
Neurologic patient, anatomic
    localization in, 6–11
  approach to, 3–11
Neuroma, acoustic, 312–313
  evoked potentials in, 43
Neuromuscular diseases, 249–269
  anatomic subtypes of, 250t
  suspected, approach to patient
    with, 249, 251
Neuromuscular junction disease,
    264
  motor and sensory deficit pattern in, 250t
Neuromuscular junction lesion,
  respiratory weakness from,
    187
Neuromuscular respiratory failure,
  185–200. See also *Respiratory
    system, failure of.*
Neuromuscular system, failure of,
  history of, 188–189
  physical examination in, 189–
    190
Neuromyelitis optica, 281
Neurontin. See also *Gabapentin.*
  for benign essential tremor, 346
  for epilepsy, 361t
  for neuropathic pain, 263–264
  information summary on, 410
Neuro-oncology, 302–379

Neuropathic pain, in multiple
  sclerosis, therapy for, 279
Neuropathy(ies)
  autonomic, 262, 264
  from antineoplastic drugs,
    323, 323t
  causes of, 262–263
    narrowing, features helpful
      in, 261t
  cranial, from antineoplastic
    drugs, 323t
  distal axonal sensorimotor, 262
  general care for patient with,
    263–264
  genetic, 263
  hereditary, 263
  HIV sensory, complicating
    AIDS, 300
  multifocal motor, 252
  optic, ischemic, fundoscopic appearance of, 144t
  radiation, 322
  painful peripheral, 222–323
  paraneoplastic, 263
  paraprotein-associated, 263
  peripheral, causes of, diagnosed
    by nerve biopsy, 262t
    from antineoplastic drugs,
      323t
  pure sensory, 317t
  sensorimotor, 317t
  sensory loss patterns in, *251*
Neuropsychologic testing, in
  epilepsy surgery evaluation,
    371
Neurosyphilis, 290–291
  cerebrospinal fluid findings in,
    287t
Neurotoxicity, of antineoplastic
  drugs, 323, 323t
Nicardipine, in increased
  intracranial pressure
  management, 158
Nimodipine, information
  summary on, 409
Nimotop, information summary
  on, 409
Nongerminomatous germ cell
  tumors, 315
Nonsteroidal anti-inflammatory
  drugs, for migraine headache,
    176, 178t
  for pain, 219
  for postconcussion headache,
    181

Nonsteroidal anti-inflammatory drugs *(Continued)*
  for tension headache, 177
Nortriptyline, for neuropathic pain, 264
  in migraine prevention, 180t
Nose, in head injury evaluation, 120
  in stupor/coma evaluation, 62
Novantrone, for secondary progressive multiple sclerosis, 278
Numb chin syndrome, 319
Nutrition, for comatose patient, 72
  in neuromuscular respiratory failure management, 193
  in severe head injury management, 123
  in stroke management, 90
Nystagmus, 121
  from peripheral or central causes, 166t
  in ataxia/gait failure evaluation, 131
  in dizziness/vertigo evaluation, 164, 166
  opticokinetic, 20
  subtypes of, 165t

O

Obturator externus muscle, 393t
Obturator nerve, *396*
Occipital condyle syndrome, from skull base metastases, 320
Occipital cortex, lesions of, visual syndromes associated with, 141t
Occipital lobe seizures, 353
Ocular bobbing, 165t
  in locked-in syndrome, 71
  in stupor/coma, 66
Ocular dysmetria, 165t
Ocular massage, for central retinal artery occlusion, 147
Ocular motility, in vision disturbance evaluation, 145, *146*
Ocular primary central nervous system lymphoma, 310
Oculocephalic reflex, in stupor/coma evaluation, 66–68
Oculomotor (III) nerve, in neurologic examination, 19

Oculovestibular reflex, in stupor/coma evaluation, 68
Olanzapine, for agitation and delirium, 108t
Olfactory groove meningioma, 311
Olfactory (I) nerve, in neurologic examination, 18
Oligodendrogliomas, 306–307
Ophthalmoplegia, internuclear, 145
Opioids, for severe pain, 219
Opponens pollicis muscle, 391t
Opsoclonus-myoclonus, 317t
Optic (II) nerve, in neurologic examination, 18–19
  ischemia of, monocular visual loss from, 139
Optic nerve sheath fenestration, for pseudotumor cerebri, 149
Optic neuritis, 280–281
  fundoscopic appearance of, 144t
  inflammatory, management of, 148–149
  inflammatory/demyelinating, monocular visual loss from, 139
Optic neuropathy, arteritic ischemic, management of, 148
  ischemic, fundoscopic appearance of, 144t
  radiation, 322
Opticokinetic nystagmus, in neurologic examination, 20
Optimization, in increased intracranial pressure management, 158–159
Orap, for movement disorders, dosage of, 341t
  for Tourette's syndrome, 348
  information summary on, 411–412
Orbital syndrome, from skull base metastases, 320
Organ donation, 244–245
Orientation, in head injury evaluation, 121
  in mental status examination, 15
Oropharynx, in neuromuscular respiratory failure evaluation, 189
Orthostatic hypotension, syncope from, 203
Osmitrol, information summary on, 414

Otorrhea, cerebrospinal fluid, in stupor/coma evaluation, 62
Oxacillin, for brain abscess, 293–294
  for epidural CNS infection, 295
Oxcarbazepine, for epilepsy, 363t
  information summary on, 409
Oxybutynin, for bladder dysfunction in multiple sclerosis, 278
  information summary on, 409–410

P

P450 enzyme inhibitors and inducers, 370t
Pain, in multiple sclerosis, therapy for, 278–279
  medications causing, 217t
  sites of origin of, *214*
Pain syndromes, 213–327
  bedside evaluation of, 216–219
  chart review in, 216–217
  complex regional, 219–220
  differential diagnosis of, 215
  elevator thoughts on, 215
  history of, selective, 216–217
  major threat to life in, 216
  management of, 219
  neurologic examination in, 218–219
  phone call on, 213, 215
  physical examination in, 217–219
  selected, 219–327
Painful peripheral neuropathy, 222–323
Pallidotomy, stereotactic, for Parkinson's disease, 345
Pallinopsia, 141t
Palmaris longus muscle, 391t
Palmomental reflex, 27
Palsy, Bell's, 255–256
  facial, 255–256
  progressive supranuclear, treatment of, 237
Pamelor, in migraine prevention, 180t
Panic disorder, syncope in, 212
Papillary ependymomas, 307
Papilledema, *18*
  in stupor/coma evaluation, 65

Paradoxical respirations, 188, *188*
Paralysis, Brown-Séquard's, 99t
  in increased intracranial pressure management, 158
  periodic, 269
  respiratory, 198, 200
Paraneoplastic disorder, ataxia from, treatment of, 136
Paraneoplastic neuropathy, 263
Paraneoplastic syndromes, 317t
Paraphasias, in delirium, 106
Paraprotein-associated neuropathy, 263
Paraprotein-mediated diseases, causing peripheral polyneuropathies, 259t
Parasellar syndrome, from skull base metastases, 320
Parenchymal contusion, from head injury, 118–119
Parenchymal hematoma, from head injury, 118–119
Paresis, in neurosyphilis, 290
Paresthesia, medications causing, 217t
Parietal lobe seizures, 353
Parkinsonian gait, 29t
Parkinsonism, gait failure features in, 128t
Parkinson's disease, 344–345
  treatment of, 237
Parlodel, for movement disorders, dosage of, 341t
  for Parkinson's disease, 344
  information summary on, 406
Parsonage-Turner syndrome, 227
Patient management, on call, 3–4
Pectoral nerves, *395*
Pediatric neurologic emergency(ies), 378–388
  birth trauma as, 378, 380–381
  brain death as, 387–388
  cerebrovascular complications of prematurity as, 381
  child abuse as, 386–387
  CNS infections as, 383
  febrile seizures as, 383
  head injury as, 386
  neonatal seizures as, 382–383
  tumors as, 385
  ventriculoperitoneal shunt malfunction as, 384–385
Pediatric patient, CNS infections in, 383

448 Index

Pediatric patient *(Continued)*
  developmental milestones in, 380t
  febrile seizures in, 357–358, 383
  muscle tone in, examination for, 378, *379*
  Rolandic epilepsy in, 357
PEEP. See *Positive end-expiratory pressure (PEEP)*.
Pelvis, in head injury evaluation, 120
Pemoline, for fatigue in multiple sclerosis, 279
  information summary on, 410
Pendular nystagmus, 165t
Penicillamine, for movement disorders, dosage of, 341t
  for Wilson's disease, 349
  information summary on, 410
Penicillin, benzathine, for neurosyphilis, 291
  procaine, for tetanus, 200
Penicillin G, for brain abscess, 293–294
  for leptospirosis, 293
  for Lyme disease, 291
  for neurosyphilis, 291
Pentobarbital, for status epilepticus, 54t
  in increased intracranial pressure management, 160
  information summary on, 410–411
Perceptions, in mental status examination, 14t
Pergolide, for movement disorders, dosage of, 341t
  for Parkinson's disease, 345
  for restless leg syndrome, 349
  information summary on, 411
Periactin, in migraine prevention, 180t
  information summary on, 407–408
Perineal muscles, 393t
Periodic alternating nystagmus, 165t
Periodic paralysis, 269
Peripheral deafferentation, gait failure features in, 128t
Peripheral nerve(s), lesions of, respiratory weakness from, 186–187
  tumors of, radiation-induced, 322

Peripheral nervous system toxicity, of antineoplastic drugs, 323
Peripheral neuropathy(ies), from antineoplastic drugs, 323t
  painful, differential diagnosis of, 215
  syncope in, 211
Periventricular hemorrhagic infarction, complicating prematurity, 381
Periventricular leukomalacia, complicating prematurity, 381
Permax, for movement disorders, dosage of, 341t
  for Parkinson's disease, 345
  information summary on, 411
Peroneus brevis muscle, 393t
Peroneus longus muscle, 393t
Persistent vegetative state (PVS), 73, 75
PET. See *Positron emission tomography (PET)*.
Phenelzine, in migraine prevention, 180t
Phenobarbital, for epilepsy, 363t
  for neonatal seizures, 382
  for seizures, 53
  for status epilepticus, 54t
  information summary on, 411
Phenoxybenzamine, for bladder dysfunction in multiple sclerosis, 279
  for reflex sympathetic dystrophy, 220
Phenytoin, for epilepsy, 364t
  for herpes simplex encephalitis, 297
  for myotonic dystrophy, 268
  for perioperative seizures, 374–375
  for status epilepticus, 54t
  for trigeminal neuralgia, 183
  information summary on, 411
Physical therapy, chest, for neuromuscular respiratory failure, 193
Physiologic nystagmus, 165t
Pimozide, for movement disorders, dosage of, 341t
  for Tourette's syndrome, 348
  information summary on, 411–412
Pindolol, for vasovagal syncope, 209

Pineal region tumors, 315–316
Pinealoblastomas, 315
Pinealomas, 315–316
Pineoblastoma, 309
Pineocytomas, 315
Pinprick, in sensory examination, 28
Piroxicam, for migraine headache, 178t
Pitressin, in organ donor management, 245
Pituitary adenomas, 313–314
  binocular visual loss from, 139
Plantar reflex(es), in neurologic examination, 25–26
  in stupor/coma evaluation, 69
Plasma exchanges, for multiple sclerosis relapses, 278
Plasmapheresis, for chronic inflammatory demyelinating polyneuropathy, 263
  for Guillain-Barré syndrome, 195
  for myasthenia gravis, 197
  for paraprotein-associated neuropathy, 263
Plavix, information summary on, 407
Plexopathy, 253, 254
  motor and sensory deficit pattern in, 250t
Poisons, causing peripheral polyneuropathies, 258t
Poliomyelitis, respiratory failure in, 200
Polymyalgia rheumatica, in temporal arteritis, 182
Polymyositis, 266
Polyneuropathy, 257–264
  acute demyelinating, complicating AIDS, 301
  chronic inflammatory demyelinating, 262–263
  clinical approach to, 258–260
  critical illness, 263
  laboratory testing for, 260
  management of, 260
  motor and sensory deficit pattern in, 250t
  peripheral, causes of, 258t–259t
Polyradiculopathy, 253
  motor and sensory deficit pattern in, 250t
Pons, lesion localization in, 9

Pontomedullary junction, lesion localization in, 9
Porphyria, seizures in, 376
Positive end-expiratory pressure (PEEP), for neuromuscular respiratory failure, 191
Positron emission tomography (PET), in amnesia/dementia diagnosis, 236
  in epilepsy surgery evaluation, 371
Postanoxic myoclonus, seizures and, 368
Postconcussion headache, management of, 181
Posterior cord syndrome, 99t
Posterior fossa meningioma, 311
Postherpetic neuralgia, 221–222
Postinfectious encephalomyelitis, 281
Postural hypotension, syncope from, 203
Postvaccinal encephalomyelitis, 281
Pramipexole, for Parkinson's disease, 345
  information summary on, 410
Praxis, in mental status examination, 14t
Praziquantel, for cysticercosis, 296
Prednisone, for arteritic ischemic optic neuropathy, 148
  for Bell's palsy, 256
  for brachial neuritis, 227
  for chronic inflammatory demyelinating polyneuropathy, 263
  for Duchenne muscular dystrophy, 268
  for herpetic neuralgia, 222
  for idiopathic intracranial hypertension, 182
  for multiple sclerosis relapses, 278
  for optic neuritis, 281
  for paraprotein-associated neuropathy, 263
  for polymyositis, 266
  for temporal arteritis, 182
  in cluster headache prevention, 181
  information summary on, 412
Pregnancy, seizures and, 365–366
Prematurity, cerebrovascular complications of, 381

Presyncope, 201
Primidone, for benign essential tremor, 346
  for epilepsy, 365t
  for movement disorders, dosage of, 341t
  information summary on, 412
ProAmatine, information summary on, 408
Pro-Banthine, for bladder dysfunction in multiple sclerosis, 279
  for myasthenia gravis, 197
  information summary on, 412
Prochlorperazine, for migraine headache, 176
Prodrome, 352
Progressive multifocal leukoencephalopathy (PML), complicating AIDS, 299
  diplopia from, 141
Progressive supranuclear palsy, treatment of, 237
Pronator drift, in head injury evaluation, 121
  in screening for hemiparesis, 23
Pronator teres muscle, 328
Propantheline bromide, for bladder dysfunction in multiple sclerosis, 278
  for myasthenia gravis, 197
  information summary on, 412
Propofol, for status epilepticus, 54t
  in increased intracranial pressure management, 158
Propoxyphene, for restless leg syndrome, 349
Propranolol, for benign essential tremor, 346
  for movement disorders, dosage of, 341t
  for tremor in multiple sclerosis, 279
  for vasovagal syncope, 209
  in migraine prevention, 180t
  information summary on, 412
Proprioception, in sensory examination, 28
Prosopagnosia, 141t
Prostigmin, for myasthenia gravis, 199t
  information summary on, 409
Protein density images, 35
Pseudocoma states, 71–72
Pseudotumor cerebri, 144t
  management of, 149, 181–182
Psychiatric complications, of multiple sclerosis, therapy for, 279
Psychiatric disorders, syncope from, 204
Psychogenic coma, 71
Ptosis, in neurologic examination, 19
Pull test, in neurologic examination, 30
Pupils, Argyll Robertson, in neurosyphilis, 290
  in ataxia/gait failure evaluation, 131
  in delirium evaluation, 106
  in head injury evaluation, 121
  in neurologic examination, 19–20
  in neuromuscular respiratory failure evaluation, 190
  in stupor/coma evaluation, 65–66
  reactivity of, in vision disturbance evaluation, 143
Pure sensory neuropathy, 317t
PVS (persistent vegetative state), 73, 75
Pyramidal system, lesion localization in, 7
Pyrazinamide, for tubercular meningitis, 289
Pyridostigmine, for myasthenia gravis, 197, 199t
  information summary on, 413
Pyridoxine, for tubercular meningitis, 289
Pyrimethamine, for toxoplasmosis, 296

Q

Quadriceps femoris muscle, testing, roots, and innervation of, 393t
Quick look test, in acute stroke, 78–79
  in amnesia, 230
  in ataxia/gait failure, 127
  in delirium, 104–105
  in dementia, 230
  in dizziness/vertigo, 162

Quick look test *(Continued)*
in head injury, 119
in headache, 172
in increased intracranial pressure, 151
in neuromuscular respiratory failure, 187
in pain syndromes, 216
in seizures/status epilepticus, 50
in spinal cord compression, 96
in syncope, 204–205
in vision disturbance, 142

R

Rabies virus encephalitis, 298–299
Race-ethnicity, in neurologic history, 5
Radial nerve, *395*
Radiation myelopathy, 322
Radiation necrosis, 321–322
Radiation optic neuropathy, 322
Radiation therapy, for brain metastases, 318
for craniopharyngioma, 315
for ependymomas, 308
for glioblastoma multiforme, 304
for leptomeningeal metastases, 319
for pineal region tumors, 315–316
for pituitary adenoma, 314
for primary central nervous system lymphoma, 310
for primitive neuroectodermal tumors, 309
toxicity from, 321–323
Radiography, chest, in ataxia/gait failure evaluation, 135
in spinal metastases diagnosis, 321
Radioisotope cerebral imaging, in brain death confirmation, 243
Reasoning, abstract, in mental status examination, 14t
Recombinant tissue plasminogen activator (rt-PA), in ischemic stroke management, 335, 336b
Rectum, in syncope evaluation, 207
Reflex(es), cold caloric, 68
corneal, 21, 68

Reflex(es) *(Continued)*
deep tendon, 69
gag, 68
in ataxia/gait failure evaluation, 133
in delirium evaluation, 107
in neurologic examination, 25–27
in neuromuscular respiratory failure evaluation, 190
in spinal cord compression evaluation, 100
in stroke evaluation, 82
in vision disturbance evaluation, 147
oculocephalic, 66–61
oculovestibular, 68
plantar, 25–26, 69
Reflex asymmetry, in seizure evaluation, 55
Reflex sympathetic dystrophy, 219–220
Reflex vasodepressor syncope, 206
Reflex vasodilatation, syncope from, 202
Relaxation techniques, for tension headache, 177
Renal failure. See *Kidney failure.*
Repetition, in mental status examination, 16
Requip, for Parkinson's disease, 345
information summary on, 413
Reserpine, for Huntington's disease, 347
for movement disorders, dosage of, 341t
for Tourette's syndrome, 348
Respirations, in stupor/coma evaluation, 64–65
paradoxical, 188, *188*
Respiratory alkalosis, in stupor/coma, 65
Respiratory rate, in neuromuscular respiratory failure evaluation, 188
Respiratory system, failure of, 185–200
bedside evaluation of, 187–190
elevator thoughts on, 186–187
general care for, 193
in Guillain-Barré syndrome, 185, 193–195

Respiratory system (*Continued*)
  in myasthenia gravis, 185, 195–198
  in poliomyelitis, 200
  in tetanus, 200
  major threat to life in, 187
  management of, 191–193
  phone call on, 185–196
  uncommon causes of, 198, 200
  in neuromuscular respiratory failure evaluation, 190
Restless leg syndrome, 349
Retina, ischemia of, monocular visual loss from, 138–139
Retinal artery, central, occlusion of, management of, 147–148
  occlusion of, fundoscopic appearance of, 144t
Retinoblastoma, 309
Retinopathy, carcinoma-associated, 317t
Retrobulbar mass lesion, 148
  monocular visual loss from, 139
Retrograde amnesia, 228
  from head injury, 121
Rhabdomyolysis, in metabolic myopathies, 268
Rheumatoid arthritis, spinal cord compression from, 95
Rhinorrhea, cerebrospinal fluid, 62
Rhomboideus minor muscle, 390t
Rhythmic alternating movements, rapid, 24
Rhythmic muscle twitching, in stupor/coma evaluation, 63
Rifampin, for tubercular meningitis, 289
Rigidity, description of, 343
  in neurologic examination, 23
Rilutek, information summary on, 413
Riluzole, for amyotrophic lateral sclerosis, 252
  information summary on, 413
Rinne test, 21–22
Risperdal, for agitation and delirium, 108t
Risperidone, for agitation and delirium, 108t
Rizatriptan, information summary on, 413
Robinul, for myasthenia gravis, 197
  information summary on, 411

Rofecoxib, for migraine headache, 178t
Rolandic epilepsy of childhood, 357
Romazicon, for ataxia from sedative intoxication, 136
  for coma, 59
Romberg's test, 30
Root compression, cervical or lumbosacral, 223–227
  clinical features of, 226t
  clinical presentation of, 223–224
  diagnosis of, 224
  treatment of, 224, 227
Root reflex, in neurologic examination, 27
Ropinirole, for Parkinson's disease, 345
  information summary on, 413

S

Saccadic eye movements, in neurologic examination, 20
  in stupor/coma, 66
Saint Louis encephalitis virus, 298
Sansert, in migraine prevention, 180t
  information summary on, 414–415
Sarcoidosis, 266, 283–284
Sartorius muscle, 393t
Scapular nerve, dorsal, *395*
Schwannoma, vestibular, 312
Sciatica, 224
Scissor gait, 29t
Sedation, in increased intracranial pressure management, 158
Seizure(s), 47–57. See also *Status epilepticus.*
  absence, 351
  alcohol-related, 367
  bedside evaluation of, 50
  chart review in, 55–56
  classification of, 350–353, 351t
  complex, 47
  delirium from, 104
    treatment of, 112
  elevator thoughts on, 48–49
  evaluation of, 53–54
  febrile, 357–358, 383
  focal, 47

Seizure(s) *(Continued)*
  following head injury, 125
  from brain metastases, 316
  from head trauma, 366
  from stroke, 366–367
  frontal lobe, 353–354
  generalized, 47
    tonic, 352
  grand mal, 350–351
  history in, selective, 55–56
  in hepatic failure, 367–368
  in porphyria, 376
  in renal failure, 367
  major threats to life from, 50
  management during, 359–360
  management of, 50–54, 56–57
    initial, 53–54
  medications causing, 49t
  myoclonic, 351
  neonatal, 382t, 382–383
  neurological examination in, 55
  new-onset, 358–360, 359t
    evaluation of, 357, 358t
  occipital lobe, 353
  ongoing, treatment of, 50–52
  parietal lobe, 353
  partial-onset, 352–353
  perioperative, 366
  phone call on, 47–48
  postanoxic myoclonus and, 368
  precautions for, 51t
  pregnancy and, 365–366
  prevention of, in increased intracranial pressure management, 157
  primary generalized, 350–352
  recurrence of, risk of, 358–360
  simple, 47
  syncope from, 210–211
  temporal lobe, 352
  thresholds for, drugs lowering, 373t
  tonic-clonic, 350–351
Seizure disorder, EEG in, 40
Selegiline, for movement disorders, dosage of, 341t
  for Parkinson's disease, 345
  information summary on, 413
Semimembranosus muscle, 393t
Semitendinosus muscle, 393t
Sensation, in neuromuscular respiratory failure evaluation, 190
  in vision disturbance evaluation, 147

Sensorimotor neuropathy, 317t
Sensorimotor syndrome, 332
Sensory ataxia, gait failure features in, 128t
Sensory dermatome map, 397
Sensory function(s), in ataxia/gait failure evaluation, 133
  in delirium evaluation, 106
  in neurologic examination, 27–29
  in spinal cord compression evaluation, 100
  in stroke evaluation, 82
Sensory responses, in stupor/coma evaluation, 69
Serotonin, for migraine, 179t
Serratus anterior muscle, 390t
Serum sickness, in pediatric patient, 384
Shaken-baby syndrome, 386
Shingles, 221–222
Shoulders, pain syndromes involving, 215
Shy-Drager syndrome, syncope in, 211
Sinemet, for movement disorders, dosage of, 341t
  for Parkinson's disease, 344
  information summary on, 413
Single photon emission computed tomography (SPECT), in amnesia/dementia diagnosis, 236
  in epilepsy surgery evaluation, 371
Situational syncope, 206
Skin, care of, in neuropathies, 264
  in stupor/coma, 73
  in ataxia/gait failure evaluation, 134
  in pain syndrome evaluation, 218
  in stupor/coma evaluation, 62
  rashes of, in neuromuscular respiratory failure evaluation, 190
Skull, fracture of, 119
  metastases to, 319–320
Skull base metastases, 319–320
Snout reflex, in neurologic examination, 27
Soleus muscle, 393t
Solu-Medrol, information summary on, 414

Somatosensory evoked potentials, 42–43
Spasticity, in multiple sclerosis, therapy for, 278
 in neurologic examination, 22–23
Spatial hemineglect, 14–15
SPECT. See *Single photon emission computed tomography (SPECT)*.
Speech, in neuromuscular respiratory failure evaluation, 190
Sphenoid wing meningioma, 311
Sphincters, perineal, 393t
Spinal accessory (XI) nerve, in ataxia/gait failure evaluation, 131
 in neurologic examination, 22
Spinal block, complete, complicating lumbar puncture, 33
Spinal cord, compression of, 92–101
 bedside evaluation/management of, 96–101
 chart review in, 100
 differential diagnosis of, 94–96
 elevator thoughts on, 94–96
 history in, selective, 100
 major threat to life in, 96
 management of, 96–97
 neurologic examination in, 98, 100
 phone call on, 92–93
 physical examination in, 97–100
 surgical intervention for, 101
 cross section of, *98*
 injury to, as birth trauma, 380–381
 evoked potentials in, 43
 gait failure features in, 128t
 lesion localization in, 10–11
 lesion of, respiratory weakness from, 186
 metastases to, 320–321
 primary central nervous system lymphoma involving, 310
Spinal epidural abscess, 295
Spinal headache, complicating lumbar puncture, 32–33
Spinal muscular atrophy, 252
Spinal tap, 310

Spine, cervical, radiographs of, in head injury, 114
 in spinal cord compression evaluation, 98
 metastases to, 320–321
Station, in neurologic examination, 30
Status epilepticus, 47. See also *Seizure(s)*.
 drugs for, *52*, 54t
 nonconvulsive, 112
 treatment of, 52–53
Status migranosus, 176
Stelazine, for agitation and delirium, 108t
Steppage gait, 29t
Stereognosis, in neurologic examination, 29
Stereotactic pallidotomy, for Parkinson's disease, 345
Stereotactic thalamotomy, for Parkinson's disease, 345
Stereotaxic radiosurgery, for brain metastases, 318
Sternal rub, in stupor/coma evaluation, 69
Sternocleido-mastoideus muscle, 390t
Steroids, in head injury management, 124
STIR sequences, 35
Straight leg raise test, 218, *218*
Streptomycin, for tubercular meningitis, 289
Stroke, acute, 76–91
 airway in, 79
 bedside evaluation of, 78–82
 causes of, 77–78
 elevator thoughts on, 77–78
 history in, selective, 80–81
 major threat to life in, 78
 management of, general care in, 90–91
  with hemorrhage, 82–85
  with infarction, 85–90
 neurologic examination in, 81–82
 phone call on, 76–77
 physical examination in, 81
 presentations of, 76t
 diplopia from, 141
 ischemic, 330–337
  cardioembolic, 331–332
  clinical presentation of, 330–334

Stroke *(Continued)*
  diagnosis of, 330–334
  from artery-to-artery embolus, 333
  from large-vessel stenosis, 332–333
  lacunar, 333
  management of, 335, 336b, 337
  seizures from, 366–367
Stupor, bedside evaluation of, 61–69
  causes of, 59–60, 60t
  diagnostic testing in, 69, 71–72
  elevator thoughts on, 59–60
  history of, selective, 61–62
  major threat to life from, 60–61
  management of, 72–73
  neurologic examination in, 62–69
  phone call on, 58–59
  physical examination in, 62
  prognosis in, 73–75
Subarachnoid hemorrhage, 325–330
  as threat to life, 171
  clinical grading of, 326, 327t
  clinical presentation of, 325–326
  diagnosis of, 326–327
  management of, 327–330
  radiographic assessment of, 82, 83
  stroke from, 78
  syncope and, 206, 211
Subclavian nerve, *395*
Subclavian steal syndrome, syncope from, 210
Subdural empyema, 294–295
Subdural hematoma, from head injury, 118
  tentorial, as birth trauma, 381
Subgaleal hemorrhage, from birth trauma, 381
Subluxations, spinal, surgical intervention for, 101
Subpial transections, for epilepsy, 372
Subscapular nerves, *395*
Suck reflex, in neurologic examination, 27
Sulfadiazine, for toxoplasmosis, 296
Sulindac, for migraine headache, 178t

Sumatriptan, for cluster headache, 177
  for migraine headache, 176, 179t
  information summary on, 414
Supinator muscle, 391t
Suprascapular nerve, *395*
Suprasellar meningioma, 311
Supraspinatus muscle, 390t
Supratentorial tumors, in pediatric patient, 385
Supraventricular tachycardia, in syncope evaluation, 205
Surgery, for acoustic neuroma, 312–313
  for brain metastases, 318
  for craniopharyngioma, 315
  for ependymomas, 308
  for epilepsy, 370–272
  for glioblastoma multiforme, 304
  for meningiomas, 311–312
  for pineal region tumors, 315
  for pituitary adenoma, 314
  for primitive neuroectodermal tumors, 309
  for skull metastases, 320
  for subarachnoid hemorrhage, 328
Swallow test, in neuromuscular respiratory failure evaluation, 190
Symmetrel, for movement disorders, dosage of, 341t
  for Parkinson's disease, 345
  information summary on, 404
Symptom characterization, in neurologic history, 5
Synchronized intermittent mandatory ventilation, for neuromuscular respiratory failure, 191
Syncope, 201–212
  bedside evaluation of, 204–207
  carotid sinus, 206, 210
  causes of, 202–204
  diagnostic testing in, 207–208
  disorders causing or mimicking, 274–277
  drugs causing, 203t
  elevator thoughts on, 202–204
  history of, selective, 205–206
  major threat to life in, 204
  management of, 208–209
  neurocardiogenic, 209

456 Index

Syncope *(Continued)*
  neurologic examination in, 207
  phone call on, 201–202
  physical examination in, 207
  reflex vasodepressor, 206
  situational, 206
  vasovagal, 209
Synthroid, for ataxia from hypothyroidism, 136
Syphilis, complicating AIDS, 300
  meningovascular, 290
Syprine, for movement disorders, dosage of, 341t
  for Wilson's disease, 349
Systemic lupus erythematosus, in pediatric patient, 384

T

T2 images, 34
Tabes dorsalis, 133
  in neurosyphilis, 290
Tachycardia, supraventricular, in syncope evaluation, 205
  ventricular, in syncope evaluation, 205
Tachykinesia, description of, 343
Tacrine, information summary on, 414
Tandem gait, in head injury evaluation, 121–122
Tasmar, for Parkinson's disease, 345
  information summary on, 415
Tegretol. See also *Carbamazepine*.
  for epilepsy, 360t, 368
  for idiopathic torsion dystonia, 347
  for movement disorders, dosage of, 341
  information summary on, 407
Temperature, in headache evaluation, 172
  in neuromuscular respiratory failure evaluation, 188
  in sensory examination, 28
  in stroke evaluation, 80
  in syncope evaluation, 205
  management of, in severe head injury management, 124
Temporal arteritis, management of, 182–183
Temporal artery, biopsy of, in temporal arteritis evaluation, 182–183
Temporal course, of disease, in neurologic history, 5
Temporal lobe epilepsy, 357
Temporal lobe seizures, 352
Tenormin, in migraine prevention, 180t
Tensilon, information summary on, 409
Tension headache, management of, 177
Tensor fasciae latae muscle, 393t
Tentorial herniation, complicating lumbar puncture, 33
Tentorial subdural hematoma, as birth trauma, 381
Teres major muscle, 390t
Teres minor muscle, 390t
Territorial infarction, 85–86, *87*
Tetanus, respiratory failure in, 200
Thalamotomy, stereotactic, for Parkinson's disease, 345
Thiamine, for coma, 59
  for delirium tremens, 110
  for hypoglycemia, 110
  for seizures, 52
  for Wernicke-Korsakoff syndrome, 239
  information summary on, 414
Thoracic nerve, long, *395*
Thoracodorsal nerve, *395*
Thought content, in delirium evaluation, 106
  in mental status examination, 14t
Thought form, in mental status examination, 14t
Throat, in head injury evaluation, 120
  in stupor/coma evaluation, 62
Thrombosis, deep vein. See *Deep vein thrombosis (DVT)*.
Thymoma, malignant, in myasthenia gravis, 196
Tiagabine, for epilepsy, 365t
  information summary on, 414
TIAs (transient ischemic attacks), 331b
  syncope in, 210
  vertebrobasilar ataxia from, treatment of, 136
Tibialis anterior muscle, 393t
Tibialis posterior muscle, 393t
Ticlid, information summary on, 414–415

Ticlopidine, information summary on, 414–415
Tics, description of, 343
in Tourette's syndrome, 348
Tissue plasminogen activator (t-PA), in stroke management, 87, 88
information summary on, 415
recombinant, in stroke management, 335, 336b
Tizanidine, for idiopathic torsion dystonia, 347
for spasticity/pain in multiple sclerosis, 278
Tolcapone, for Parkinson's disease, 345
information summary on, 415
Tongue, biting of, in stupor/coma evaluation, 62
Tonic seizures, generalized, 352
Tonic-clonic seizures, generalized, primary, 350–351
secondary, 352
syncope from, 210
Topamax, for epilepsy, 365t
information summary on, 415
Topiramate, for epilepsy, 365t
information summary on, 415
Toradol, for migraine headache, 178t
Torsion dystonia, idiopathic, 347
Touch, light, in sensory examination, 27–28
Tourette's syndrome, 347–348
Toxic disorders, causing peripheral polyneuropathies, 258t
delirium from, 103
Toxic encephalopathy, acute, in pediatric patient, 384
Toxic myopathies, 267–268
Toxicity, chemotherapy, 323, 323t
radiation, 321–323
Toxoplasmosis, 295–296
complicating AIDS, 299
Tracheostomy, in neuromuscular respiratory failure management, 191
Transcortical motor aphasia, 17t
Transcortical sensory aphasia, 17t
Transcranial Doppler (TCD) ultrasonography, 36
in ataxia/gait failure evaluation, 135

Transcranial Doppler (TCD) ultrasonography *(Continued)*
in brain death confirmation, 243
Transducer, epidural, in intracranial pressure monitoring, 153
Transient global amnesia, treatment of, 238–239
Transient ischemic attacks (TIAs), 331b
syncope in, 210
vertebrobasilar, ataxia from, treatment of, 136
Transplantation, bone marrow, toxic effects of, 323–324
Transsphenoidal surgery, for pituitary adenoma, 314
Trapezius muscle, testing, roots, and innervation of, 390t
Trauma, birth, 378, 380–381
delirium from, 103
head, 113–125. See also *Head, injury to.*
spinal cord compression from, 94
spinal cord injury from, management of, 96–97
Tremor(s), action, in benign essential tremor, 345
benign essential, 345–346
description of, 343
in multiple sclerosis, therapy for, 279
in neurologic examination, 22
wing-beating, in Wilson's disease, 348
Triceps brachii muscle, 391t
Tricyclic antidepressants, for migraine headache, 176
for pain syndromes, 219
in migraine prevention, 180t
Trientine, for movement disorders, dosage of, 341
for Wilson's disease, 349
Trifluoperazine, for agitation and delirium, 108t
Trigeminal neuralgia, 220–221
management of, 183
Trigeminal (V) nerve, in neurologic examination, 20–21
Trihexyphenidyl, for idiopathic torsion dystonia, 347
for movement disorders, dosage of, 341

Trihexyphenidyl *(Continued)*
  for Parkinson's disease, 345
  information summary on, 415–416
Trileptal, for epilepsy, 363t
  information summary on, 409
Trochlear (IV) nerve, in neurologic examination, 19
Tubercular meningitis, 289
  cerebrospinal fluid findings in, 287t
Tumor. See *Neoplasms.*
Tylenol. See also *Acetaminophen.*
  for migraine headache, 178, 178t

U

Ulnar nerve, *395*
Ultrasonography, Doppler, 35–36. See also *Doppler ultrasonography.*
Upper motor neuron system, lesion localization in, 7
Urecholine, information summary on, 406
Uremia, neuropathy from, 262
  with renal failure, treatment of, 112

V

Vagal nerve stimulator, for epilepsy, 365
Vagus (X) nerve, in ataxia/gait failure evaluation, 131
  in neurologic examination, 22
Valium. See also *Diazepam.*
  for agitation and delirium, 108t
  for delirium tremens, 109
  for idiopathic torsion dystonia, 347
  for movement disorders, dosage of, 341
  information summary on, 408
  rectal, for epilepsy, 368
Valproate, in cluster headache prevention, 181
  IV, for epilepsy, 368
Valproic acid, for epilepsy, 361
  for status epilepticus, 54t
  in migraine prevention, 180t
  information summary on, 416
Vancomycin, for bacterial meningitis, 288t

Vascular disorders, delirium from, 103
  spinal cord compression from, 96
Vasculitis, cerebral, 334b
Vasculopathy, radiation-induced, 322
Vasodepressor syncope, 209
Vasodilatation, reflex, syncope from, 202
Vasospasm, treatment of, 330
Vasovagal syncope, 209
Venereal Disease Research Laboratory (VDRL) test, in neurosyphilis diagnosis, 290
Venography, MR, 35
Ventilation, mechanical, for neuromuscular respiratory failure, 191–193
  reassessment of, in severe head injury management, 123
Ventilatory reserve, in neuromuscular respiratory failure evaluation, 190
Ventricular catheter, in intracranial pressure monitoring, 152–153
Ventricular tachycardia, in syncope evaluation, 205
Ventriculoperitoneal shunt malfunction, in pediatric patient, 384–385
Verapamil, in cluster headache prevention, 181
  in migraine prevention, 180t
Versed, information summary on, 408
Vertebral artery dissection, 333
Vertebral body, blood supply to, metastases and, 320
Vertebrobasilar insufficiency, 206
Vertebrobasilar stenosis/occlusion, syncope from, 210
Vertebrobasilar TIAs, ataxia from, treatment of, 136
Vertical nystagmus, 165t
Vertigo, 161–169
  bedside evaluation of, 162–166
  benign positional, management of, *168,* 169
  chart review in, 162–163
  differential diagnosis of, 161–162
  elevator thoughts on, 161–162
  history in, selective, 162–163

Index **459**

Vertigo *(Continued)*
  major threat to life in, 162
  neurologic examination in, 164, 166, *167*
  phone call on, 161
  physical examination in, 163–166
Vestibular schwannoma, 312
Vestibulocochlear (VIII) nerve, in ataxia/gait failure evaluation, 131
  in neurologic examination, 21–22
Vibration, in sensory examination, 28
Vioxx, for migraine headache, 178t
Viral encephalitis, 297–299
Viral meningitis, 286, 289
  cerebrospinal fluid findings in, 287t
Vision, acute disturbances of, 137–149
  bedside evaluation of, 142–147
  binocular visual loss as, 139, *140*
  chart review in, 142–143
  differential diagnosis of, 138–142
  diplopia as, 139, 141
  elevator thoughts on, 138–142
  history in, selective, 142–143
  major threat to life in, 142
  management of, 147–149
  monocular visual loss as, 138–139, *140*
  neurologic examination in, 143–147
  phone call on, 137–138
  physical examination in, 143–147
  color, in neurologic examination, 18–19
  loss of, from idiopathic intracranial hypertension, 182
Visual acuity, in neurologic examination, 18
  testing of, in idiopathic intracranial hypertension, 182
Visual evoked responses, 42
  in ataxia/gait failure evaluation, 135
Visual fields, in neurologic examination, 18

Visual fields *(Continued)*
  in stupor/coma evaluation, 65
  in vision disturbance evaluation, 144
  lesions of visual pathway and, *140*
  testing of, in idiopathic intracranial hypertension, 182
Visuospatial ability, in mental status examination, 14t
Vital capacity, serial measurements of, for neuromuscular respiratory failure, 193
Vital signs, in ataxia/gait failure evaluation, 130
  in delirium evaluation, 102, 105–106
  in head injury evaluation, 119–120
  in headache evaluation, 172
  in neuromuscular respiratory failure evaluation, 185, 187–188
  in pain syndrome evaluation, 216
  in spinal cord compression evaluation, 92–93, 97
  in stroke evaluation, 79–80
  in stupor/coma evaluation, 62
  in syncope evaluation, 205, 207
Vitamin B_{12}, deficiency of, 133
Vitamin deficiency states, causing peripheral polyneuropathies, 258t
Voltaren, for migraine headache, 178t

W

Wada test, in epilepsy surgery evaluation, 371
Waddling gait, 29t
Wallenberg syndrome, signs and symptoms of, 9–10
Warfarin, in ischemic stroke management, 335
  information summary on, 416
Wasting, in motor neuron disease, 251
Watershed border-zone infarction, 86, *87*
Waveforms, ICP, 154, *155*, 156
Weakness, fluctuating, in myasthenia gravis, 195

Weakness *(Continued)*
  generalized, causes of, 186–187
  neuromuscular respiratory failure from, 185
  in motor neuron disease, 251
  in myasthenia gravis, drugs exacerbating, 198t
Weaning, from mechanical ventilation, 192–193
  criteria for, 193b
  trial protocol for, 192b
Weber's test, in neurologic examination, 21
Wernicke-Korsakoff syndrome, ataxia in, 233
  treatment of, 239
Wernicke's aphasia, 16, 17t
West Nile virus, 298
Wigraine, information summary on, 409
Wilson's disease, 348–349

X

Xanax, for agitation and delirium, 108

Z

Zanaflex, for idiopathic torsion dystonia, 347
  for spasticity/pain in multiple sclerosis, 278
Zarontin, for epilepsy, 361t
  information summary on, 409–410
Zidovudine, for AIDS dementia complex, 238
Zolmitriptan, for migraine headache, 176, 179t
  information summary on, 416
Zomig, for migraine headache, 176, 179t
  information summary on, 416
Zonegran, for epilepsy, 366t
  information summary on, 417
Zonisamide, for epilepsy, 366t
  information summary on, 417
Zostrix, information summary on, 406–407
Zyprexa, for agitation and delirium, 108t